UNDERSTANDING THE SOCIOLOGY OF HEALTH

SAGE was founded in 1965 by Sara Miller McCune to support the dissemination of usable knowledge by publishing innovative and high-quality research and teaching content. Today, we publish over 900 journals, including those of more than 400 learned societies, more than 800 new books per year, and a growing range of library products including archives, data, case studies, reports, and video. SAGE remains majority-owned by our founder, and after Sara's lifetime will become owned by a charitable trust that secures our continued independence.

Los Angeles | London | New Delhi | Singapore | Washington DC | Melbourne

CONTENTS

ABOUT THE AUTHORS

Anne-Marie Barry is a research consultant in Edinburgh and former lecturer in health sociology at Robert Gordon University, Aberdeen. Her research interests primarily focus on social inequalities and health and wellbeing and have also included alcohol and drug use, sexual health, mental health and bereavement.

Chris Yuill is a lecturer at Robert Gordon University, Aberdeen. In addition to *Understanding the Sociology of Health* he has co-authored other textbooks on health and on sociology with SAGE, including *Key Concepts in Health Studies* (with Iain Crinson and Eilidh Duncan) and *Sociology for Social Work* (with Alastair Gibson), both published in 2010. Chris has additionally published a variety of journal articles exploring the relationships between alienation and health, and aspects of urban experience. He is also a member of the British Sociological Association and until recently has sat as a member of both its national council and national executive, where he held responsibility for the publishing activities of the association.

ACKNOWLEDGEMENTS

We would like to thank all the people at SAGE, who, as always, make the writing of a new book a much easier and lighter task. We would also like to thank the anonymous referees who took the time and effort to provide invaluable feedback for this edition. We hope that we meet your expectations.

We would like to thank Catherine Wills and Kate Weiner for their advice on health technologies (but if we have misconstrued anything in that chapter, then it is our fault and not theirs).

Chris would like to thank various people. Firstly, he would like to thank Sophie, Jo and Ruth for their support and kindness. Secondly, he would like to thank his students for their enthusiasm and commitment.

COMPANION WEBSITE

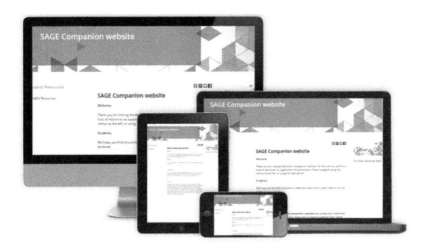

Understanding the Sociology of Health, 4th edition is supported by a wealth of online resources for both students and lecturers to aid study and support teaching, which are available at http://study.sagepub.com/barryandyuill4e

For students

- Videos: Watch and learn! Videos featuring discussion of key topics to give you deeper insight into selected concepts.
- Online readings: A range of free, in-depth, scholarly articles are available to complement chapters of the book.
- Weblinks: These websites will help you to further explore the issues you have learned about in each chapter of the book.

- Glossary: Sociology can often present new concepts and ideas that can be a little daunting to grasp at first. This glossary is an accessible collection of key concepts and terms.

For lecturers

- PowerPoint slides: Each chapter has its own dedicated PowerPoint slide show. These can be used as they are, or adapted to meet lecturers' particular needs.

INTRODUCTION

The book you are now reading should not be regarded as being all there is to understanding the sociology of health. It is just one part of an overall package that offers web-based material, links to further reading and other learning materials (such as videos). All of the additional material just mentioned can be found on the companion website and all you have to do in order to access that material is complete the online registration. There is also an option available on the companion website that allows you, the reader, to contact us, the authors. We would be happy to hear from readers about their experiences of using the textbook and suggestions for additional material or resources that could be added to the companion website.

It will be this book, however, that will be the main resource for most readers. As with all introductory texts one has to be selective in the material that is covered. There are so many fascinating and stimulating ideas, concepts, theories and pieces of research out there being produced by medical sociologists and other social scientists that it is impossible to cover everything. What we have chosen to do instead is to try to cover what we would consider to be the essential starting points for understanding the sociology of health (for example, how class, gender and ethnicity interweave with health), plus some of the more advanced debates (for example, on income inequality) that are reshaping our understanding of health and that have a resonance beyond academia. We have also chosen to keep the style as straightforward as possible but without losing sight that ideas and learning should also be challenging and stimulating. So, hopefully, we have avoided being too conversational or lapsing into the obscure phrases of complex academic jargon. If you do wish to pursue topics in greater depth then each chapter ends with suggestions for further reading, and more in-depth readings written by leading academics on particular topics can be downloaded from the companion website.

Throughout the book you will see various features that we hope will you assist in the understanding and learning of the sociology of health. These features are found embedded in the text and in the introductions and conclusions of each chapter. The features include:

- An opening summary of the main points, issues and concepts that are covered in a chapter.
- Definitions, which provide clear and concise definitions of key concepts and terms.
- Questions, which allow the reader to reflect on issues and topics raised in the text.
- Links, which indicate where related information in other chapters can be found.

And finally, each chapter ends with a summary of the main points that were discussed in the chapter and a case study that allows the reader to apply the knowledge they have gained of a particular subject within the sociology of health to a particular situation.

The book unfolds in the following three sections. The first section, 'Theories, Perspectives and Concepts' (Chapters 1–4), provides an overview of sociological perspectives on health and how we can scientifically and objectively research and understand society. This perspective begins in Chapter 1 by exploring and defining the remit of sociology as a discipline, the various types of sociological theory and how developing a sociological imagination can open new insights into health. We then move on, in Chapter 2, to interrogate medicine as the dominant mode of understanding health. Here we discuss how medical knowledge is socially constructed and consider other modes of healing, such as alternative therapies and traditional medicines. Attention then turns in Chapter 4 to how sociology attempts to understand health and the variety of approaches and methods that sociologists adopt in their research.

The second section, 'Key Themes' (Chapters 5–11), focuses on several important issues within the sociology of health. We discuss, for example, some of the main forms of inequality in society relating to class, gender, ethnicity and sexuality and how those social processes shape and condition health. The chapters in this section have been revised to offer a more global analysis of their topics. With the world becoming a more integrated and interdependent entity, it is only right that all sociology should at least seek to reach further than the boundaries of one nation state. By also going beyond one country, various comparisons become available that allow further insights into the importance of the social and how society frames and shapes our experiences and lives. We also explore sociological insights into chronic illness and disability, mental wellbeing, and ageing.

The third section, 'Contexts' (12–16), also introduces new chapters and revisions. The scope of the health policy chapter has been broadened to include a greater consideration of global issues, while a new chapter covering health technologies explores how technology alters our approach to health.

Overall, we trust that this book is enjoyable to read and will provide you with helpful and useful resources for the study of the sociology of health.

SECTION 1

THEORIES, PERSPECTIVES AND CONCEPTS

SOCIOLOGICAL THEORY: EXPLAINING AND THEORISING

MAIN POINTS

- Sociology is a scientific approach to understanding people in society.

- Social structures can often exert more influence over our behaviour than we would expect.

- Sociological perspectives on health emphasise that it is vital to understand the social in order to fully understand health and illness.

- The sociological imagination invites us to think beyond our own subjective perceptions.

- Sociological theories are useful in moving away from common-sense understandings of society.

INTRODUCTION

The aim of this chapter is to introduce the discipline of **sociology** and to focus, in particular, on the significance of the sociological study of health, illness and medicine for health-related professions. In order to do so it is necessary to begin by establishing the scope and remit of sociology as a subject area *and* as an explanatory method.

Sociology is concerned with the study of **society**, and specifically with key issues such as explaining change and the distribution of **power** between different social groups.

The discipline of sociology also offers its students specific methods of investigation and explanation. For example, this chapter introduces you to the concept of the **sociological imagination**, asking you to adopt a critical and questioning approach to even the most mundane aspects of social life. Sociological knowledge is based on a 'scientific' approach built upon evidence to support theoretical perspectives. This chapter offers an introduction to a range of sociological perspectives.

SOCIOLOGY: A METHOD OF ENQUIRY AND EXPLANATION

The raw material of sociology is human society, the development of groups, and the ways in which social groups are organised and change over time. Sociology is, therefore, the study of society. Such a statement, however, tells us very little about sociology and does nothing to draw out what is distinctive about the discipline in relation, for example, to psychology or simply to our own observations of society and social groups. Sociology is concerned with the study of human society (Giddens and Sutton 2013: 4) in terms of the interaction between individuals and groups and the interaction between groups. It is not individuals *per se* who draw our attention, but how they interact with the social environment. Giddens and Sutton (2013: 7) use the term 'society' to refer to the 'common cultural features such as language, values and basic norms' of particular countries, but also the 'enduring patterns formed by relationships among people, groups and institutions'. Sociologists refer to society as a 'system' and our own behaviour as 'institutionalised' to draw attention to what is external to the individual that is 'society' itself. 'Society' refers to the structural factors that influence our beliefs and behaviour and that establish some predictability and regularity in our lives.

> Sociology is the study of the interaction between groups and individuals in human society. The term society refers to a range of external factors that influence our beliefs and behaviours.

What troubles many new students of sociology is the suggestion that something referred to as 'society' shapes or determines our behaviour. Such an explanation seems to take away what is individual about us and suggests that our behaviour and our beliefs are not unique but may be determined by an external force and replicated by many other individuals. On reflection, however, this process of shaping and influencing is evident in all that we do. **Socialisation** into the norms and values of a particular society enables us to predict and make sense of the behaviour of others and ourselves. 'Society' provides us with the cultural resources to live in the social world because patterns of behaviour, responses and ways of behaving are not invented anew each day but exist outside any one individual. In most human encounters within a specific society, there are roles to be played out, responses to be predicted and cues to be acted upon.

> Socialisation refers to the process whereby we become aware of the values and beliefs of society.

4

Rosenhan's classic study 'On being sane in insane places' (1973) is an excellent illustration of the potential for our identities to be imposed on us by others. Rosenhan's experiment involved eight researchers posing as 'insane' who presented themselves to mental health professionals, claiming to hear voices. Apart from the supposed symptoms, the researchers told the truth about their circumstances and background. All eight researchers were admitted to hospital. Except for the initial alleged symptoms, the researchers acted normally and upon admittance stated that they no longer had any symptoms. According to Rosenhan, it is therefore problematic to say that we 'know' what insanity is. The medical professionals in this case responded to certain cues (alleged symptoms) and interpreted the researchers' behaviour and histories in the light of their assumed insanity. This experiment is important in so far as it illustrates the way in which others can impose identities upon us. The behaviour of the researchers was interpreted in the light of a set of shared symbols and meanings. In this case, the shared symbols and meanings referred to the diagnostic categories developed and used by the medical profession. The diagnosis of insanity only had meaning in the light of these categories. This particular experience begs the question of whether patients actually present 'real' symptoms or whether the symptoms are in the minds of the people who make the diagnosis.

A further example of the way and extent to which the group influences individual behaviour can be illustrated with reference to the work of Festinger et al. (1956). In this case, the group was a cult that was prophesying the end of the world by a very specific date and time. When the prophecy was proven false, the beliefs of the group members were *not* fundamentally altered. A message from God, relayed by the group leader, indicated that the end of the world was not to happen at this point after all, since the group manifested such goodness that the world would be saved from destruction. Festinger then asks why beliefs persist even in the light of contradictory evidence. The explanation lies within the group itself and its ability to reinforce the original belief. The power to do so is greater when the group consists of a close network without any dissenters. Festinger notes that, in this case, people who had been part of the group but who had not gathered in one place prior to the alleged catastrophe did not show the same adherence to the original prophecy.

LINK

Chapter 5 provides an example of the complex relationship between structural factors and personal choice in relation to health inequalities.

The relationship between society and individuals

Thus far this discussion has been concerned with demonstrating what sociology 'is' by examining the subject matter or what has been referred to as the 'raw material' of study, namely society. However, the discussion has developed further in terms of suggesting a specific and distinct relationship between individuals and the society or **structure** in which they live. A helpful example of the way in which structure (society) influences the actions and experiences of individuals is provided by Giddens. He uses the analogy of language to illustrate the relationship that individuals have with the wider social structure. None of us has invented the language that we use, but without it social activity would be impossible because it is our shared meanings that sustain 'society'. However, as Giddens and Sutton (2013) also point out, each of us is capable of using that language in a creative, distinct and individual way, and yet no one person creates language. In the same way human behaviour is not determined in a mechanical way by the structure we call society. Later chapters discuss the significance of social **class** in determining levels of morbidity and mortality and yet not every person in each social class category will have identical experiences. There will, however, be enough similarities in patterns of health within each social class for us to justifiably place people in these specific groupings. Similarities in people's experiences can be seen in terms of income levels, of availability of local resources such as GPs, of geographical location, and of their physical environment and patterns of expenditure. The relationship and interplay between society and the individual is explained in terms of **structure** and **agency**. The latter is a concept used to refer to a cluster of ideas about the potential for individuals to determine their lives, to change their environment and, ultimately, to influence the wider structure. The concept of agency, therefore, allows us to appreciate the way in which we are shaped by society, and in turn shape society.

The term structure is similar to that of 'society' in so far as it draws our attention to those factors that help determine our experiences through the establishment of expected ways of behaving. In contrast, the concept of agency reminds us that individuals do not simply act out predetermined roles but 'interpret' those roles in a way unique to them.

If the subject matter of sociology is human society, and behaviour is explained primarily in terms of 'structure', then this logically denotes specific factors in the explanatory framework of the discipline. Sociological explanations of what determines our state of health will necessarily differ from, for example, biological explanations. Clearly, disease is a biological and physical entity experienced through the medium of the body. The causes of disease, while biological, can also be considered in terms of social and structural factors. The immediate cause of a disease may be infection but the factors that lead to this may be many and varied. If we reflect upon patterns of morbidity and mortality over the last two centuries, then it is possible to observe a significant shift away from infectious diseases to chronic conditions. In other words, when we consider the factors that influence a person's state of health, the risk of infection, an ability to fight infection and genetic predisposition are greatly important but, within sociology, these are not our main focus. Social and environmental factors such as age, social class and gender are as, if not more, important.

QUESTIONS

Gender is a good example of how structures shape our lives and how we make individual choices about how we live. As a man or a woman, what experiences do you share in common with your gender? In what do you consider yourself 'unique' and different from all other women or men?

It is possible to define what we mean by 'sociology' by sketching out the discipline's remit in terms of the study of human society. From this it is logical to conclude that the study of sociology is relevant to understanding and explaining health in so far as health and its determinants need to be explained within a social context. Within nurse education, for example, the emphasis placed on 'holistic' care can also be used to justify the study of sociology in that it provides information that places an individual within a social context. To conclude that this is all that the discipline of sociology can offer in terms of studying health, illness and medicine is mistaken and unnecessarily limiting. What sociology offers is a questioning and critical way of thinking and a distinct method of explanation. To fully appreciate this element of sociology it is helpful to understand how, why and when the discipline came into being.

A sociological understanding of health considers structural and social factors, rather than simply biological explanations of health and disease.

The historical origins of sociology

The discipline of sociology is fundamentally a modern one, bound up with attempts to explain, anticipate and alter a rapidly changing world. According to Giddens and Sutton (2013), the focuses of sociology at its inception were the structures and relationships that derived from industrialisation. An examination of the works of the founding fathers of sociology (Comte, Durkheim, Weber and Marx) suggests a preoccupation with attempts to understand a rapidly changing world and to do so in a way that was 'scientific', objective and rational. Auguste Comte, for example, believed that the development of any society was ultimately positive and progressive, and identified three different phases: the religious, the metaphysical and the scientific. Each of these phases represented a mode of thought and explanation: the religious period represented a supernatural interpretation of the world;

In historical terms, modern is a term used to refer to the time period from the late nineteenth century to the mid-twentieth century.

the metaphysical one replaced religion with a belief in forces such as nature; and the final, scientific, stage represented the most positive and rational phase of human development (Craib 1997: 23). Understanding this new and complex society meant adherence to rational, scientific and empirical methods. The underlying motivation of the discipline was to reveal the reality of social relationships. For Karl Marx, this meant making plain the 'real' relationships of power and exploitation behind social class. For Emile Durkheim, getting to the heart of the reality meant the observation and recording of 'facts' to provide a picture of the world as it is, rather than to anticipate how the world should be.

Can sociology be 'scientific'?

Sociology strives to be scientific in the sense that it seeks to evidence its findings and to ensure that explanations are consistent. A fundamental difference between the social and natural sciences is that the subject matter of the social sciences, unlike that of the natural sciences, is human beings and their behaviour.

To the extent that sociological explanations attempt to be rational and empirical, they share certain features with scientific disciplines. According to Bruce (1999), scientific explanations are consistent (that is to say they cannot contradict themselves) and must accord with the evidence; and when evidence is found to refute an explanation, the explanation itself must be changed (1999: 3). A fundamental issue for sociologists is whether sociology is a science in the same sense as the physical sciences. Bruce suggests that one crucial difference is in the methods employed to uncover evidence. Natural sciences are able to make full use of the experimental method because of the relative simplicity of their subject matter. As Bruce points out, we can explain why, how and when water boils, but because the water 'has not *decided* to boil we do not need to refer to the consciousness of the water' (1999: 12). However, any explanation of human society and human behaviour has to take into account the consciousness of the subject, because actions have meanings which derive from consciousness. For these reasons the experimental method is impractical for sociologists.

This does not mean, however, that evidence need not be sought when sociologists generate and test theories. Despite apparent difficulties in establishing the 'truth', Bruce (1999: 17) argues, it is still possible to arrive at an accurate account of people's lives. He draws an analogy between sociological evidence and evidence in a court of law: in both cases, he suggests, it is possible to establish the truth from what appear to be contradictory accounts.

QUESTION

What do you think are the main differences between sociological methods of enquiry and those associated with the natural sciences?

The 'sociological imagination'

There is little doubt that sociology is one of the most controversial of all academic sub-jects, often giving rise to hostile reactions. Sociology has been associated with a radi-cal and left-wing perspective, and despite the fact that sociologists such as Comte and Durkheim conceived the subject in terms of describing and analysing what actually exists as opposed to speculating on what ought to exist, sociology has always been strongly asso-ciated with critiques of existing societies and speculation about the possibility of change. Zygmunt Bauman recognises that this questioning approach can invoke hostility: 'In an encounter with that familiar world ruled by habits ... sociology acts as a meddlesome and often irritating stranger' (cited in Kirby et al. 2000: 43).

What critics might see as most questionable about the discipline of sociology, its prac-titioners see as its main strength. Anthony Giddens, for example, writes that the study of sociology is essentially liberating because 'it teaches appreciation of cultural variety and allows us an insight into the workings of social institutions' (cited in Kirby et al. 2000: 3). To 'do' sociology requires one to think in a specific way; fundamentally, it requires what C. Wright Mills describes as the **sociological imagination**. C. Wright Mills urges us to think outside our own experiences and look at what appears to us as 'mundane' in a new light. Using the sociological imagination means departing from what are referred to as common-sense explanations: this implies an explanation of phenomena based on limited observations of human behaviour and our own, again limited, experiences of the social world. C. Wright Mills (1970) states that the sociological imagination enables three fundamental questions to be asked: (1) What is the structure of this par-ticular society? (2) Where does this society stand in human history? (3) What varieties of men and women now prevail in this society and this period? What is important here is the questioning attitude to what is given, what is seen. Asking and answering all three questions ensures that no assumptions are made about what is being studied and that the context, both cultural and historical, is taken into account when considering any explanation of what is observed.

> The concept of the sociological imagination refers to a specific way of thinking about the world, characterised by a willingness to think beyond our own experiences and to challenge common-sense or obvious explanations of human society and human behaviour.

We seek to argue that without this critical and questioning edge, 'doing' sociology ceases to have any real purpose other than to describe, to provide background detail and a social context. Such an approach does not require one to ask the critical questions posed by C. Wright Mills, and neither, crucially, does it ask us to think about why social situations are as they are. One of the fundamental concerns of sociology is the distri-bution of power in society and its consequences. When, later in this book, you analyse inequalities in health, you will see that social class is one of the main factors influencing levels of morbidity and mortality. What Chapter 5 will describe and analyse are not simply differences but inequalities in people's chances of good health and longevity. Inequality

The sociological imagination is crucial to 'doing' sociology as it provides a critical and questioning edge, without which the discipline would be limited to simply describing social phenomena.

in terms of health is, literally, a matter of life and death. Social classes don't exist in isolation from one another, they form part of a social relationship; social disadvantage has another side, and that is social advantage. An understanding of theories of power is therefore essential to 'doing' sociology successfully.

This chapter has so far drawn out what is unique about the discipline of sociology in terms of its subject matter, the nature of sociological evidence, methods of explanation and the mindset described as the sociological imagination. The next section seeks to expand upon these themes by presenting an explanation of how sociologists explain social phenomena in terms of different theoretical perspectives.

AN INTRODUCTION TO SOCIOLOGICAL THEORY

In this section we seek to explain and illustrate how sociologists explain the social world. To do this we will examine various competing theoretical approaches. To begin, however, it is necessary to think about what is meant by the term **theory** as a method of explanation. In common-sense terms a theory refers to a set of ideas or propositions used to explain and predict social phenomena. Our explanations derive ultimately from a particular perspective or worldview. Comte, for example, as we have already seen, divided human history into three phases, each characterised by a particular mode of thought (religious, metaphysical and scientific). Each of these modes of thought permits only certain kinds of explanation. The rational and scientific phase does not tolerate explanations that cannot be evidenced.

Within the discipline of sociology, theory refers to attempts to provide systematic and consistent explanations of social phenomena. The term paradigm refers to a systematic way of thinking.

Similarly, Seale and Pattison (1994), in their study of the history of medicine, identify 'paradigms' or worldviews that characterised different stages in the development of medicine. Scientific medical knowledge is just one example of a medical **paradigm** and is based on what Seale and Pattison refer to as 'systematic investigation of all aspects of human biology ... and includes experimental manipulation of body functions and testing of treatments under scientifically controlled conditions' (1994: 28).

Sociological theory and common-sense theory

Bruce (1999: 3) argues that sociological explanations should share characteristics with scientific explanations in so far as they should be consistent, must accord with the evidence and must change if evidence can be found to refute them. To the extent that this is true, it seems that sociological explanations differ from more common-sense explanations.

It is possible to argue that the latter do not have to be supported by evidence, and when evidence *is* produced there is little or no attempt to scrutinise its validity. Common-sense theories tend to be more in the nature of opinion than of fact. So far, then, this discussion has succeeded in establishing that sociological theory is characterised by the need to be consistent and evidenced. What also distinguishes sociological theory from common-sense theories is its ability to provide an 'account of the world which goes beyond what we can see and measure' (Marshall 1998: 666). 'Doing' and using sociological theory, therefore, enables us to explain phenomena of which we have no direct experience. Such a definition highlights what is unique and exciting about the discipline of sociology: its ability to inform us of differences and to think beyond our own experiences. Understanding the nature of sociological theory is a reminder of the importance of using the 'sociological imagination' as described by C. Wright Mills. Sociology is characterised by a range of different theoretical approaches, each providing a very different way of understanding social phenomena. The purpose of what follows is to provide you with an overview and an introduction to these differing perspectives.

> Doing and using sociological theory enables us to explain phenomena of which we do not have direct experience.

Functionalism

The first approach to be examined is **functionalism**. This theoretical approach is based on an analogy between society and a biological organism. Just as the body is made up of different but interrelated and interdependent parts, so society is made up of a number of different systems and subsystems. These different parts achieve unity in so far as they function to sustain the whole, in this example the wider social structure. Therefore, functionalism is less concerned with the individual and his or her aims, beliefs and consciousness, than with how our actions and beliefs function to maintain the system as a whole. An essential element in ensuring that the system is maintained is the cultural subsystem which ensures that individual motivations are in line with the values of the system as a whole. Without this central value system society would cease to function, because its cohesiveness could not be ensured. Each person has a certain role or function to fulfil, bounded by a certain set of expectations about how they will behave and how others should respond. These social expectations are referred to as role relationships, each of which carries with it a specific set of rights and obligations. The fulfilment of these roles and relationships ensures order and continuity in society.

> Functionalism offers an explanation of human society as a collection of interrelated substructures, the purpose of which is to sustain the overarching structure of society. As such, functionalism provides a 'consensual' representation of society based, first, on an agreement to sustain society as it is and, second, on shared norms and beliefs.

> When a person takes on the 'sick role', they are excused from their normal roles and responsibilities. The medical profession determines who is legitimately 'sick'. This regulatory role ensures that not too many people are unable to fulfil their normal roles – otherwise illness would have a detrimental effect on the society as a whole.

In relation to the study of health and illness, for example, the functionalist perspective is usefully illuminated by Talcott Parsons' concept of the **sick role**. First, the concept is used to analyse sickness as a social role, not merely as a biological phenomenon and physical experience: for any society to function smoothly, 'sickness' needs to be managed in such a way that the majority of people maintain their normal social roles and obligations. This perspective is based on the assumption that if too many people were to describe themselves as 'sick' and in need of being excused from their normal range of social obligations, this would be 'dysfunctional' in the sense of being disruptive for society as a whole. Those individuals who are judged by the medical profession as genuinely ill are only temporarily excused from normal obligations, and then only if they comply with the rules of the sick role. Those people taking on the sick role do so only if they agree to comply with the regime given by the medical practitioner and if they are committed to getting well as soon as possible.

LINK

Chapter 2 provides an illustration of the functionalist explanation of the doctor–patient relationship.

The functionalist perspective is a consensual approach to understanding society, which also assumes that the latent or hidden functions of everyday activities have significance for maintaining the system as a whole. In relation to something as simple as eating, Lupton (1996) argues that the 'function' of food can be seen in broader terms than just as nutritional intake. A functionalist perspective serves to highlight the way in which 'food practices serve to support co-operative behaviour or structures of kinship in small groups' (1996: 8). Lupton has also argued that the meal is a way of illustrating the culture of a specific society in terms of the order in which food is served (savoury then sweet) and the mixing of food types and temperatures.

However, the functionalist perspective has been subject to much criticism. In relation to the sick role, for example, it has been suggested that Parsons overlooked the potential for conflict between the patient and the practitioner and that he misguidedly assumed that the practitioner would always act in the best interests of the patient. Nonetheless, the main criticism is that it is an unproven assumption that situations have a fixed, obvious and shared meaning.

Symbolic interactionism

In contrast, **symbolic interactionism** is based on the premise that there is a fundamental difference between the subject matter of sociology and that of the natural sciences. While the study of the natural world deals with physical, inanimate objects, the subject matter of sociology consists of people whose actions are motivated by human consciousness. Symbolic interactionism is, therefore, concerned with how people see and understand the social world. This theoretical approach is concerned less with the larger social system or structure than with interpreting human behaviour. As with the 'sociological imagination', the emphasis here is on looking again at the most common-sense and commonplace aspects of our culture and questioning what we assume to be 'natural' and 'normal'.

The significance of this approach can be seen in relation to understanding health behaviour that appears to be irrational. Graham (1993) examined patterns of cigarette smoking among mothers on low incomes. What was revealed were relatively high levels of spending on cigarettes in low-income households. In terms of what can be observed or assumed, this behaviour might well indicate a degree of irrationality in that it contradicts dominant health messages about the dangers of smoking, and diverts limited financial resources from the family. Graham, however, favours a theoretical approach dependent upon the symbolic interactionism tradition of interpreting human behaviour in the context of people's own beliefs and meanings. This alternative interpretation associates cigarette smoking with the maintenance of normal, caring routines in that smoking creates a 'space' between the mothers and their children, providing 'time out' from the demanding routines of caring. 'Viewed within the context of mothers' daily lives, cigarette smoking appears to be a way of coping with the constant and unremitting demands of caring: a way of temporarily escaping without leaving the room' (1993: 93).

Symbolic interactionism explains social phenomena from the perspective of its participants. An essential element of this theoretical perspective is the unique nature of the social world as made up of the actions of participants motivated by human consciousness. The meaning of human action cannot, therefore, be observed or assumed, but must be interpreted by studying the meanings that people attach to their behaviour.

What the interactionist tradition presents us with is insight into two important aspects of social phenomena. First, in terms of the emphasis placed on the disputed nature of meaning, we are clearly reminded of what is central to the discipline itself, namely the questioning of the taken-for-granted. Second, the focus is on what are referred to as the **micro** elements of society, that is, the small-scale interactions between individuals and between individuals and groups. An overview of the research based on this approach indicates both the strengths and the weaknesses of symbolic interactionism. Becker's (1974) analysis of deviance is an excellent illustration of the symbolic interactionist perspective. The definition of deviance that Becker offers does not assume that what is described as deviant is fixed for all time, or that different cultures have the same definition of what counts as deviant. Becker's analysis focuses instead on the understanding of the meaning of deviance and the way in which that definition may be considered fluid rather than static. Becker defines deviance as any act that is perceived as such. Deviance is a label attached to the behaviour of an individual, rather than a quality of their behaviour. His own research tended to concentrate on certain types of 'deviant' behaviour, such as illicit drug use and prostitution, the process that led to an individual taking on a deviant career, the factors that sustained him or her in that deviant career, and the processes whereby deviant behaviour became labelled as such. Becker's research concentrated less on the structural factors that might help explain crime

In the context of this discussion, micro refers to the small-scale aspects of human behaviour, for example why individuals embark on criminal activities. Macro refers to the larger, structural aspects of society. In terms of criminal activities, this might involve analysis of the economic circumstances of criminals, of law making and law enforcement, and of the role of the state in regulating such behaviour.

and deviance, such as poverty, and placed little emphasis on the source of power of those agencies, such as criminal justice agencies, who label some people deviant. Becker talked of 'moral entrepreneurs' as influential shapers of public morals, but made little or no attempt to place these individuals and groups within the social context of society. In other words, the **macro** elements of the social structure were given much less emphasis.

Marxism

Strictly speaking, Marx did not set out to be a sociologist, and it was mainly with the political radicalisation of the 1960s that his ideas became part of the sociological main-stream. His ideas, however, do provide powerful insights into the structure of society, suggesting that it is the economic structure of any society that determines the social relations contained within that structure. It is the distribution of the ownership of the means of production that gives rise to specific patterns of class relations, which, cru-cially, in all societies are characterised by inequalities of power. Marx described modern societies in the west as capitalist, that is to say divided between those who privately own the means of production (a minority) and those who are dependent on selling their labour power to make a living (the majority). This classic division provides a description of the two main classes, the bourgeoisie and the proletariat. The relationship between the two is unequal, primarily in that the relations of production result in the exploitation of the latter in a way that is systematic and oppressive.

Marxist theory is used to question the 'naturalness' of capitalist relations and to unmask the reality of what is fundamentally an exploitative relationship. This theoretical approach is representative of the structural analysis of society – less concerned with the micro elements and more concerned with the larger picture, the underlying factors that explain social, economic and political relationships. Marxist theory, therefore, is a distinct sociolog-ical perspective, a tool for our analysis of the social structure. It would be a mistake to assume that all that this theoretical perspective can offer us is an appreciation of the significance of economic factors on, for example, health chances. Such an approach would lose sight of what Marxist theory can pro-vide us with in terms of a critique of existing social, economic and political relationships. Vicente Navarro's analysis (1976, 2002) of the causes of ill health and the relationship between the state and the medical profession is based on such insights. What Navarro provides us with is an explanation both of the causes of inequalities of health between different social classes and of why this situation continues and is, as he argues, main-tained by the medical profession (Moon and Gillespie 2005).

Marxism explains social phenom-ena as primarily determined by the economic structure of society. Social change, it is argued, is the product of changes in economic relationships. In the context of the modern period the advent of cap-italism and industrialisation pro-duced social divisions based on the ownership or non-ownership of property. The economic ine-qualities that result from owner-ship or non-ownership of property are the starting point for under-standing why there are inequali-ties in health between the middle and the working classes.

The key to this situation is, Navarro suggests, to be found in the alliance of interests between the ruling classes and the medical profession; each, for different reasons, derives power from the continuation of these conditions of inequality. For the ruling classes, health inequalities are an indication of the difference in life chances that exist between themselves and the working classes in particular. The provision of health care through a system such as the National Health Service is largely about maintaining a reasonable level of health among the working classes, sufficient to ensure that people are able to work and be returned to work following illness. Navarro in part explains the medical profession's alliance with the ruling classes in terms of their shared willingness to perpetuate the belief that the principal causes of ill health are personal and physical rather than social. Such a situation in turn strengthens the position of the medical profession in explaining illness to the lay population, but also, significantly, fosters a dependency on medicine to cure illness and disease. To admit that patterns of disease and illness are largely determined by economic and social factors would be to rob the medical profession of ideological dominance, which is founded on the claim that it is medical advances and medical technology that have produced the most startling improvements in the health of the nation. Therefore, the alliance between the ruling classes and the medical profession serves the interests of both by maintaining the professional dominance of the latter and by sustaining a reasonably healthy working population for the former.

Feminism

Marxist theory has been criticised in particular for its almost exclusive emphasis on the economic determinants of social relationships and for the resulting primacy of social class in any analysis of inequality. **Feminist theory** from the 1960s onwards sought to challenge what was seen as the invisibility of gender in sociological theory. Giddens suggests that sociology has as its main focus 'the study of the social institutions brought into being by the industrial transformations of the past two or three centuries' (1986: 9). Feminist critics argued that the founding fathers of sociology were concerned with a narrow range of topics such as social class, the division of labour in industrial society and the role of the state.

Feminism is a broad concept that explains social structures as fundamentally based on inequalities between women and men. In general, feminist sociologists have challenged the traditional preoccupation of the discipline with the effects of industrialisation and the world of paid work and institutional politics. Such an approach, it is argued, has ignored significant elements of society, such as the family and gender relationships.

It is possible to argue that two essential elements of this social transformation were largely overlooked. The first relates to the way in which industrialisation impacted specifically upon women, compared to men. According to Ramazanoglu (1989), one of the most significant changes for women related to the shift of work for remuneration from the home (or near the home) to a separate and distinct space, such as the factory. Such a split set up for the first time the dilemma of how to combine 'work' and childcare. The second element illuminates the practical changes in women's lives as well as conceptual shifts in explanations of social phenomena. The modern era is associated with a perceived split between the 'public' and the 'private' spheres. It was assumed that the natural area of study for sociology was the 'public' world of paid work, politics and the state. Since these were also the areas where men were dominant, it was this aspect of the social world that came to be associated with them. Women, on the other hand, remained within the 'private' sphere of the home, family and unpaid work. The former sphere was clearly seen as open to change, while the latter was assumed to be unchanging and 'natural'. The result of this conceptual split was an unquestioning acceptance of women and men as fundamentally different from one another and an assumption that these 'natural' differences could not be altered.

As a challenge to these assumptions, feminist theory can make a substantial contribution to our understanding of the social world in general and to the study of health and illness in particular. Feminist theory provides, for example, an analysis of gender relations on the basis of the way in which female inequality has been structured and maintained in society. One rather controversial concept used to explain this inequality is that of **patriarchy**, literally meaning the rule of men over women and of older men over younger men. In terms of uncovering what is distinct about women's lives as compared to men's, the concept of patriarchy provides a unique insight into many aspects of women's lives. Writers such as Oakley (1984) have argued that women's lives have been subject to far greater control and regulation by the medical profession than have men's. Particular examples can be seen in relation to pregnancy and childbirth, where what was previously seen as a 'natural' event attended by women rapidly became the focus of medical intervention, and now principally takes place in hospital, with the profession of obstetrics being dominated by men.

Postmodernism

The final theoretical approach to be discussed in this chapter is less a school of thought than part of a recent critical and challenging questioning of traditional sociological theory. **Postmodernism** refers to the present historical period, which is characterised by the globalisation of the economy and culture, and by a fragmentation of individual identity such that old certainties of class and national and gender identity are called into question. The term 'postmodern' also refers to a particular paradigm or worldview. In this case, what is being challenged is the certainty of our knowledge about the world, the ability of sociological theory to uncover the 'truth' about the social world, and the desirability of this. Thus, the emphasis of this particular approach is less on producing an all-embracing theory which explains all aspects of the social structure, and more on enquiring into the nature of knowledge itself.

Michel Foucault argued that in order to understand science and medicine we have to think about them as 'discourses' about the body, health and the natural world, rather than accepting these disciplines as objective descriptions of reality. The concept of **discourse** is an important one within contemporary sociology and represents a distinct way of thinking, seeing and conversing about particular phenomena, all of which create a virtual 'arena', ruling some ways of thinking as legitimate and others as not. Medicine is often described as a dominant discourse in relation to the study of health, disease and the body because western biomedicine has become the accepted, and therefore legitimate, way of thinking, talking about and seeing these aspects of human experience. Medicine represents one discourse on health, disease and the body and Foucault draws our attention to previous, non-scientific explanations of disease and perceptions of the body. Postmodernist theory makes two main contributions to the study of health and disease. First, we are offered a way of challenging the dominance of medicine and questioning what appears to be scientific, true and objective. Second, we can appreciate the way in which knowledge discourses can be used to discipline us. According to Bilton et al. (1996: 424), medicine cannot be seen, then, as merely and actively associated with clinical healing: 'the medicalisation of the body ... has to be understood as a process of social control'. We have seen from the earlier example of feminist theory and the critique of the regulation of pregnancy and childbirth that the application of medical techniques and knowledge often results in the control and regulation of patients.

Postmodernist theories veer away from all-embracing theories such as those described above that attempt to explain all social phenomena. Instead, the emphasis is on the impossibility of uncovering the 'truth' about society. Postmodernism draws our attention to how our knowledge of the social world is constructed, and offers a critical and questioning approach to understanding the world around us. Medical knowledge is an example of an established body of thought that is challenged by postmodernism as just one interpretation of reality. In other words, the 'truth' of medical knowledge is challenged.

Discourse refers to a specific way of thinking about and conceptualising a particular subject. The essence of a discourse is the language used to express thoughts. Science is an example of a discourse that rules out some kinds of explanations (for example, spiritual) and only allows for others (for example, rational and evidenced 'facts').

CONCLUSION

This chapter has sought to establish the nature of the discipline of sociology by detailing what is distinctive about its subject matter and method of enquiry. You have also been introduced to various theoretical explanations of social phenomena. Only by having such theoretical perspectives are we able to glimpse what is beneath the common-sense surface perceptions. In the rest of the book you will see how this distinctive way of looking at the world helps to bring about an understanding of health in its fullest and widest sense. What will emerge is that health is clearly bound up with the social world, with some of the main inequalities and patterns of health and illness only explainable by reference to sociology.

SUMMARY POINTS

- Sociology is concerned with the study of society and specifically with key issues such as inequalities in life chances.

- Sociology offers what Bruce (1999) terms a 'scientific' method of enquiry, characterised by the search for valid evidence.

- The study of sociology requires us to think outside our own experiences and to employ the 'sociological imagination'.

- Sociological theory can be distinguished from 'everyday theory' by its requirement to resort to reasoned, evidenced and coherent explanations of social phenomena.

TAKING YOUR STUDIES FURTHER

This chapter will have helped you understand many of the key terms, concepts, theories and debates relating to sociological theory. Listed below are books that will provide deeper and more detailed discussions of the points raised in this chapter. You will also find additional resources on the companion website, including downloads of relevant material, links to useful websites, videos and other features. Please visit the companion website at https://study.sagepub.com/barryandyuill4e

RECOMMENDED READING

Benton, T. and Craib, I. (2010) *Philosophy of Social Science: The Philosophical Foundations of Social Thought*, 2nd edn. Basingstoke: Palgrave.

Bruce, S. (1999) *Sociology: A Very Short Introduction*. Oxford: Oxford University Press.

Craib, I. (2004) *Classical Social Theory: An Introduction to the Thought of Marx, Weber, Durkheim and Simmel*. Oxford: Oxford University Press.

Scambler, G. (2002) *Health and Social Change: A Critical Theory*. Buckingham: Open University Press.

UNDERSTANDING HEALTH

MAIN POINTS

- The medical model of health stresses a mechanistic view of the body and a reliance on biological causation to explain illness.

- The social model provides a holistic approach, stressing that health and illness can only be explained by analysing the social.

- There are limits to the social model too, as it can overemphasise the role of the social and forget that health is experienced in the human body.

- Traditional medicine and alternative therapies provide other models and ways of thinking about health and wellbeing.

INTRODUCTION

The previous chapter introduced the vital concept of the 'sociological imagination' necessary for the practice of sociology, where we try to think about the society in which we live in new and different ways, putting aside stereotypes and trying to acquire new insights into what is being studied. When we turn to health the sociological imagination urges us to think of health in a radically different manner from what we are perhaps used to. Guided by the sociological imagination, health ceases to be limited to the horizons of biology and individual choice, but is placed into the context of how embodied social agents live in a society that enables or denies the material, emotional and symbolic resources to live a life that is fulfilling and meaningful.

This chapter develops the points made above in greater depth and detail. First, how sociology understands health is discussed. Here we examine two different perspectives or models of health, the medical and the social, and how they contrast with each other. The main point to be raised here is that we should not wholly dismiss biomedicine, the dominant model of understanding health, but maintain a critical distance from some of its claims as to how effective and complete it is in fully addressing all aspects of health. Attention then turns to a deeper examination of biomedicine, where we discuss core aspects of how it operates. The way in which its knowledge of health is constructed is critiqued, followed by a discussion on how that knowledge creates certain power relationships in society. The final sections of this chapter focus on opposing and different approaches to health: alternative medicine and traditional medicine. Here we explore how people engage in health practices that are quite different from orthodox biomedicine in different parts of the world.

MODELS OF HEALTH

On the companion website: Chris Yuill talks about why it is important to think through what we mean by health.

Biomedicine is the principal way of understanding health and illness in global culture, being widely accepted not just by the medical profession but also by the lay (non-professional) population. There is general agreement among contributors to debates in medical sociology that the medical model of explanation of health has a number of defining characteristics. Nettleton (2013), for example, describes five features:

Mind–body dualism. This refers to an acceptance that when one is treating disease the mind and the body can be considered as two separate entities. The physical body rather than the more problematic 'mind' is the subject of medicine. Medicine's appropriation of the body is such that, until recently, there was very little written by sociologists about the body; this was the domain of the medical profession.

Mechanical metaphor. Nettleton uses this concept to draw our attention to the way in which medicine is said to view the body as a machine, the functioning of which is determined by biological and scientific laws. Having knowledge of how the body functions allows medical practitioners to 'repair' any dysfunction.

Technological imperative. This refers to the significance attached to medical methods of intervention, whether pharmacological or surgical, in treating the body. As we shall see, there is often a tendency to overemphasise the curative element of biomedicine and underplay the beneficial contributions made by, for example, changes in diet or environment. While the development of medical technology brings with it considerable benefits, these developments also have a cost, for instance in terms of the harmful consequences either of medicines or of medical intervention. We discuss in Chapter 3, for example, that some of the major advances in the overall health of people in the United Kingdom was achieved by engineering and the creation of public sanitation.

Reductionist tendency. Biomedicine is described by Nettleton as 'reductionist' in that there is a tendency to reduce all explanations to the physical workings of the body. There is an echo of this reductionist tendency in the dualistic nature of medicine as well as in the significance attached to the 'technological imperative' in the primary role attached to all things physical. One of the major criticisms of the medical model stems from its apparent unwillingness to acknowledge that both social and psychological factors influence health.

Doctrine of specific aetiology. This refers to the belief that all disease originates from specific and knowable causes.

Another criticism levelled at the **medical model of health** is that as well as doing good it can do harm. The concept of **iatrogenesis**, associated with Ivan Illich, refers to an illness caused by a doctor; that is to say, harm would not have been caused without the medical intervention. Illich argues that the 'damage done by medicine to the health of the individuals and populations is very significant' (1993). This is referred to as 'clinical' iatrogenesis and Illich cites drug therapies, doctors or hospitals as the cause of harm. A second aspect is 'cultural' iatrogenesis, which denotes a dependence on medicine to cure and to care for people. Illich argues that cultural iatrogenesis means that people no longer take responsibility for their own health problems and the diagnosis of their symptoms. Illich asserts that 'medical practice sponsors sickness ... reinforcing a morbid society that encourages people to become consumers of curative, preventative, industrial and environmental medicine' (1993: 158). The result of this dependency is a situation of 'medical nemesis', where the harm caused by medicine is difficult to eliminate except by recourse to further medical intervention, which in itself results in further harm. Illich paints a picture of an inevitable decline into an increasingly unhealthy world, where the provision of health care ultimately has a negative effect on our wellbeing.

> Iatrogenesis literally means harm caused by doctors. In its most literal sense it refers to the harmful consequences of medical intervention. Illich also uses the concept to draw our attention to our cultural dependence on medicine and medical practitioners, such that we do not seek alternative explanations or alternative remedies for ill health.

QUESTION

What examples can you give of instances where medical intervention has had negative effects?

A balanced account of the harm resulting from health care would also, clearly, have to take into account positive developments in medicine. Hardley (1998) characterised the 1950s and 1960s as a period of great optimism about the potential of medicine to cure and care for people, and evidences this with reference to mass vaccination programmes that eradicated diseases such as polio and smallpox. At one end of the spectrum medicine can save and prolong life through radical interventions such as organ transplants, while at the more mundane end of the spectrum the symptoms of minor ailments such as headaches and menstrual pain can be eliminated by readily available pain relief. It is hardly surprising, therefore, that lay people may have a sense of dependency on medicine. Compared to people's experiences of health in the past, our own ill health may well seem trivial. Giddens comments that a glance at those experiences 'provides graphic evidence of the level to which illness and the prospect of an early death haunted the lives of individuals in the eighteenth century. Infectious diseases were rampant and the ordinary person suffered from a range of chronic complaints which many of us in modern social conditions would find intolerable' (1997: 47–8).

In the eighteenth century in particular, deadly fevers – contemporaries called them 'spotted', 'miliary', 'hectic', 'malignant', etc. – struck down hundreds of thousands, young and old alike, while the so-called 'new' diseases gained ground – some crippling, such as rickets; some fatal, such as tuberculosis. Today's minor nuisance, like flu, was yesterday's killer. 'The Hooping Cough is yet with us', wrote George Crabbe in 1829, 'and many children die of it.' And all this against a backdrop of endemic maladies, such as malaria and infantile diarrhoea, and a Pandora's box of other infections (dysentery, scarlatina, measles, etc.) that commonly proved fatal, above all to infants, to say nothing of the 101 other pains, eruptions, swellings, ulcers, scrofula and wasting conditions, not least the agonising stone and the proverbial gout, which threatened livings and livelihoods, and all too often life itself (Porter and Porter 1985, reprinted in Giddens 2001: 116).

THE MEDICAL MODEL AND THE CONSTRUCTION OF MEDICAL KNOWLEDGE

The medical model is a specific way of thinking about and explaining disease based on biological factors. Such a description of the medical model may well strike you as rather rigid, and as a far more accurate account of medicine and medical practice in the past rather than today. We would argue, however, that central elements of medical knowledge remain but that medicine is a dynamic body of thought, capable of changing and adapting in the light of new discoveries. The fluid nature of medical knowledge means that some elements of the medical model may be more or less important now than they were in the past.

This fluidity of medical knowledge and the reason it changes over time is in part due to the socially constructed nature of medical knowledge. **Social constructionism** is characterised by an emphasis on the extent to which 'society' is actively and creatively produced by human beings. The world is portrayed as made or invented, rather than as a given or taken for granted: 'Social worlds are interpretive nets woven by individuals and groups' (Marshall 1998: 609). The extent to which medical knowledge can also be said to be socially constructed, that is, the degree to which medical knowledge is a product of those engaged in its practice, can be illustrated by Jewson's (1976) concept of paradigms of medical knowledge. The term paradigm (introduced in Chapter 1) refers to a model or mode of thought, a particular way of seeing the world, that sets boundaries to what we see, how we might measure and record that information, and which factors are significant and which are not.

> Social constructionism is a theory that emphasises the extent to which 'society' is actively and creatively produced by human beings.

Paradigms of knowledge shift and change over time, as illustrated by the earlier discussion of the medical model, and therefore offer us a way of conceptualising the fluid and dynamic nature of medical knowledge.

Table 2.1 represents a simplification of the three paradigms. It is a useful starting point in the analysis of the social construction of medical knowledge and raises the following significant points:

- Medical knowledge has changed and developed over time. What was once held as a reasonable explanation may later be disputed and cast aside. Early medical theories of **hysteria**, for example, maintained that the womb of 'hysterical' women moved around the body.
- Medical knowledge and, more generally, knowledge about health and disease has become increasingly specialised, first focusing on the 'whole' person, then examining specific parts of the body, and finally analysing the construction of cells. Theoretical knowledge of the body, learned knowledge, has taken precedence over experiential knowledge. Medicine and medical practice have increasingly become the preserve of those educated and trained by current practitioners and registered with their professional bodies. Lay practitioners, such as lay midwives, were systematically excluded from the practice of medicine.

Table 2.1 Jewson's three paradigms of medical knowledge (Seale and Pattison 1994)

Bedside medicine	Clinical medicine	Laboratory medicine
• Disease as a total 'psychosomatic' experience • Lay and 'medical' practitioners • Place of treatment: home	• Specific aetiology of diseases • Specialist practitioners in possession of specialist knowledge about the body • Place of treatment: hospital	• Disease as a 'biochemical disturbance' • Specialist practitioners, knowledge of cellular construction of the body • Place of treatment: laboratory

- Each paradigm shift in thought has entailed a shift in the nature of the relationship between the practitioner and the patient. The 'bedside manner' paradigm suggests that, at least in the case of the wealthy, practitioners (physicians or doctors) were 'patronised' by clients. Clients paid directly for the service and those providing it were often considered their social inferiors; power lay with the patient.

AWAY FROM THE MEDICAL MODEL AND TOWARDS THE SOCIAL MODEL

It is perhaps easier to see the relevance of such a model in the past, when infectious diseases were the main cause of morbidity and mortality. The major killers of the twentieth and twenty-first centuries are long-term, chronic illnesses – not only in the high-income countries of Europe and North America, but also increasingly in the middle-income countries, such as South Africa. What distinguishes these conditions from diseases of the past is that their causes are 'social'. This emphasis on the social as the cause of disease is the major theme that runs throughout this book. What we mean by claiming that the causes of disease and poor wellbeing are social is that various aspects of the societies in which we live are not good for our health and wellbeing. Those aspects include inequality, sexism and racism, and how living in a society where you experience a lack of control, purpose and meaning damages your health. This is a different way of understanding health that moves away from a focus on biology, or what are seen as risk factors (poor diet, smoking, lack of exercise or drinking too much). These risk factors are important, but they are not the whole story in understanding health, nor are they the only causes of poor health. As Marmot (2012) has claimed, perhaps up to one-third of our health is attributable to these factors, while the rest is down to the kind of society in which we live. To help understand that wider context of health, and how it is not just biology and risk factors that are important in understanding health, sociologists have developed what they call the social model of health.

The main aim of the social model of health is to place health into a social context and to understand health as emerging out of many different processes and influences that include but definitely go beyond the purely biological. By doing so, health is no longer separated from the lived experiences of everyday life. Sociologist James Nazroo (2012) provides a useful way into the social model of health. He asks us to think about health in a different way. Instead of saying that is it about what individuals do that causes them to have good or poor health, we should, he suggests, ask what it is about society that causes good or poor health. Most people are used to thinking of health in individualistic terms (What does that person eat, or how much exercise do they take?) and it is an approach to health that is repeated and supported in popular culture, witnessed in popular dramas or in fiction. By shifting the emphasis onto the social, a whole raft of new questions and new approaches opens up. As we shall encounter throughout this book, various social processes create the context in which we exist and which in turn provides the resources, opportunities and challenges that either enable or prevent us from leading a life that is healthy, rewarding and fulfilling.

As we mentioned in the previous chapter, sociologists do not claim that society operates with rigid iron laws or that people lack the agency to make decisions concerning their lives. Rather, what we must appreciate is that not everyone has equal access to a range of resources that can enable them and the communities in which they live to lead the lives that they want, and allows them to make the decisions and adopt the conditions in which to lead healthy lives.

However, sociologists and people using sociology should be mindful, as Williams (2001) warns us not to uncritically accept the social model of health. It too can lapse into problems that are almost the mirror opposite of the medical model of health. The medical model of health can be found short on focusing solely on the biological, and sometimes sociologists following the social model can overemphasise the social to the point where they forget that there are fleshy biological bodies out there where pain, discomfort and illness are experienced. What Williams and other writers, such as Shakespeare (2006), emphasise is that we need to develop more nuanced models of thinking about health that capture the richness and depth of all the multiple processes which ultimately shape our health.

> The concept of power is the subject of much debate within sociology. In the context of this discussion, however, the concept refers to (a) the ability to ensure that a particular point of view prevails in a disputed situation, (b) the capacity to ensure that someone acts in a certain way, and (c) the ability to stifle opposition to a particular perspective.

Another point raised by the likes of Williams is that the social model of health can be overly critical of the medical profession. While many of the criticisms hold true, and we encounter them throughout this book, the medical profession is also not as powerful as it once was, and it now faces various pressures that challenge the **power** and influence it once held. Challenges to the medical profession have come from a variety of sources. Patients are generally better informed about their condition than in the past, and those with chronic long-term conditions can accumulate an impressive level of knowledge and understanding of their illness. Cultural and political developments have encouraged us to see ourselves as consumers of health care, with resulting rights to adequate treatment and recourse if we feel that the treatment has not been appropriate. A second challenge has come from alternative practitioners (more of which later in this chapter), who have raised serious questions about the effectiveness of conventional treatments and their potentially damaging long-term effects. A third challenge to **clinical autonomy** can come from governments as they seek to regulate medical and other health professionals. A final, fourth challenge can be found in how private pharmaceutical corporations can influence and set the health agenda. A useful example of the latter is provided by the introduction of drugs such as Viagra, used to treat sexual dysfunction in men, where pharmaceutical companies (as opposed to the medical profession) contribute to creating a narrative of what needs can be treated in order to create a market for their products (Marshall 2010).

OTHER WAYS OF HEALING: ALTERNATIVE THERAPIES AND TRADITIONAL MEDICINES

Here we consider two paradigms of health that are quite different from orthodox medicine and the biomedical approach to health. The first is **traditional medicine**, the type of health care that vast numbers of people rely on mainly in the global south, which is steeped in the traditions and history of a particular nation. The second is **alternative medicine** or complementary therapies, which appear typically in the global north. The appeal of alternative medicine lies in a form of health care where the centrality of the patient is much more pronounced than in conventional medical practice.

TRADITIONAL MEDICINE

Both traditional and alternative medicines share a holistic understanding of the causes of poor and good health, focusing on the unity of the mind and body, and how that unity is affected by the circumstances in which one lives. They do, however, differ in other regards. Traditional medicines are typically found in the global south and draw deeply on the experiences, beliefs and culture of a particular society. Alternative medicines are typically found in the global north and are popular among people who are dissatisfied with conventional medicine. They are also often drawn from or appropriate traditional medicines but lack the cultural roots in the society in which they are adopted.

The general line of discussion has emphasised biomedicine as the globally dominant perspective on health, and in many respects that is true, which is why it is important to be able to understand and critique it sociologically. Thinking of the world in this way, however, ignores the stubborn fact that for a considerable number of people globally it is traditional medicines that are turned to and utilised in times of illness instead of, or alongside, biomedicine or forms of healing that are regarded as orthodox in the global north. The use of traditional medicine adds a further dimension to our discussion here on understanding health: that what occurs in the global north (so-called western countries, such as those in Europe and North America) does not always apply to other parts of the world. Care must be taken not to be what is called Eurocentric, where ways of thinking and behaving are assumed to be the only way of being, or are thought of as being superior to cultures and traditions elsewhere.

It is very difficult to identify an exact figure either in terms of actual people or in monetary terms, but the World Health Organisation (WHO) (2013: 26) suggests that in China there were 907 million visits to providers of traditional medicine in 2009 and that in Lao People's Democratic Republic 18, 226 traditional health practitioners form the basis of health care for 80% of the population. Traditional medicine can be defined as follows:

> Traditional medicine is the sum total of the knowledge, skills, and practices based on the theories, beliefs, and experiences indigenous to different cultures, whether explicable or not, used in the maintenance of health as well as in the prevention, diagnosis, improvement or treatment of physical and mental illness. (World Health Organisation 2013: 15)

The form traditional medicine takes varies by country and region, though often an emphasis on some form of holism is present, or a belief in magic or the presence of spirits. As Busia (2005: 919) notes from an African perspective, 'Unlike a medically trained doctor, the traditional African healer looks for the cause of a patient's misfortune/illness in the context of the social, natural and spiritual environment'. Often traditional medicines predate the arrival of the western colonial powers, who introduced early forms of biomedicine. Ayurveda, a traditional medicine practised in India, can, for instance, be traced back to the Bronze Age (Gupta et al. 2014).

Actual remedies used in traditional medicines are derived from medicinal plants and herbs or from animal sources. Writing about traditional medicines in South Africa (*umuthi*), Williams and Whiting (2016) identify that a wide range of plants are used in that approach to health, and also a range of therapies and medicines derived from vertebrate and invertebrate animals, such as pythons, starfish and ostriches. They note that the use of animal-derived medicines is often driven by social, personal and cultural considerations.

Some cross-over and overlap can exist between alternative medicines and traditional medicines. So, for example, Ayurvedic medicine, which emphasises a holistic approach to life and the importance of balancing life forces with exercise and diet, is highly popular in India, from where it originated. Because it belongs to Indian culture and exists within deep historical roots, it is classed as traditional. When people who do not have Indian heritage in countries in Europe and North America use Ayurvedic medicine it is not part of their traditions or culture and therefore is an alternative or complementary medicine. It is the traditional use of the medicine that is important.

CHOOSING TO USE TRADITIONAL MEDICINES

Different reasons exist as to why people choose to access traditional medicine and to be treated by traditional therapies. In addition to cultural reasons, accessibility and cost are other prompts for people choosing traditional medicines. In Africa, the ratio of traditional healers to members of the population is substantially lower than that of orthodox medical doctors: 1:500 compared to 1:40,000 (World Health Organisation (WHO) 2013: 27). In some places, accessing the services of medical doctors is impossible for a variety of reasons, but can include infrastructure, in that there are no roads or transport services that people can utilise in order to reach a medical doctor. Therefore, in time of need, someone who practises traditional health care may be the only choice available. Cost, too, can be a reason for choosing traditional medicine. In an economic analysis of why people choose traditional health care in Ghana, Sato (2012) identified a relationship between socio-economic status and healthcare usage. She found that while people of all socio-economic groups preferred to use orthodox medical health care, as level of income decreased people were more likely to opt for traditional care. However, as she points out, it is quite common for people to use both traditional and orthodox health care simultaneously.

INTEGRATING TRADITIONAL MEDICINES AND ORTHODOX MEDICINE?

The relationship between traditional medicines and orthodox medicine need not be one of separation or opposition. Given that for many traditional health care is the only option available to them, perhaps it makes sense to attempt to develop traditional medicine as a resource. The World Health Organisation has proposed that traditional medicine could play a vital role in providing health care. In their *WHO Traditional Medicine Strategy 2014–2023* (2013: 11) they recommend:

- harnessing the potential contribution of TM to health, wellness and people-centred health care;
- promoting the safe and effective use of TM by regulating, researching and integrating TM products, practitioners and practice into health systems, where appropriate.

Research by sociologists also suggests that traditional medicine and traditional health providers could be integrated into an overall healthcare system. Work by Rishworth et al. (2016) in Ghana found that for women giving birth in the Upper West Region of that country, skilled birth attendants (doctors, nurses or midwives) could not always be accessed due to the geographic remoteness of the area, and that in times of need women turned to traditional birth attendants as the only alternative. However, those traditional attendants are technically not allowed to assist with a delivery unless accompanied by a skilled birth attendant at an appropriate facility. This policy was implemented with the intention of meeting international health policies advanced by the WHO. The intention is that all women should have a skilled attendant with them when giving birth as a means of reducing neonatal mortality rates. Despite developing policy to meet this objective, neonatal death rates have not been significantly reduced. In countries such as Ghana, the infrastructure and the skilled health workers are not always there and in more remote areas issues of poor transport and access are difficult to resolve. Perhaps, as Rishworth et al. suggest, providing support, training and resources for traditional birth attendants is one way forward.

QUESTIONS

Think about the integration of traditional birth attendants into orthodox healthcare systems. What advantages and disadvantages can you identify? What is your view on this matter?

ALTERNATIVE THERAPIES

Alternative, or complementary, therapies embrace many philosophies and methods, but collectively represent a challenge to the concepts of health and disease articulated in the medical model. This part of the discussion begins by defining what is meant by 'alternative' practices and provides specific examples.

In their broadest sense, the terms **alternative medicine** and **complementary medicine** can be used to describe any practices that fall outside the boundaries of conventional medicine. West (1993) acknowledges that it is problematic to try to define such a diverse body of practices, but offers the possibility of categorising different types. The main categories are identified as physical, psychological and paranormal. She suggests a further distinction between practices that demand a high level of training and those she describes as virtually 'do-it-yourself'. For others, the principal distinction between 'alternative' medicine and biomedicine is the former's 'holistic' emphasis. Saks suggests that in 'orthodox' medicine, the overwhelming emphasis is on the physical, with the mind and the spirit 'still typically regarded as relatively peripheral to health care' (Saks 1998: 198). In contrast, and despite their apparent diversity, most alternative therapies deal 'with the unity of the mind, body and spirit' (1998: 198). The following are examples of two alternative approaches to understanding health and illness.

- Alternative medicine embraces any medical practice that falls outside the boundaries of conventional medicine.
- Some commentators use the term complementary medicine to imply that non-conventional medicine can be used in conjunction with western biomedicine rather than as a radical alternative.

ALTERNATIVE CONCEPTS OF HEALTH

The following discussion requires you to draw on the examples of specific practices outlined above. The central elements of alternative medicine are detailed in Table 2.2.

Attempts to describe particular alternative practices and to detail what is specific about the concepts of health underpinning this approach reveal the essential differences between alternative medicine and the biomedical model. The discussion has sought to draw your attention to differing conceptions of health, disease and the relationship between mind, body and spirit. Biomedicine has sought to emphasise a further distinction between itself and alternative practices by asserting the supremacy of science over superstition. Previous discussions of biomedicine have dealt with its commitment to scientific methods free from social or political bias (British Medical Association, cited in Saks 1992). The scientific observation of natural phenomena allows for the development of laws governing such

Table 2.2 Alternative medicine: concepts of health (Aakster 1993)

Alternative medicine	Biomedicine
Health as a balance of opposing forces within the body.	Health as the absence of disease.
Disease understood as indicating the presence of negative, disruptive forces within the body. Symptoms are the product of the body's attempts to rid it of toxic substances.	Disease as defined in relation to a specific part of the body. Essentially, disease is understood as a deviation from normal functoning.
'Reading' the body, examining dietary habits, lifestyles and constitution types to achieve diagnosis.	Diagnosis achieved by examining the form and structure of specific organisms and the degree to which the presence of a disease indicates a deviation from normal functioning.
Therapy is based on an attempt to strengthen vitalising, positive forces within the body.	Therapy consists of attempts to destroy or suppress disease.

phenomena and, perhaps most significantly, such laws and the resulting 'facts' can be said to be valid because the results can be reproduced repeatedly, proving their validity. This reproducibility of results, it is argued, cannot be matched by alternative medicine.

The juxtaposition of 'scientific' medicine and 'unscientific' alternative practices leaves little scope for debate, as both sides appear to base their arguments on criteria not accepted by the other. It is biomedicine, however, that enjoys the dominant position as *the* established form of medicine. An essential element of this dominance can be traced back to a wide acceptance of the validity of science and scientific methods during **the Enlightenment**. The practice and philosophy of alternative medicine are, arguably, at a distinct disadvantage because science has reached the status of 'truth'. In the opening chapter, you were introduced to some of the basic elements of a postmodern critique of society and knowledge. Postmodernism is critical and sceptical of attempts to offer single, monolithic explanations of any phenomenon and so the whole basis of rational scientific knowledge has been questioned. Saks (1998: 204) argues that this critique of 'science, reason and enlightenment' provides a useful tool with which to reappraise the philosophical basis of alternative medical practices. Since postmodernism is characterised by 'the acceptance of multiple realities and coexisting narratives' (1998: 204), it is possible to appraise the relative merits of alternative medicine and biomedicine in such a way that both are accepted as different but equally valid conceptions of the body, health and disease. Interestingly, the British Holistic Medical Association also draws attention to changes in modes of thinking and in particular to an acceptance of the non-scientific in terms of recognising the significance of the human spirit and conscience. It argues that medicine in the twenty-first century will increasingly come to recognise the significance of the relationships between the mind, body and spirit and the human capacity to alter both the internal and the external environment (www.bhma.org).

CHOOSING TO USE ALTERNATIVE MEDICINE

Alternative medicine clearly demonstrates the possibility of a philosophical challenge to the dominance of orthodox medicine. It should also be evident from the critique of medicine presented in the preceding chapter that the practice of orthodox medicine is also ripe for criticism. Looking at the reasons for the increasing use of alternative and complementary health care, McQuaide (2005) points to several trends in wider society. These indicate a growing individualism and dissociation from civic society and mainstream medicine, and tie in with Putnam's (2000) ideas on the decline of civic society in the USA. Contemporary Americans are less likely to direct their efforts towards communal goals and activities and instead seek private solutions to their problems. Alternative health care fits this trend, as often the individual seeks out an alternative therapy for themselves as opposed to engaging with something like the National Health Service, with its communal orientation to health.

In relation to mainstream medicine, McQuaide (2005) makes the point that it is the unequal power relationship that puts people off using such services. More equal and participatory relationships are sought in alternative therapies and that appears to be one of their main attractions. Earlier work by Sharma (1992) and more recently by Pedersen et al. (2016) found that in general people used alternative medicine because they placed a high value on what they found to be the more equal and informed relationship between practitioners and patients, and because of the importance attached to the consideration of the personal circumstances of their illness. Further to this point, Coward (1993) argues that biomedicine not only has medicalised many aspects of human existence, but has done so in an inhumane way. The examples of iatrogenic practices discussed earlier included a consideration of the harmful side-effects of drugs as well as examples of medical interventions, such as surgery, that have resulted in harm to the patient. The later discussion of mental health (Chapter 8) will also illustrate that the practice of medicine, as well as specific forms of treatment, has been uncaring and inhumane. The supposed neutrality of biomedicine, its ability to see disease as a purely biological entity, may not always be perceived as beneficial. As Coward comments, a purely rational explanation of disease as arbitrary does not, perhaps, satisfy a more fundamental need to understand why our own life has been affected in this way.

In addition to these individualistic currents, McQuaide (2005) also notes the influence of the baby boomer generation (those born between 1945 and 1960). As a generation, they grew up with counter-cultural ideas strongly influenced by the 'hippie' idealism of the 1960s, where nature and all things natural enjoyed a strong profile. Alternative health care, with its associations of being natural, neatly mirrors the culture that this generation were part of in their youth. This preference for all things natural, coupled with a desire to maintain health by purchasing that health care, has opened up a considerable market for alternative health care. This has to be tempered by acknowledging that it is only really a viable option for those with a disposable income. Other reasons for the popularity of alternative medicine are identified in Table 2.3.

Table 2.3 Explaining why people use alternative medicine (Sharma 1992; Coward 1993; Lupton 2012a)

- **The limits of biomedicine**

Biomedicine is unable to 'cure' certain conditions.

Biomedicine does not place enough emphasis on the causes of illness and is preoccupied with relieving symptoms.

The side-effects of biomedical treatment are potentially harmful.

Biomedical treatment is often too drastic and too invasive.

- **The benefits of alternative medicine**

Provides an explanation of the causes of ill health and disease in the context of a person's individual lifestyle.

Provides a more egalitarian relationship between patient and practitioner.

Offers an alternative to 'high-tech' medicine.

Treats the whole person.

Encourages individuals to take greater responsibility for their health.

- **The use of alternative medicine as an expression of postmodern society**

Expresses a greater desire for self-determination and choice.

Challenges the cultural dominance of biomedicine.

Reflects a more general trend for maintaining the body through the purchase of consumer goods and services.

We have highlighted the assumed advantages of alternative practices over orthodox medicine. However, these practices themselves have been subject to critical scrutiny. Commentators such as Coward (1993) have emphasised the individualistic assessment of health underpinning many alternative practices. Such an approach can be contrasted with the **social model of health**, which draws our attention to the social, economic and cultural determinants of health. Chapter 5, examining inequalities in health, seeks to place patterns of morbidity and mortality in a social context. There is widespread acceptance within the discipline of sociology that economic and social factors have a significant impact upon health outcomes. Sociologists of health do not deny the importance of agency (that is to say, the capacity of individuals to act rather than be acted upon), but maintain that agency has its limitations. In contrast, Coward (1993) argues, alternative medicine stresses the extent to which individuals can determine their health status and offers an explanation that leads almost inevitably to the conclusion that individuals are responsible for their own health regardless of their social circumstances.

This appeal to the individual is, Coward suggests, part of a cultural obsession with the performance and appearance of the body. It is important to note, however, that a central theme in the world of the 'worried well' is an obsession with appearance in terms of the body as a project, something owned by the individual and open to change and development by them. The widespread popularity, for example, of diets to lose weight, fitness to tone the body and cosmetic surgery to alter it, is evidence of the new significance attached to the body. Working on the body to alter or enhance its appearance is represented as a matter of choice and self-determination. Good health and poor health, therefore, become matters of personal responsibility and, as Lupton (2012b) reminds us, contain strong moral overtones of how we ought to care for the body.

Coward argues that part of the attraction of alternative medicine is its association with the natural world and the healing power of nature (cited in Lupton 2012b: 128). Like the concept of 'science', with its association with the values of rationality, objectivity and progress, 'nature' is closely linked to ideas of virtue, goodness and purity (Lupton 2012b: 134). Such an association suggests that nature and natural remedies are implicitly good for you and inevitably are preferable to artificial substances such as pharmacological drugs. Lupton argues that it is impossible to support such a clear-cut distinction between natural and artificial substances since 'many naturally occurring substances can be toxic, and many chemicals are derived from naturally occurring substances' (2012b: 134). Many freely available herbal remedies carry the potential to be harmful when not taken in an appropriate manner. One such example, for the treatment of depression, would be the use of St John's Wort, available over the counter and capable of being used even when a diagnosis of depression has not been made. It is perhaps ironic to note that, at a time when the use and efficacy of drugs are subject to more stringent regulation, and when there is a requirement for pharmaceutical manufacturers to provide detailed patient information, natural remedies are not subject to the same degree of regulation. Most herbal remedies are in fact not classified as medicine and, therefore, are not subject to the same requirement for testing and regulation as artificial substances.

CONCLUSION

This chapter has attempted to raise questions and perhaps challenge commonly held notions of what health is and how it can be understood. What we have stressed here is that the usual, accepted way of thinking about health as being about our biology and as being affected by the kinds of behaviours we engage in (whether that is smoking or exercising) is only one aspect of health. As Marmot (2015) states too, it is not the whole picture. What we should do instead is try to think of health as being much wider than that, and to place it in the context of the society in which we live, and how that society enables or prevents people being as healthy as they can be. The barriers that prevent many people from living as healthy as life as they can are often beyond their control, and lie in how a society is structured. What those barriers are and how they shape and influence health are explored in greater depth throughout this book.

SUMMARY POINTS

- Health is more than our biology and what we do in terms of eating, smoking and exercising.

- The social model of health emphasises that health emerges out of a variety of social causes and social processes.

- Some people in high-income nations have rejected or questioned the medical model of health and have. They feel that orthodox medicine does not fully embrace their individuality, whilst alternative medicine offers a more person-centred approach.

- Ideas of what constitutes health and health care are often dominated by western models of health and health care. Many parts of the globe have their own traditional forms of health care that are ignored and undervalued, and can add to the health of local populations.

TAKING YOUR STUDIES FURTHER

This chapter will have helped you understand many of the key terms, concepts, theories and debates relating to models of health. Listed below are books that will provide deeper and more detailed discussions of the points raised in this chapter. You will also find additional resources on the companion website, including downloads of relevant material, links to useful websites, videos and other features. Please visit the companion website at https://study.sagepub.com/barryandyuill4e

RECOMMENDED READING

Bradby, H. (2008) *Medical Sociology: An Introduction*. London: SAGE.

Gabe, J. and Monaghan, L.F. (eds) (2013) *Key Concepts in Medical Sociology*. London: SAGE.

Lupton, D. (2012a) *Medicine as Culture: Illness, Disease and the Body*, revised 3rd edn. London: SAGE.

A BRIEF HISTORY OF
HEALTH AND HEALING

MAIN POINTS

- Humans have throughout history and pre-history sought to be healthy and to heal the sick.

- The causes of disease emerge out of how humans interact with others and change the environment around them.

- Ideas about health and healing relate to society, whether it 'allows' or enables people to think in a certain way.

- Mortality from infectious disease in Britain was greatly reduced not through biomedicine but by changes to society.

- Despite the many innovations and advances that have made a difference to health, ill health and early mortality remain prevalent in high-income countries.

INTRODUCTION

One way of better understanding the present is to explore the past in order to work out how and why we arrived at the place we are in. Doing so raises many interesting questions, paradoxes and points on which to reflect. That is the task of this chapter: to take stock not just of how medicine as we encounter and understand it today came into being, but also of the wider social and historical influences that frame, inhibit or enable certain developments to take place. One key lesson to highlight here in the introduction is that when we look through time at the rise of medicine, what we find is that the broader social and cultural context is much more important in many respects than the activities and endeavours of a few individuals making discoveries or formulating new drugs. In fact, medicine as a distinct profession based on a particular understanding of the human body is actually a historical late arrival on the health and healing scene. That particular point alone actually begs the question of why humans (in high-income nations at least) were becoming much healthier and living longer before the arrival of the various drugs, therapies and procedures that biomedicine makes claims about in order to privilege its place in society. So any history of health and healing has to range more widely than simply cataloguing who did what and when; by just focusing on the 'Great Men' of medicine we may ignore the much richer and more interesting circumstances that gave humans their understanding of the body, illness and disease and what it is to be healthy. That is why this chapter is called 'a history of health and healing' as opposed to 'a history of medicine', in order to capture those wider dynamics.

Trying to include all of the history of health and healing in a single chapter would be almost impossible. It is such a varied and complex topic. We focus instead on a few important points in time that illustrate either how diseases and illnesses came into being or how humans went about understanding disease and developing methods of healing. So what we find is that many of the diseases that have affected humans over time arise out of how people shape the world around them, whether this is to switch to farming and settled living or to found vast cities that, for example, allow diseases to jump species or create conditions that make it easy for bacteria to spread. We also find that the development of ideas on health and healing requires societies that permit and provide certain stable and accepting social conditions that allow individuals to think, to experiment and to write about health, the body and healing. Finally, we also find that many of the great leaps forward in improving human health are not down to the innovations of biomedicine, but are the results of changes to the social and environmental conditions in which we live.

The McKeown thesis

McKeown (1976) is widely credited with pointing out that the reason for the health advantage (albeit one riddled with inequality) that people in high-income western countries can expect is not the brilliance of medical science, but much more the improvements in living standards. McKeown contended that between the 1750s and 1914 the advances made by medical science had an almost negligible influence on the general health of the population. Changes to and improvements in diet and housing in particular and other broader social and economic changes instead ensured that the life expectancy of the British population increased. The decline of tuberculosis (TB) provides the classic example that is indicative of his overall approach. He charts how the death rate attributable to the disease went from 4000 per million in the 1830s to almost zero in the 1960s. What is notable about TB is that by the time the main treatments and inoculations had been developed in the 1940s and 1950s the disease was almost over.

As a thesis, this exerted a considerable influence when it was published in the 1970s and helped to shake up thinking on what it is that makes people ill and what contributes to health. Various other commentators have challenged the detail of what McKeown put forward and queried him on methodological grounds, ranging from a less than critical acceptance of older and more modern approaches to categorising and classifying disease, to not appreciating the sizeable contribution of public health officials in the late 1800s in combating infectious disease, and to attaching too much importance to wider social and economic changes (Colgrove 2002; Szreter 1988, 2002). The fact that his thesis has been critiqued does not mean that the general assumption of widening our search for the causes and cures of disease beyond the domain of biomedicine is incorrect; as Harris (2004) has argued, the broad lesson of McKeown's work, that health is enmeshed in social and economic change, is clearly defensible. It is in this spirit of charting the wider influences that society exerts on health and healing that the rest of this chapter proceeds.

HEALTH AND HEALING IN DEEP HISTORY

Humans have always sought to keep themselves healthy and to heal the members of their community who fall ill. The roots of medicine and the healing arts are commonly associated with antiquity and the ancient civilisations of Greece and Rome (approximately 3000 years ago) and the writings of Galen and Hippocrates (both of whom are covered in the next section), but we can extend the historical narrative further back in time. The archaeological record speaks of many interesting instances where humans in the *Neolithic period* (or the New Stone Age, approximately 5000 years ago) attempted to practise various forms of healing crafts and even surgical procedures. The most obvious (and perhaps dramatic) ancient form of healing was trepanation or trepanning; this procedure involved using a sharp flint tool to bore a hole in the skull in order to remove bone. Though trepanning may have evolved as part of some ritual, to release a malignant spirit trapped in the skull for example, it definitely also exhibited medical uses. As primitive as trepanning may appear to the modern mind – using a piece of stone with none of the technology and the facilities we would associate with contemporary cranial surgery – a reasonable number of people apparently did survive the procedure.

The Neolithic period began roughly 9500 BC, and refers to a time that witnessed a sudden increase in human technology using natural materials such as stone and flint.

The Neolithic Revolution refers to the transition away from hunting to farming and a settled way of life that allowed for early villages and towns to emerge. It began around 9500 BC in the Middle East and reached Britain around 5000 BC.

There is also recent archaeological evidence that the necessary surgical skills required to amputate limbs were present in the Neolithic period. An excavation in 2005 found the grave of a young male whose left forearm bones were missing (Buquet-Marcon et al. 2009). No other explanation for why those particular bones were missing could be identified, and close examination of the upper arm strongly suggested that an operation had taken place; this had proven successful, as fresh bone growth on the amputated bone indicated that the man possibly lived a number of years following the removal of his lower arm. Not only does this example imply that our Neolithic ancestors could exercise surgical skills, it also suggests that they possessed knowledge concerning the skills of pain management and infection control to complement and make the removal of a limb successful.

What is possibly of more interest in exploring health and healing in the Neolithic period is that many of the various diseases that have affected human health for thousands of years have their origin in this deeper history. The Neolithic period witnessed an important historical transition for human beings: the ending of a nomadic hunter-gatherer lifestyle and the adoption of a settled agricultural lifestyle. This development is known as the *Neolithic Revolution*. So instead of the main source of food being what was made available through hunting big game, scavenging the carcasses of dead animals and foraging for wild fruits, nuts and berries, there was a switch to what could be produced by domesticating wild animals and wild plants in a process we now call agriculture. Where this process began is hard to formally identify, and it is probable that the shift to a settled lifestyle occurred reasonably simultaneously across different regions and for different and unique regional reasons. However, an area known as the Fertile Crescent in the Middle East, spanning the northern regions of present-day Egypt, Palestine, Israel, Iraq and Iran, can credibly claim to demonstrate the first instances of a move away from the old nomadic hunter-gatherer lifestyle to the new fixed and settled farming culture.

Zoonosis or zoonotic disease refers to diseases that are prevalent in one species and transfer to another, where often the new host has very little resistance to the new disease.

The taking up of a fixed-place lifestyle carried substantial implications for health. By domesticating wild animals (the ancestors of cattle, pigs, chickens and sheep in particular), human beings came into contact with animals on a regular basis, often in close proximity in living and sleeping quarters. That high level of contact, alongside the build-up of animal waste products near domestic settlements, created the opportunity for diseases to transfer from one species to another. Thus an influenza that was originally only found in pigs, for example, could be picked up by humans in a process known as *zoonosis*, coming from the Greek *zoo* meaning animal and *nosis* meaning ailment. Being infected by such a virus was bad news for the new human hosts as they had very limited immunity to the new viruses.

Endemic refers to a disease that is constantly present in a particular community but at a low frequency, while epidemic refers to the outbreak of a disease that is new to a particular community.

Another change in people's health was that sufficient populations existed in the new settlements for disease to become *endemic*. Bands of hunter-gatherers comprised too few individuals to constitute a viable and stable population for certain viruses to exist and proliferate. Quite simply, the virus itself would die out as its hosts died out, and being nomadic, such small groups would rarely come into contact with other groups of humans to allow the virus to spread to a new group of hosts. By living in larger numbers and in greater concentration with others, humans created the ideal conditions for viruses and new diseases both to spread and to become endemic within a population. Measles is an example of such an endemic disease and first appears in the historical records as the Antonine Plague in AD 165–180.

What is emerging here is that there is something about the way that humans go about being social and creating new social forms and societies that leads to disease and illness. Even at a bacterial level there is a strong social aspect in the emergence of those pathogens that are harmful to human health.

QUESTIONS

The history of zoonotic disease stretches deep into time. Can you identify more recent examples of zoonosis? Also, think of the social reasons that have created the conditions for a disease to jump between animals and humans.

ANCIENT GREECE: PHYSICIANS AND PHILOSOPHY

No history of health and healing can ignore the developments in Ancient Greek medicine attributed to Hippocrates (*c.* 460 to *c.* 370 BC) and the body of work later developed by Galen (AD 129–216). Hippocrates is an interesting figure in the history of healing as he is popularly credited with being the first great physician, and he was responsible for penning the more than 60 texts gathered together in what is known as the *Hippocratic Corpus*. Today we often think of Hippocrates in relation to the Hippocratic Oath, even though very few doctors actually take this oath. Doctors in the UK instead agree to uphold a set of ethical principles defined by the General Medical Council.

There is one slight problem with Hippocrates as a living breathing historical man: there is very little evidence that he actually existed. Textually, the same author does not write the works that are attached to his name, and close reading of the texts indicates that they are collections of material by a variety of authors, taken from different sources and covering quite a diverse subject range. In effect, the Corpus is akin to a wiki document, which is multiply and anonymously authored, like an entry in Wikipedia, except over a much longer period! Differences and contradictions exist within the Corpus too: the most notable is that not all the texts agree on exactly what substances constitute the various fluids or humours (more of which soon) that are responsible for health and illness and which form the basis of Ancient Greek medicine.

Ancient Greece or Classical Greece refers to Greek society from the eighth century BC to 146 BC (the Roman conquest). This period in Greece is characterised by the building of the Parthenon in Athens and the rich philosophical traditions of Plato, Aristotle and Sophocles.

Regardless of the exact historical details, what emerged out of Greece in the ancient period was one of the world's first recognisable systematic approaches to health and healing. It was a system that basically shaped not only how the Ancient Greek world understood medicine but also the medieval world, and it still resonates today, though more likely in alternative therapies rather than in mainstream medicine. The system of medicine that the Ancient Greeks formulated was centred on the *four humours*, as outlined in the Hippocratic text *On the Nature of Man* (likely to have been written by the physician Polybus, *fl. c.* 400 BC). These four humours were vital life-giving substances *internal* to the body but they were additionally and importantly associated with other *external* characteristics. This internal/external relationship meant that the humoral system was essentially holistic, perceiving health as being an outcome of different forces, of processes directly connected both with the person and with the world in which they lived. The various relationships between the humours, the person and the world needed to be in balance for a person to be healthy. Should the humours become unbalanced then illness would follow.

The four humours consisted of blood, phlegm, yellow bile and black bile. The first two humours (blood and phlegm) are fairly easy to identify, with the blood obviously being the blood that flows through the body and phlegm being mucus. The two biles, on the other hand, are a little more complex and it is harder to find a modern-day equivalent. Yellow bile is foam associated with the formation of blood, while black bile is a darker, heavier substance also produced during the formation of blood and most likely to be found in the dark matter of excrement. Both biles are present in blood and flow in the blood around the body. One of the reasons for the inclusion of the two biles is that by having four humours it was easier to produce a symmetrically neat philosophical system that could be related to other qualities that were already established in Ancient Greek thought. Each humour was therefore in turn connected to a primary quality of hot, cold, dry or wet; to a type of behaviour of sanguine (extroverted and 'red blooded'), phlegmatic (calm and on an 'even keel'), choleric (ambitious and 'go getting') or melancholic (introverted and kind); and to a season of spring, summer, autumn or winter. The easiest way to understand the relationships between the humours and their various other attributes is diagrammatically, and this can be found in Figure 3.1.

The restoration of balance was the critical element in the practice of Ancient Greek medicine. It relied upon the physician making careful observations of the patient, not just of their signs and symptoms, but of how those signs and symptoms related to the life of the patient, the context in which they lived, the part of town in which they resided and so on – basically, as full a determination of all aspects of the patient's life as possible. There was also no division between the mind and the body in Ancient Greek medicine; the two were regarded as being intrinsically related to each other, and therefore separating out a physical malady from a mental malady simply did not make any sense for the Ancient Greek physician. So after a prolonged period of gathering observations the physician would have to decide, based upon his judgement, intuition and reference to the Hippocratic texts,

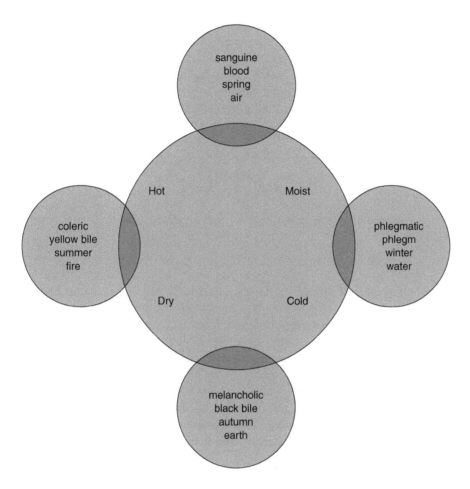

Figure 3.1   The Greek humoral system

which humour was out of balance and what course of action was required to bring that humour back into line. So, for example, if someone was judged to be too hot, then this related to excess blood and too much exercise. To restore balance, blood might be let and drained from the body while a period of rest and little activity would be also be recommended, as would foods that were thought to be cooling. Diet was an important part of Greek medicine and much of the physician's advice given to a patient would have been dietary, as foods were also ascribed humoral properties.

Some of these 'cures' may appear today to be a little bizarre, offering very little chance of actually healing anyone, and this low probability of success raises the question: why did ordinary people go along with them? Any success of the humoral system was possibly due to the very personal basis of treatment, whereby an ill person received lengthy one-to-one attention from a well-read and respected member of the community, and so could feel better as a result of some form of 'placebo' effect. The humoral system was also relatively easy to understand and appealed to common-sense notions of balance that most people would find intuitively believable. Finally, in the short term at least, the blood-letting could provide relief from high blood temperature and could also assist with sleep.

QUESTION

What advantages do you think Ancient Greek medicine may have over current biomedicine in terms of the relationship between physicians and patients?

What is important about Ancient Greek medicine is that it is very much a product of the society from which it came. The Ancient Greek world was a highly philosophical society, with philosophy pervading every aspect of thought, producing such philosophers as Plato and Aristotle, whose philosophy forms the bedrock of much contemporary western thought. Ancient Greek medicine was part of that philosophical culture and tradition. It was bound up in the philosophical quest to find the basic elements from which all life arose and to advance a complete and integrated model of how everything worked. The four humours fitted this bill, with the substances of the four humours being the building blocks of life, while the overall neatness of the humoral system met the Ancient Greek quest for a system of philosophy that could explain everything.

HEALTH AND HEALING IN EARLY MEDIEVAL ISLAM: PRESERVATION AND INNOVATION

The Ancient Greek system of medicine was to become a highly pervasive body of thought, defining and informing discourses and practices of health and healing for centuries to come. It was not until the 1700s that it finally began to fall out of favour, to be replaced by germ theory, as developed in the 1800s. Even today the presence of the four humours is still very much evident in alternative and complementary medicine. In addition to the influence of the humours in systems of healing, another reason for their continued longevity was their absorption historically into everyday culture. Shakespeare in his plays, for example, often wrote the main characters to reflect a particular humour, such as the sanguine Falstaff or the melancholy Hamlet.

The dominance of humoral medicine over such a long period did not mean that the system did not go without any further development. It was in the early medieval period (*c.* AD 500–1000) and in the Islamic world that most of the enriching and progressing of Greek medicine occurred, and this is what is considered next.

Early medieval Islam (or the Golden Age of Islam) was broadly speaking a period between CE 750 and 1250, when Islamic countries across the Middle East, North Africa and Spain made advances and innovations in art, philosophy, literature, engineering, mathematics and medicine.

Particular features of Islamic society at this time are crucial in understanding why ideas of health and healing advanced among the Islamic countries and not in Northern and Western Europe. In the early Middle Ages the Islamic and Arabic countries were, in so many respects, leading global civilisation, exhibiting innovative developments in architecture, technology, mathematics (algebra, for example, is derived from the Arabic word *Al-jabr*, reflecting its origin in Islamic science), art, philosophy and medicine. Western Europe was living through what until recently was commonly referred to as the 'Dark Ages', a violent episode of Viking raids and Anglo-Saxon invasions that followed the collapse of Classical Roman and Greek civilisation. Any traditions of formal medicine in Europe were in a critical state. Instead of being widely used and part-and-parcel of everyday life, any of the Ancient Greek texts to have survived into this period were safely locked away in monasteries, out of sight and out of mind of the general populace. Even when life became a little more peaceful, the power of the Church and the centrality of Christian religion tended to restrain and inhibit any substantial advances in healing. Christianity did not completely forbid the practice of medicine, since much of what took place as healing activity was overseen by the Church, but they preferred and privileged their divine mission to save souls over any mundane matters of health. Medical historian Roy Porter neatly captures this mindset as follows: 'Thus in the case of the dying, it was more important that they should be blessed by a priest than bled by a doctor' (1999: 110). The Church and religion held further control over matters of health and healing by ensuring that hospitals were in the hands of monks and that healing shrines dedicated to saints who were associated with some divine act of healing were the main port of call for most ill people. Porter also notes the continued role of superstition and folk medicines among lay notions of healing. The cure for epilepsy, for example, was for the sufferer to be in contact with the herb oak-mistletoe.

In comparison the Islamic countries to the south were more peaceful, but it was not just the absence of war and violence that made a difference. The geographic reach of Islam was sizeable, encompassing not just the Middle East, which we most often associate with Islam today, but also North Africa, India and Spain. It was this vast reach around southern Europe, the southern Mediterranean and India, and the connections with China, that allowed Islamic scholars to preserve, gather and translate the various works and books of Ancient Greek medicine that had survived the decline of the ancient period around the fourth century.

Islamic society also exhibited openness to other cultures, which provided another social reason as to why medicine in the Islamic world flourished. Given the historical period, Islamic societies were *relatively* tolerant of other cultures, allowing Christians

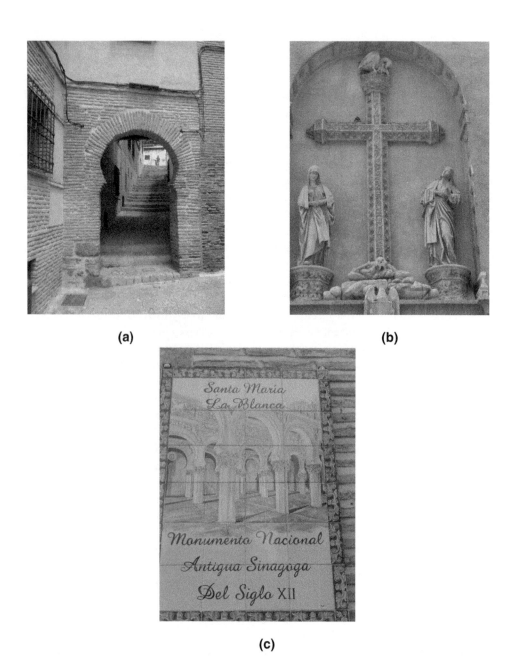

(a)

(b)

(c)

Figure 3.2 Details from the medieval Spanish city of Toledo. Left to right: an Islamic arch, a Christian cross and a street sign for a Jewish synagogue, indicating something of the cosmopolitan history of religious and ethnic coexistence in the city, whether under Islamic or Christian rule, in the early and high Middle Ages

and Jews to practise their religious beliefs and to practise as physicians too. This tolerance also promoted the sharing of ideas, and the multicultural towns of the Arab world, like Toledo in central Spain, became places of vibrant creativity and innovation, with Northern Europe by comparison being nowhere near as dynamic (Figure 3.2). It was not until the Renaissance of the twelfth century that the arts, science, medicine and philosophy in European society were to flourish.

Although, drawing extensively on the Greek traditions of the four humours, the Islamic scholars held onto and retained the knowledge generated by the Greeks, they also added and considerably developed that knowledge. Most Arabic scholars began by translating the Greek originals, but in doing so they began to adapt and augment them by including material from their own Arabic traditions and, more importantly, their own discoveries. Ophthalmology (anatomy, physiology and diseases of the eye) provides a useful example of the process just mentioned. While this practice was based on Greek originals, the Islamic scholars identified new diseases and developed new treatments, some of which were surgical. For example, in the *Memorandum Book for Oculists*, 130 eye diseases are detailed, and in Khalīfah's *The Sufficient Book on Ophthalmology*, various intricate instruments for eye surgery are identified and guidance is given on their use. Other examples of Islamic innovation include the work of Ibn Sīnā (*c.* 980–1037), or Avicenna as he is more commonly referred to in the west. He compiled and wrote the formidable *Canon of Medicine*, a pinnacle document of Islamic medicine. This work is a highly structured summary and synthesis of the philosophy of medicine. Other works by the likes of al-Kaskarī in his *Compendium* recorded case histories and examples of the practice of medicine (Pormann and Savage-Smith 2007).

Many of these texts were to find their way into Western European culture around the 1100s and onwards as the 'Golden Age' of medieval Islam came to an end. The main route for these texts into Western Europe was through translation into Latin, with the Latin versions being warmly received in the nascent university systems of Europe. As Pormann and Savage-Smith (2007) relate, the rigour of the Islamic texts was highly appreciated and Ibn Sīnā's *Canon* was still used by European universities during the 1500s.

What we can gather from Islamic ideas on health and healing is that for ideas to develop and to grow the social circumstances have to be right. In this case a reasonably open society, where ideas and thoughts could be exchanged and debated, was vital for both the retention of older healing systems and their subsequent development. This brief survey of Islamic medicine also indicates that medicine as we understand it today is not purely the invention of the west and that its genesis is much more global, drawing on a variety of cultures and traditions.

THE 1700s: THE ENLIGHTENMENT AND REVOLUTIONS

The 1700s saw the beginnings of modern medicine. Before discussing ideas of health and healing in this period, it is useful to summarise what was happening in the 1700s.

This was the beginning of a new historic epoch, one that was markedly different from the feudal period preceding it. Much of the understanding of life was tied into religion, and all explanations of both the natural and the social worlds related to God, religion and the monarchy in some way. We encountered some of the limitations that religion in Western Europe placed upon medicine in the previous section. For example, even up to the early 1700s it was still widely believed that the King or Queen had a divine relationship with God, and with that relationship came supernatural powers to cure the sick just by his or her touch. An illustration of the extent to which religion dominated everyday life was the trial and execution in Edinburgh of 18-year-old Scottish theology student Thomas Aikenhead in 1697. His crime was to question the existence of God and the truth

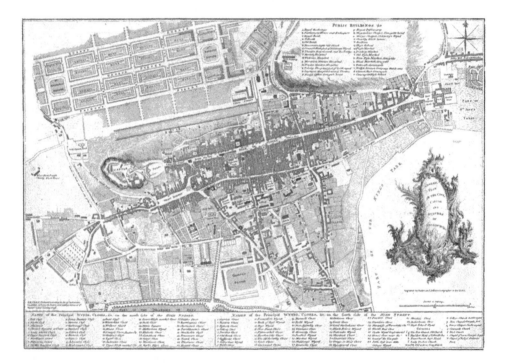

Figure 3.3   A map of Edinburgh from 1773. The street layout of the city captures the differences between the old feudal society and the modern society brought in by the Enlightenment. The New Town, near the top of the map, is formal, rational and scientifically laid out in accordance with Enlightenment principles, while the Old Town towards the bottom of the map consists of rambling unplanned streets, with the two main sources of power, the Monarchy and the Church, dominating the high ground in the middle of the map

Source: Faden, William, Jeffereys and Thomas (1773) 'General Plan of the City Castle and Suburbs of Edinburgh'. London. Available at: www.rsgs.org/ifa/gems/mapped1773.html

of the Bible. In such an intolerant society it was difficult to envisage any form of thinking that broke with religious conformity, let alone developed new ideas about medicine. But within a few years of his death and in the same city, all sorts of new ideas were coming to the fore that fundamentally changed how people think. What occurred in the 1700s (though some trends had begun in the 1600s) was a period of social change and substantial transformation (Figure 3.3). This period of change was prompted by three interweaving historical events: the Enlightenment, the Industrial Revolution and the French Revolution. The three events swept aside the old society, which was religious and monarchic, and replaced it with one that was scientific and modern, and one where people could develop new ideas without fear of the hangman's rope – the fate of Aikenhead – being the reward for thinking differently.

The Enlightenment: thinking scientifically

The Enlightenment was a historic period that changed how humans interpreted and understood the natural world in which they lived and the social worlds that they created. This change in human thinking was led by various Scottish and French philosophers in the 1700s, people such as David Hume (1711–76), Adam Smith (1723–90), Lord Kames (1696–1782) and Adam Ferguson (1723–1816) (in Edinburgh and Glasgow) and Jean-Jacques Rousseau, Voltaire and Montesquieu (in France), though German philosophers, such as Immanuel Kant, also figure prominently. The Enlightenment was also a period of intense optimism: that human beings could not only understand the world on their own terms but were now capable of changing the world for the better, and were in a position to sweep aside all the barriers that had restrained previous generations. One of those barriers was disease, and the new scientific methods of understanding that allowed the human body to be understood in a depth and a detail never known before held the promise of allowing humans to free themselves from the fear of disease and pain.

The work of David Hume is significant both within the story of the Enlightenment and for how he helped pave the way for the experimental science with which we are familiar today. As a philosopher, he developed the empiricist ideas of the English philosopher John Locke. The main contribution of Hume's work, as laid out in *An Enquiry Concerning Human Understanding* published in 1748, was to develop a method or process whereby events that occurred in the natural world could be scientifically understood. He emphasised the importance of repeated observation of whatever was under study as a method of grounding an understanding of that object of study in scientific terms. His influence is evident in how people went about understanding the body and disease. Observation (or sense impressions as he called them) and experimentation were the keys to unlocking the secrets of the body, as was a dismissing of religious and supernatural interpretations of what one found.

Albrecht von Haller (1707–77) provides a useful example of how medicine progressed during the Enlightenment in line with the 'new' scientific methods advocated by the likes of Hume. He was a prodigious if not precocious scholar, publishing numerous volumes.

47

His most important works include the *Primae lineae physiologiae* (1747) and all eight volumes of the *Elementa physiologiae corporis humani* (1757–66). These two works would be very recognisable to anyone who studies physiology and anatomy today; they are filled with detailed and rigorous depictions and annotated illustrations of the inner workings and composition of the human body (Figure 3.4).

Recording the human body in a series of two-dimensional illustrations, such as von Haller and others had done, changed how the body is perceived. Instead of it being a rounded, integrated living entity, the various body parts were just that: a series of parts, similar to what may be found in any other machine. Though not intended, the mapping of the human body in this way resulted in a separation of the mind from the body, and the person from their social context. Such a move led to healing being markedly less holistic than in previous times; the whole person was gone, to be replaced with an unfeeling machine but made of flesh instead of metal.

This tendency within the Enlightenment to strip away all the wonder of being, as some saw it, and replace it with a mechanistic account of what it is to be human, was not, however,

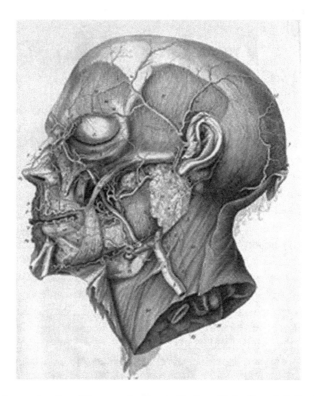

Figure 3.4 An example of the work of von Haller. Note the detail of this illustration of the muscles and veins beneath the skin of the human head

accepted by all. In Germany, for example, the Romantic movement, consisting of artists, writers and the exponents of *Glaubensphilosophie* or *Gefühlsphilosophie* (philosophers of faith or feeling), such as Schiller and Goethe, sought in their works to bring back the wholeness, if not the magic and enchantment, of life (Banning 2010). Some medical people of the time were also influenced by this Romantic backlash against the over-rationalism of the Enlightenment; they attempted to create a form of medicine that kept the insights into the human body gained by the new scientific approaches, but did not lose sight of the whole person. The influence of the German Romantic philosophers was evident, for example, in the work of German physiologist Johannes Müller (1801–58). He was very much imbued, at least as a younger man, with the Romantic philosophical ideals of unity and meaning. Such ideas led to a rejection of the fragmenting tendencies of French and English rationalist science, which disconnected one part of the body from another and, in the process of separating the person into her constituent parts, lost all sense of the total human being. Instead, Müller wanted to fuse together his studies of physiology with his knowledge of philosophy so that physiology was not just the examination of isolated and separate systems within the human body but the study of the complete person (Shryock 1979: 197). Had this approach, as advanced by Müller, become more popular and not been eclipsed by more materialist and fragmentary approaches to the body, then contemporary medicine *might* have become more holistic and less reductionist than it is – a tantalising thought!

The Industrial Revolution: preventing disease on an industrial scale

If the Enlightenment fundamentally affected what people think, then the Industrial Revolution fundamentally changed what people do. Prior to the Industrial Revolution the bulk of the production of household goods, for example, was on a small-scale craft basis, involving skilled workers labouring on an object from beginning to end, often based in their own home or in a local workshop. Whatever was made, be it a table, an iron pot or a piece of cloth, was also a one-off, and likely to be unique in many respects. What the Industrial Revolution did was to sweep this form of craft industry aside and replace it with large-scale homogenised factory production, resulting in the manufacturing of vast volumes of goods on a scale never known before in human history. The Industrial Revolution also reshaped society in two other important ways that had a profound influence on health.

The first is, in many ways, obvious: the massive expansion of urbanism (living in cities) that occurred from the late 1700s and into the late 1800s. The new urban centres, such as Manchester in England and Glasgow in Scotland, which had been relatively small market towns or quiet coastal towns, experienced considerable growth in a very short period. People abandoned rural life for a variety of reasons, such as poverty, shifts towards less labour-intensive agricultural production or the collapse of traditional feudal ways of life, and headed towards the newly expanding industrial cities. On arrival they would seek work in the new factories, but they would also live in conditions of absolute squalor created by the pollution of the smoke-belching factories in which they worked and the overcrowded insanitary housing that was their only choice (Figure 3.5). Urban historian Tristram Hunt (2005) claims that it is hard to overemphasise just how bad early Victorian city life really was. In addition to the smoke, soot, noise and dirt that were byproducts of industrialisation, people kept domestic livestock (pigs, sheep and cows, plus their faeces, were common in cities); sewage was frequently dumped into rivers; and, as the main means of transporting both people and goods about the new cities was horse-drawn carriages, the streets were filled with horse manure. This was squalor on a grand scale.

It is little surprise to find that life expectancy was low and early death commonplace. In the great cities of Manchester, Liverpool and Glasgow, the average life expectancy in the 1840s for most people was somewhere in their middle twenties. All the filth, pollution and cramped living conditions ensured frequent outbreaks of cholera, typhoid and typhus. The young Friedrich Engels (2009: 67–8), future associate of Karl Marx, provides a contemporary account of the effects of this urban privation on the health of working-class people in Manchester:

> These courts were built in this way from the beginning, and communicate with the streets by means of covered passages. If the totally planless construction is injurious to the health of the workers by preventing ventilation, this method of shutting them up in courts surrounded on all sides by buildings is far more so. The air simply cannot escape; the chimneys of the houses are the sole drains for the imprisoned atmosphere of the courts, and they serve the purpose only so long as fire is kept burning. Moreover, the houses surrounding such courts are usually built back to back, having the rear wall in common; and this alone suffices to prevent any sufficient through ventilation. And, as the police charged with care of the streets does not trouble itself about the condition of these courts, as everything quietly lies where it is thrown, there is no cause for wonder at the filth and heaps of ashes and offal to be found here. I have been in courts, in Millers Street, at least half a foot below the level of the thoroughfare, and without the slightest drainage for the water that accumulates in them in rainy weather!

Again, the causes of ill health and early death outlined above are to be found in how human beings have interacted with their environment and each other. Essentially, it is all down to human activity. Yes, there are naturally occurring bacteria at work in the form of *Vibrio cholerae* (cholera), *Rickettsia* (typhus) and *Salmonella enterica enterica* (typhoid), but there is no intrinsic capability within the bacteria by which they can spread themselves unassisted. The devastating death tolls required humans to shape the world around them in a particular way (unhealthy, in this instance) that allowed the bacteria to infect so many people.

What is caused by human action can also be undone by human action. It was not the intervention of biomedicine that came to the rescue of people dying from communicable

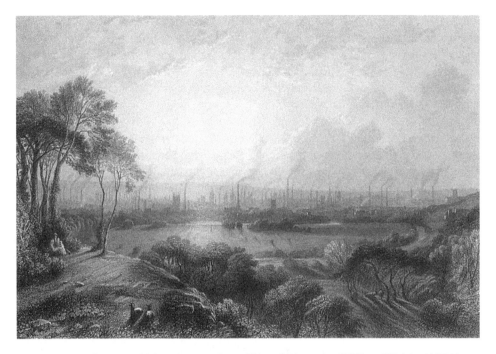

Figure 3.5 A view of Manchester from Kersal Moor, by William Wylde (1852). The stark difference between the rural countryside and the polluted smoke-filled city is evident in this mid-nineteenth-century painting

diseases in the Victorian city, but rather people intentionally deciding to reshape their environments and social interactions in ways that dealt with the conditions that allowed cholera, typhus and typhoid to spread.

The reshaping of cities took place from the mid-1800s onwards in Victorian Britain. New sewage systems were constructed, clean water supplies were introduced, and attempts were made to clear away the worst of the living conditions in many of the major cities across Britain. It was these innovations in city life that were responsible for the increases in the health and life expectancy of people living in cities. There are many figures, not connected with the medical profession or medical establishment, who greatly contributed to the health of British cities but whose contribution is not fully appreciated. One example is the civil engineer Joseph Bazalgette (1819–91). In 1858 an event that was known as the Great Stink overwhelmed London, when the fetid smell of raw human waste that had been discharged into the Thames became utterly unbearable. The stench was so profound that the Houses of Parliament were almost shut down for four weeks as MPs could not work in the smell. Bazalgette was charged to overhaul London's sewage system in order to tackle the stench and to deal with the ever-increasing volumes of human waste. The hundreds of miles of sewers, the pumping houses and the sizeable alterations to the Thames riverbank which he designed, and whose construction he oversaw, all dealt with the sewage and saw off the stink. As the sewage and waste were directed out of the city, the drinking water supply became free from contamination; outbreaks of cholera, like the Broad Street episode in 1854 that claimed over 600 lives, were to be consigned to history. Thousands of lives were potentially saved not by an innovation of medical science but by an act of civil engineering (Barnett 2008).

The work of Florence Nightingale on hospital wards provides the second useful example of how changes in social organisation can lead to better health. Her approach to hygiene and cleanliness may appear to be obvious and commonsensical, but at the time it was highly innovative, saving many lives by avoiding unnecessary infection. Perhaps more effective, however, in treating the ill than her work as popular 'lady of the lamp' and ministering angel in the wards, as her image holds her to be, was her powerful grasp of statistics (Figure 3.6). Through innovative and in many respects ground-breaking use of statistics she was able to demonstrate the links between good sanitation and good health, a relationship not readily accepted by male medical doctors of the time. Her work was additionally powerful in contesting male domination of health, by establishing a professional vocation for women that offered social status within both the hospital and wider society.

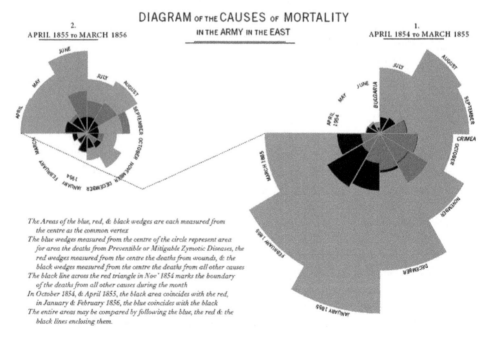

Figure 3.6 Florence Nightingale's 'Diagram of the Causes of Mortality in the Army in the East'

We have seen great advances in health and in understanding of the body emerging from the 1700s into the 1800s. It is, once more, to the wider social perspectives that we must turn to explain these developments. Had the Enlightenment not occurred then the social conditions for people to think about health and healing in a more secular and scientific manner might not have come into existence; and even when people did formulate more scientific approaches to health, these alone were not as effective as changes made to the fabrics of cities or the organisation of hospital wards, for example.

The final comment to be made here is that it was in 1858 with the Medical Registration Act that the medical profession became the legally dominant group in society in relation to health and healing. Many of the breakthrough techniques to cure and help ill people also came along at that time too, with the formulation of germ theory by Louis Pasteur in the 1860s and Robert Koch in 1890. The medical profession as we understand it today arguably arrived late in the day after many of the main causes of illness and death had been dealt with.

BRINGING IT UP TO DATE

The last few pages have covered a great deal of historical time. In the course of moving through that time we have noted that many of the diseases that have faced humans over the centuries have resulted, in some way, from human impact on the environment, whether switching to farming or to building waste-filled cities; and we have seen that the means of curing or preventing those diseases relate to broader and wider social developments.

When we arrive at the beginning of the twentieth century, what we find is that the main killers of the preceding centuries, such as TB, cholera and typhus, were pretty much over in high-income countries like Britain. Infectious disease generally, with the notable exception of the Spanish flu outbreak following the First World War, was no longer a major source of mortality. There is a 'however' coming into play here. Despite the many advances in discovery and development, such as germ theory, penicillin and various diagnostic procedures, and in public health measures like the National Health Service in the United Kingdom or private health care in the United States, people still experience pain, distress and illness and ultimately die.

So in some respects things have not really changed that much. A great many of the illnesses that humans encounter are created by their actions and how they arrange their societies. In the Neolithic period it was the shift to farming and living with animals that was responsible for many historically new health problems; in the Victorian city it was the filth of society; and in the twenty-first century it is the complexity and inequalities of modern life (Wilkinson and Pickett 2010). As discussed in Chapter 5, inequalities do not have to exist, at least to the extent that they do; there are particular political and social reasons why so many experience sizeable differences, not just in their health and wellbeing but in many other aspects of their lives. So it is not cholera that kills people in the twenty-first century but cancer, stroke and heart disease – conditions that emerge out of artificial social inequality. The actual type of disease may have changed but the deep causes remain embedded in human society, and it is on that level that we need to focus in order to understand the deeper meanings of health and wellbeing.

SUMMARY POINTS

- Humans have exhibited for long periods of time a desire to heal ill and sick fellow humans.

- The best way of understanding the history of health and healing is to explore the wider dynamics of the society you are studying. Doing so reveals why certain health issues exist in the first place and why certain forms of healing come into being.

- Modern scientific medicine is very effective at curing people, but (a) this capability has existed only comparatively recently in human history and (b) the major gains in human health have been made by how humans organise and reorganise the societies in which they live.

- The development of modern medicine, for example, required not just people to perform experiments, but deeper changes to be made in society that allowed people to develop scientific approaches.

CASE STUDY

Kallinos has been feeling unwell for some time. His temperature is very high, it is a hot summer and it does not matter whether he sits on his rooftop, where he can catch some of the cooling breeze coming across the plain from the sea, or in the shade of his house. His wife, Althaia, has sent for the physician, who lives in a nearby village, to come and visit to see if he can practise his arts, skills and judgement in order, the Gods willing, to cure the malady that is affecting Kallinos. She is worried that he may die – she had lost her brother last year at this time, and the burden of so much grief would be too great for her to bear.

The physician arrives, and Althaia welcomes him into her house. She is glad to see him and his presence is very reassuring. He has deep, wise eyes and asks after her, how she is coping with her husband's illness. He then sits with Kallinos. He is there for a long time. Althaia listens and notes that the physician does not simply ask about the illness but enquires into so many aspects of Kallinos's life, how often he exercises, what he eats, how often he lies down with his wife, how angry he gets when something does not go the way he wants, and what he thinks about life in general. By the end of the consultation, Kallinos appears to be slightly better; he is laughing and smiling for the first time in several weeks. Thinking deeply, and rubbing his head as if he is turning the pages of a book, the physician decides that Kallinos is not too ill; he has just been eating too many rich foods. So for a cure he must eat as much simple, plain food as possible, with each meal containing lettuce and with a little coriander to finish, as this will help Kallinos sleep. It would also be good to keep him as cool as possible but on this occasion he thinks bleeding Kallinos would not be for the best, something he would normally prescribe given that heat and blood are so closely aligned. The change in Kallinos's diet maybe sufficient to help.

QUESTIONS

1. The above case study is set in Ancient Greece. Which knowledge base is the physician drawing upon in order to heal his patient? Outline its basic concepts and approaches.
2. How does this knowledge base relate to wider aspects of ancient Greek society?
3. In what ways is the Ancient Greek system different from contemporary approaches to health and healing? Is there anything in the Ancient Greek approach to healing that could potentially be superior to contemporary medicine?
4. Why did this particular system survive as a healing discourse for so long in history and why is it now making a comeback in certain forms of alternative therapies or complementary therapies?

TAKING YOUR STUDIES FURTHER

This chapter will have helped you understand many of the key terms, concepts, theories and debates relating to the history of health and healing. Listed below are books and articles that will provide deeper and more detailed discussions of the points raised in this chapter. You will also find additional resources on the companion website, including down-loads of relevant material, links to useful websites, videos and other features. Please visit the companion website at https://study.sagepub.com/barryandyuill4e

RECOMMENDED READING

Barnett, R. (2008) *Sick City: Two Thousand Years of Life and Death in London*. London: Strange Attractor.

Pormann, P.E. and Savage-Smith, E. (2007) *Medieval Islamic Medicine*. Edinburgh: Edinburgh University Press.

Porter, R. (1999) *The Greatest Benefit to Mankind: A Medical History of Humanity from Antiquity to the Present*. Hammersmith: Fontana.

EVIDENCE AND ENQUIRY: AN OVERVIEW OF SOCIOLOGICAL RESEARCH

MAIN POINTS

- Research is integral to sociology, as it both provides evidence for existing claims about society and prompts new ways of thinking and theorising about society.

- Research is a practical activity, which needs careful planning and coordination to realise its aims.

- There are two main methodological traditions: quantitative and qualitative.

- Quantitative methods focus mainly on statistical relationships, as gathered through surveys.

- Qualitative methods focus mainly on experiences, as gathered through interviews or focus groups.

- Research has to be ethically sound in order to prevent distress or harm for the people who participate in the research.

INTRODUCTION

Research is integral to sociology and it is vital for the following two reasons. First, without research many of the insights and observations that sociologists put forward about society would have no validity or evidence to support the claim being made. So, for example, sociologists make claims that health is distributed unevenly across society, according to class, gender and ethnicity. If you turn to the various chapters on those social structures in Section 2, then you will find summaries of some of the evidence that sociologists use to give credence to those statements. Second, research makes sociologists think about society in new ways, with the result either of challenging existing ways of thinking about something or of raising questions that have never been posed before. A useful example here is Bury's (1991) work on chronic illness. Following his interviews with young people with rheumatoid arthritis, Bury drew attention to the social aspects of chronic illness. His research helped to generate the concept of 'disrupted biography', which enables sociologists to gain insights and explain the challenges that chronic illness can present to people with conditions such as multiple sclerosis or Parkinson's disease.

In this chapter, we will be exploring some of the main issues concerning the focus of sociological research and the various methods that are involved in trying to find out about society. We will begin by considering whether or not sociology is a science, before moving on to some of the nuts and bolts of going about developing a research project. Attention will then turn to reflecting on types of research method and how they reveal different aspects of society and how people experience society. Finally, a review of ethical issues will examine why it is important to provide safeguards for the people who participate in a research project and some of the steps necessary to do so.

SOCIOLOGY AS A SCIENCE

As discussed in Chapter 1, sociology shares many of the characteristics of other sciences. These characteristics include using rigorous and systematic methods during research and developing from that research logical and theoretically informed discussions and conclusions. To that extent sociology is a science, but it does have one quite notable difference in contrast to the natural sciences. That difference is in what sociologists study. Sociologists have as their object of study *people* in a *society*. Studying people is quite different from, let us say, looking at how two different chemicals combine in a test tube. Chemicals are not aware of themselves, nor are they capable of acting on their own volition and making their own decisions. People, on the contrary, are self-aware, are conscious, and can make up their own minds and purposefully act accordingly. Therefore, we have to be alert not just to recording and observing what transpires when people interact and engage in activities, but also *why* they interact and the motives and thinking behind their engagement with certain activities. So, for example, in Chapter 2 we looked at the increasing uptake of alternative

Research question refers to the aspect of the social world that is to be investigated.

Literature review refers to a systematic analysis of all published material that is of interest or relevant to the research.

Method refers to the way in which the actual data are gathered.

Analysis means making sense of the data and deriving conclusions that inform the research question.

Dissemination refers to making the results and conclusions of the research known to a wider audience.

58

therapies. Much of the research in that area explores why people are opting for such therapies and the motives and reasons that lie behind their actions. What it reveals is that many people opt for alternative therapies because of disillusionment with mainstream medicine and a desire to be treated in an individual and holistic manner.

LINK

See Chapter 1 for more information on sociology as science.

DOING RESEARCH

Engaging in research requires a great deal of planning and prior thought. Getting the planning right (or as right as possible) before any actual fieldwork is carried out can make a decisive difference to the success of the final project. There is a great deal to organise and think about. Building the research project on a firm foundation is essential if the research is to be able to answer the questions that it sets out to examine. Research is very much a practical activity shaped by a variety of constraints and considerations, where the researcher has to be aware of and attuned to what they can deliver rather than what they might wish to do. Let us now look at what the planning stage involves.

Research question

First, it is crucial to work out what the **research question** is, and to be absolutely clear about what the research is trying to find out. A research question is what the research seeks to do, and what aspects of the social world need to be understood. What initially prompts a research question is quite varied. Sometimes the research question is posed by theoretical concerns to prove or disprove an existing theory, sometimes by a knowledge gap that is noted in the literature, or sometimes because a funding body (for example, a local authority or a charity) needs information on some aspect of its service.

Once the research question has been formulated, you have to be aware of the practical limitations of what you are seeking to do. Research is very much the 'art of the possible' – understanding what resources one has to put into play and how much time is available to do the research. A potential trap in all research is that the initial ambition of a research project is too big and to realise the aims would require excessive amounts of time, funding and people. Often, planning research involves honing the research question down to a very tight set of aims that can actually be answered and can be practically pursued.

So, for example, you might wish to research how having a chronic illness has impacted on all of the sufferers' sense of self, changed the dynamics of family and personal relationships, and so on. This would involve perhaps interviewing everyone in the UK about what differences and experiences they have encountered in their lives since the onset of, let us say, multiple sclerosis, HIV/AIDS or Parkinson's disease. Undoubtedly, if this could be done, it would be a very valuable piece of research. However, given the numbers of people to be interviewed (potentially tens of thousands), the time (months, if not years) needed to do it, and the army of research assistants and interviewers necessary to carry out the interviews, plus the no doubt astronomical cost, it simply could not happen. Instead, it would be much more practical to select just one chronic illness, for example multiple sclerosis (MS). Again, one would not be able to interview everyone with MS, for the same reasons as before, given the numbers of people with the condition and the time and financial implications. This in turn means reducing the intended number of people who could be asked to participate in the research. The main point is that one always has to be practical in what can be achieved and to make sure that the research question can be addressed in a relevant and meaningful way.

Literature review

The next stage involves going through the literature that already exists on the subject – **the literature review**. It is highly unlikely that any piece of research is entirely novel or unique. A great deal (if not all!) of research follows on from and is informed by other pieces of research. It is therefore essential to consult and read all the other existing relevant material. Doing so will aid the researcher in many ways. It will provide an awareness of the main findings and issues that have been put forward so far and how new research can contribute to this body of knowledge. Sometimes this contribution will illuminate gaps in the previous research or offer different or critical counterpoints to what other researchers have found and discussed.

Choosing an appropriate research method

Once the research question has been posed and the literature reviewed, attention turns to how to actually do the research. This requires the selection of an appropriate **method** to answer the research question. In some respects, this will involve choosing between quantitative and qualitative methods. The differences between the two approaches will be explored later in this chapter, but essentially quantitative methods tell us about 'how many' and 'how much', while the qualitative methods answer questions of 'what', 'how' and 'why' (Green and Thorogood 2014: 5).

Analysing the data

Data unfortunately do not 'speak' for themselves and they require further work to produce meaningful information. The actual type of data collected determines the type of **analysis** that is required. For statistical data, one of the most common approaches is to use some form of software package such as SPSS. This allows the researcher to model any relationships and variables that the research set out to find. Qualitative data, on the other hand, require a different approach; they are the spoken words of the research participants. They have to be fully transcribed (typed out) before themes can be identified in the various participants' responses.

Disseminating research findings

Gathering, analysing and interpreting data and reaching a conclusion or raising important issues as a result of research is not the end of the process. Of equal importance is what one does with the research when it is complete and how results are conveyed to the wider world – the **dissemination** of research findings. In terms of reaching a wider audience, Burawoy (2004) has made an appeal for what he terms 'public sociology', arguing that sociologists should strive to make their research and ideas relevant and understandable to the wider society. It is not only academics who are interested in what research has to say; other people, such as user groups, those involved in the study, policy makers and indeed the public at large, are also concerned.

QUANTITATIVE AND QUALITATIVE METHODS

As outlined above, it is important to select the correct method to help you answer your research question. Within sociological research it can be useful to distinguish between two broad methodological approaches. These are **quantitative research** and **qualitative research**. Within these approaches, each method has its own orientation to the ways in which we can investigate society. On a very simple level, quantitative research methods place an emphasis on statistics and on measuring the differences between, relationships among and extent of various social phenomena, while qualitative research methods place an emphasis on how people experience and make sense of the society in which they live.

Quantitative research refers to mainly statistics-based research that is useful for answering research questions that focus on measuring the extent and range of particular phenomena.

Qualitative research refers mainly to interview-based research that seeks to find out the meanings that people attach to their experiences and actions.

We shall look at specific examples of qualitative methods shortly, but first it is useful to look at some of the debates that have surrounded both approaches as they can help us to understand their relative advantages and disadvantages. Much of the debate over the years concerning methods has centred on which approach is the more 'effective' and the more 'scientific'. Qualitative research has often been criticised for being unscientific in that it is closer to a form of journalism, given its emphasis on interviews as opposed to, for example, the randomised control sampling and statistical techniques prevalent in certain quantitative research. Other criticisms are that qualitative researchers lack the impartiality and the objectivity that are supposedly part of quantitative research.

Quantitative research, on the other hand, has been taken to task on many grounds. Even though quantitative methods can tell us a great deal of useful information and are ideal for establishing predictive information, various problems and drawbacks have been identified. For example, much of the survey work on class and health inequalities clearly indicates that one can predict that people found in the lower social classes will have a greater chance of increased morbidity and early mortality. While this is very valuable, this form of research only tells us about one level of social reality. What is missing are insights into how people experience and construct their worlds. The reliance that quantitative methods have on statistical modelling can also be problematic. In compiling and cross-referencing statistics some of the important features of the social world are lost, such as context and the power relationships between people.

Even though there are strong arguments for and against both methods, they should be thought of as complementary. It is the strengths of each that should be appreciated and those strengths in turn should be matched with the research question in hand. So, for example, if the purpose of the research is to investigate the frequency of consultations on a certain condition (for example, depression) by social class in a certain area, then a quantitative method, such as a survey, would be useful. If, on the other hand, the research seeks to explore what it means to be a working-class person with depression, then a qualitative method, such as an in-depth interview, would be the preferred option.

The discussion above has presented the choice of quantitative and qualitative methods as being an either/or option, where one has to be selected rather than the other. Increasingly we are seeing the use of mixed methods, where both methods are used in the same piece of research.

Quantitative method: surveys

If a very large population is to be researched, then a survey can be a useful way to do this. Surveys can take a variety of forms. Traditionally, they have involved the distribution of postal questionnaires or the conducting of structured interviews (either in person or by telephone), though with current technology surveys can be completed using websites or other online media. A defining characteristic of the survey approach is the way in which questions are asked. Questions are tightly *structured*, involving a specific set of questions, asked in a designated order, usually with a limited range of answers. The purpose of such a fixed set of questions and answers is to allow information to be collated and compared across a distinct population. Variables (for example, age, class, ethnicity and gender) can therefore be identified and various associations can be made.

Survey questions: examples

- Please circle which of the following responses is closest to what you thought overall of the Middlefield Wellman Project.

  o   Very satisfied   Satisfied   Happy   Dissatisfied   Very dissatisfied

- How often did you attend the Middlefield Wellman Project? Circle as appropriate.

  o   On one occasion   On two or three occasions   On four or more occasions

Qualitative methods: interviews

One very common research approach in the sociology of health and illness is the in-depth interview. Typically, this is carried out on a one-to-one basis where highly detailed information and data are elicited by talking with someone who meets the criteria of the research project. Most interviews last between one and two hours and are usually recorded using a tape or digital recorder. This recording is then transcribed so that the interview can be analysed.

In many respects, one can think of an interview as a purposeful conversation where the actual data collected are in the form of what someone says (Green and Thorogood 2014). It is up to the interviewer to guide or facilitate the conversation. This can be done in two ways. There is a *structured* approach (as in the survey approach outlined above), but more commonly in interviews one follows a *semi-structured* approach. This is very much a 'looser' and more open technique. The interviewer will have certain topics she will wish to explore, with the emphasis being on allowing the interviewees to express and communicate what they feel or have experienced about what is being researched. So, instead of having a fixed agenda of questions, the interviewer will have an outline of areas or issues to be addressed and will raise those areas or issues as and when appropriate during the interview. This can mean being flexible and not rigidly adhering to a preset order or question format or style.

Conducting a semi-structured interview requires certain skills, techniques and styles of approaches. One should remember that someone is giving up their time to discuss what can be quite intimate and personal details of their life, and due respect should be accorded. It also entails behaving and acting in certain ways before, during and after the interview. Before the interview takes place it is important to identify and create a non-threatening and relaxed atmosphere for the interviewee. This can involve identifying a venue that is familiar to the person who is being interviewed; this could include many different places, such as their home or place of work, so long as they are comfortable there. During the interview the interviewer should be attentive to what the interviewee is discussing and always appear interested. This can be achieved in a variety of ways. Often, the most effective are quite subtle actions such as nodding one's head or briefly commenting on how useful or important something is that the interviewee has said. Engaging with someone in this way also makes it more likely that the interview will elicit the information that the research requires. Questions should always be open (that is, not questions that have yes or no responses) and allow the interviewee room to explore issues they regard as being important.

Semi-structured questions: examples

- How did you feel about having physiotherapists and occupational therapists coming into your home?
- Could you tell me more about how you felt when you heard the diagnosis from the specialist?

Importantly, the interview is not about obtaining some form of universal 'truth', nor should it necessarily match an 'objective reality'. This is one possible objection to the interview approach: that it may not be able to gather accurate data, and therefore any conclusions reached may be invalid. This could be because the interviewee is unable to recall specific events, or has a particular view (or bias) about the research topic. However, it is how the person sees *their* world that is sought in an interview, and not whether or not this matches some other view of the world (for example, the researcher's or that of a powerful social group, such as the medical profession).

Focus groups

Another highly popular method is the focus group approach. This involves a small interactive group of people discussing and commenting on issues and questions prompted by the researcher. As with interviews, a focus group will also be recorded and then transcribed for subsequent analysis and, as with in-depth interviews, the group session can last anywhere between one and two hours. Who actually populates the focus group is dependent on the research questions and aims. Sometimes this can be a wide range of people if the researcher wishes to explore, let us say, how take-up and perception of alternative therapies differ by social class. Other times it can be people who share a particular characteristic, for example depression, if the research is investigating the day-to-day experiences of people with mental health problems.

Focus groups can be very useful research tools in a number of ways. First, unlike interviews, where there is a one-to-one conversation between the interviewer and the interviewee, talking with a group of people is much closer to how people interact in the rest of their lives and therefore creates a more 'natural' and 'commonplace' environment, hopefully making it easier for people to contribute what they want. For the researcher, this natural aspect of the focus group also allows insights into group dynamics and the ways in which people express their ideas and relate to others. Second, the views and experiences of a number of people can be accessed in a relatively short period. Given the time and financial considerations that affect most research, this can be a very appealing option.

There can be some problems with a focus group, and these relate to the very fact that it is a group. As in any social situation, where a group of people are gathered together to discuss a particular subject, some people will be more vocal than others, while some people may feel too nervous to contribute. It can be difficult to keep everyone on track and it is usually necessary to set ground rules, such as asking group members not to interrupt someone who is making a contribution. The points made about successful interviewing also apply here in that the interviewer needs to be attentive and interested throughout, while creating a relaxed and participative atmosphere.

Ethnography and participant observation

Wogan (2004) playfully refers to ethnography as 'deep hanging out'. This remark is not as flippant as it sounds, since ethnography is about spending a great deal of time with a group of people in order to discover how they see the world, while observing, sharing and participating in their everyday experiences. Sometimes this can involve just witnessing what is going on or perhaps (though this can be problematic) going 'under cover' and attempting to become one of the group which is being studied.

One of the best-known examples of ethnography in sociology is Goffman's *Asylums* (1961). In this study, Goffman adopted the role of assistant to an athletic director (similar to what we would call a physiotherapist today) and spent as much time as possible talking to and interacting with patients in St Elizabeth's, a hospital for people with mental illnesses. The aim of the research was to investigate the effects that institutional life had on the identities and experiences of those patients. Famously, he identified the processes that lead to institutionalisation, a state of being where an individual's own identity is replaced by an identity that suits the requirements of an institution. Reflecting on the usefulness of ethnography after he had completed the research, Goffman noted:

> It was then and still is my belief that any group of persons – prisoners, primitives, pilots or patients – develop a life of their own that becomes meaningful, reasonable, and normal once you get close to it, and that a good way to learn about any of those worlds is to submit oneself in the company of the members to the daily round of petty contingencies to which they are subject. (1961: 8)

What Goffman is putting forward here is that only by being with a group of people for a length of time can one come close to understanding the contours and rhythms of their lives. This is unlike the other methods that were discussed above, as they only capture a snapshot – albeit what can be a fairly detailed snapshot – of the lives and experiences of certain groups of people. Ethnography can help to get into the nitty-gritty of social life and reveal how people construct and produce their day-to-day lives.

One issue that all researchers face before embarking on ethnographic research is how much information to divulge about themselves to the group or **community** they are going to be studying. This is an issue because there are two approaches that one can adopt during ethnographic research: covert or overt. A covert approach entails a certain level of concealment and deception. This could mean pretending that you are one of the group or someone who would normally be associated with the group. For some research projects this may be entirely appropriate, but this approach can be challenging for a number of reasons. Let us take a slightly exaggerated example to illustrate what a covert ethnography might entail. If one were to do an ethnographic study of the stresses and strains facing junior doctors, one could pretend to be a junior doctor. This would allow the researcher first-hand observations of the actual experiences of junior doctors as they work through their various shifts. One would be able to witness the rhythms and contours of what causes the most stress and the various coping strategies junior doctors may employ. On one level this would appear to be an excellent method of gathering some very detailed and accurate information. There are, however, certain drawbacks associated with this covert approach: most importantly, would the researcher have the necessary skills to pass himself off as a doctor? This is highly unlikely, given the number of years required to amass such specialised knowledge, and most sociologists simply would not have time to do that. There are also ethical issues (of which more later in this chapter). If you were pretending to be a junior doctor, then this would inevitably require the treating of patients, which is where such an approach would run into severe problems, as it would be utterly irresponsible to do this.

An overt approach, on the other hand, requires the researcher to disclose their identity as a researcher and be up-front as to what they are doing. This may avoid some of the ethical issues outlined above but it can lead to other problems, the main one being that the naturalistic flow of events is disrupted. Having someone observing (or 'hanging out') and recording what is happening is highly unusual (unless they are a medical student, for example) and this can make people reflect on what they are doing and interact in uncharacteristic ways.

An important feature of ethnography is to keep a detailed account of what one observes and encounters. As Crang and Cook (2007) point out, keeping a thorough, detailed notebook (though this could include all sorts of digital media) is an essential part of the ethnography. It is where observations, thoughts and conversations are recorded for future analysis. In effect, the notebook *is* the data and what is recorded in the notebook becomes the basis for the conclusions or conjectures that are advanced from the research.

Analysing qualitative data

As we discussed earlier, one of the defining attributes of qualitative research is the collection of the spoken word during an interview or focus group. This forms the data of the research. Analysing such data requires a distinctive approach in that the researcher is not applying mathematical formulae or models to the data, as is usual with quantitative data. Rather, one of the most common approaches is for the researcher to identify themes within the data. This involves going through the transcripts from the interviews and 'coding' what is said. Unlike slotting numbers into a software package or into equations, this is not always a 'neat' task. It often means scribbling notes and annotations on transcripts, cutting up those transcripts or attaching stick-on notes, and keeping memos. Crang and Cook capture this part of the research project well:

> It is a process that involves doing nitty-gritty things with paper, pens, scissors, computers and software. It's about chopping up, (re)ordering, (re)contextualising and (re)assembling the data we have so diligently constructed. It's about translating a messy process into a neat product. (2007: 133)

Let us now turn more closely to this 'messy process'. If we follow what is referred to as a 'grounded theory' approach (one of the most commonly used in health research) we begin with what Strauss (1987) calls 'open coding'. Here the researcher reads though the transcript and begins to note down what she or he deems to be significant or what crops up several times. There is a certain amount of 'trial and error' in doing this. Some codes will work and emerge throughout the transcripts while others will not. The codes one attaches could be those that the researcher sees emerging in the transcripts or could be *in vivo* codes: these are the ways that the participants involved in the research see the world in which they live and how they think about their own experiences. There is a cyclical process at play here, with the researcher going back through the transcripts continually refining and 'neatening up' the codes that have been previously identified. This cyclical process stops either when no new concepts emerge out of the data or when the existing concepts cannot be refined any further.

Once no new codes can be generated or further honed from existing codes, the next stage involves trying to make sense of all the different codes and seeking out ways of making them meaningful by looking for connections and relationships. This is referred to as *axial coding*.

After all the relationships have been worked out and identified, attention can turn to the final stage. This is where you try to work out the one central or *core category* that helps to explain what all the other codes and themes mean. Essentially, this entails taking an overview of those codes and themes and seeing what commonality runs through all of them. This may involve a more theoretical or abstract code than the other themes that have been discussed so far.

In the example given in Table 4.1, we can see how this might take place. This is a transcript of research on the psycho-social health of workers in a Scottish call centre. The research sought to investigate the link between how the requirements of performing emotional labour all day to people down a telephone line created certain emotional states that in turn had possible health consequences.

Table 4.1 Example of coding themes on a transcript of an interview

Line	Interview	Themes
101	*Int*: So, what really gets you down at work?	
102	Steve: Gets me down? Aye, heaps of things!	
103	Mainly, it's that they're always looking at you,	Surveillance
104	you know, always got their nose in what you're	
105	doing. It's like, you know, they dinnae trust you.	Trust
106	Hate that!	Anger
107	*Int*: Anything else?	
108	Steve: As I said – heaps! The other thing is that	
109	you are not allowed to make your own	Lack of autonomy
110	decisions. If it does not fit their perceived little	
111	wee plans, then ye cannae just go ahead and do	
112	it. Everything is controlled, and worked out to	
113	so minute a degree. And you've got to stick to it,	
114	even if it doesnae work or takes longer, know	
115	what I mean? They just don't trust you with	Trust
116	anything!	
117	*Int*: How does that make you feel?	
118	Steve: Well, angry again, but pretty depressed as	Anger/depression
119	well. It's all day with your heid against the	
120	same brick wall.	Lack of job fulfilment

ETHICS

Invariably, with research into health, sociologists encounter ethical issues. This applies especially when the research is investigating issues that are quite personal and intimate for the subjects of the study, or potentially involves accessing confidential medical and clinical information. Sociologists often have to seek ethical approval for their research due to the very real possibility of causing either distress or upset. This can include, for example, unintentionally making information public concerning diagnosis of chronic illness, or revealing someone's sexuality or their views on other people in a user group. All of this could cause embarrassment but could also seriously damage and hinder relationships or future courses of treatment and care for the subject.

> Ethics refers to guiding principles and considerations concerning the conduct of the researcher in ensuring that no harm is done to the physical and emotional well-being of those who participate in the research.

To avoid causing problems, the researcher is required to follow two courses of action. The first is to adhere to a code of **ethics**. In the United Kingdom all sociologists should consult and follow the British Sociological Association's (BSA) code of ethics, which outlines the considerations that sociologists should follow when engaging in research activity. Part of the guidelines, on relationships with participants in this instance, is shown below. A neat summary of the code, as well as good all-round advice when engaging in research with people, is 'to do no harm'.

Relationships with research participants

- Sociologists have a responsibility to ensure that the physical, social and psychological well-being of research participants is not adversely affected by the research. They should strive to protect the rights of those they study, their interests, sensitivities and privacy, while recognising the difficulty of balancing potentially conflicting interests.

- Because sociologists study the relatively powerless as well as those more powerful than themselves, research relationships are frequently characterised by disparities of power and status. Despite this, research relationships should be characterised, whenever possible, by trust and integrity.

- In some cases, where the public interest dictates otherwise and particularly where power is being abused, obligations of trust and protection may weigh less heavily. Nevertheless, these obligations should not be discarded lightly.

- As far as possible participation in sociological research should be based on the freely given informed consent of those studied. This implies a responsibility on the sociologist to explain in appropriate detail, and in terms meaningful to participants, what the research is about, who is undertaking and financing it, why it is being undertaken, and how it is to be disseminated and used.

- Research participants should be made aware of their right to refuse participation whenever and for whatever reason they wish.

www.britsoc.co.uk/ (search for equality and ethics)

Some ethics codes

The Economics, Social and Research Council:
www.esrc.ac.uk/ (search for framework for research ethics)

The College of Occupational Therapists:
http://www.cot.org.uk/ (search for ethics)

The Chartered Society of Physiotherapy:
http://www.csp.org.uk/ (search for research ethics)

Many other bodies have their own ethical codes and they too are worth consulting. Overall, these ethical codes share similar concerns about maintaining professional standards in terms of behaviour and not exposing participants in research to any harm or distress.

The second course of action involves submitting a proposal to an ethics committee. This could be an internal body, such as a university ethics committee, or an external body, such as the local NHS ethics committee. Due to heightened – and very real – concerns about people's rights, these have become increasingly common and, in some ways, increasingly demanding. In the proposal the researcher will outline what the study is about, what the possible risks to the people involved in the study are, and what measures will be taken to avoid creating or encountering ethical problems. This can be quite complex and the ethical considerations and safeguards of the NHS in particular can be very demanding and thorough. Once clearance has been obtained from the committee, or the researcher has acted on their recommendations to enhance the protection of the people in the study, then the research can go ahead.

One very common ethical consideration, and something of vital importance when involving people in research, is that the researcher must obtain informed consent from those taking part in the research. This will involve providing them with an outline of what the research is about, what they will be asked to do in the research, and how the information they provide will be handled, stored and disseminated. Consent is usually sought by asking those who are taking part to sign a form that lays out the points just made. It is vital that at all times communication is understandable to the respondent. When the research involves people who may not be able to understand what is being required of them, such as children, then some form of proxy consent is required.

CONCLUSION

Research is an essential part of the sociological project and provides both questions and answers in our attempts to understand society. The focus of sociological research, though, differs from that of the natural sciences. Sociologists are faced with the dynamic flow of an ever-changing world animated by the actions of thinking and purposeful human beings. Understanding their motives, interpretations and experiences therefore forms a great deal of what sociologists do. This in turn affects and influences the research methods that are used in the pursuit of knowledge. In addition to the statistical profiles of the more familiar quantitative approaches, sociologists employ qualitative approaches, which seek to access and bring forward the motives and narratives of people in everyday life.

SUMMARY POINTS

- Research is a vital part of sociology.

- Sociological research is scientific like the natural sciences, but deals with purposeful, self-aware people as opposed to inanimate objects.

- Research is a very practical activity and requires the researcher to be realistic in what they can do in order to meet their research question.

- Quantitative methods include surveys and mass questionnaires and are useful for establishing the size and extent of particular social phenomena.

- Qualitative methods include focus groups, in-depth interviews and ethnography and are useful for understanding the experiences and motives of people.

- Interviewing people requires certain skills so as to create an environment in which research participants feel at ease, where they can discuss and comment on their experiences.

- Ethical considerations are an important aspect of research. Care must be taken not to physically, psychologically or emotionally harm people who participate in the research.

CASE STUDY

The following tasks could be useful for you to consider in relation to the points raised above. Read the tasks and then reflect on the questions below.

TASK A

Students are often young people who, when they move away from home for the first time, have to adapt quickly to being independent. Often universities find that the first year is very stressful for students. As is discussed in this book, stress can be a cause of ill health. How would you research the issues that students face at this stage in their college or university career and the effects these issues have on their health?

TASK B

Most universities have a range of students on a variety of courses. Intuitively, one would think that students on health-related courses would have better or wider knowledge of health and have a healthier lifestyle than students on non-health-related courses. How would you research this comparison between different cohorts of students?

For each task, think about the following:

1. What would a suitable research question be?
2. Where would you look for previous literature on student experiences away from home?
3. What method would you use – quantitative or qualitative?
4. What problems might you encounter in doing the research?
5. What ethical issues would you have to be aware of? What permissions and consents would have to be obtained?

TAKING YOUR STUDIES FURTHER

This chapter will have helped you understand many of the key terms, concepts, theories and debates relating to sociological research. Listed below are books that will provide deeper and more detailed discussions of the points raised in this chapter. You will also find additional resources on the companion website, including downloads of relevant material, links to useful websites, videos and other features. Please visit the companion website at https://study.sagepub.com/barryandyuill4e

RECOMMENDED READING

Bryman, A. (2001) *Social Research Methods*. Oxford: Oxford University Press.

Crang, M. and Cook, I. (2007) *Doing Ethnographies*. London: SAGE.

Green, J. and Thorogood, N. (2014) *Qualitative Methods for Health Research*, 3rd edn. London: SAGE.

Hugman, R. (2005) *New Approaches in Ethics for the Caring Professions*. London: Palgrave Macmillan.

Mason, J. (2002) *Qualitative Researching*. London: SAGE.

Richards, L. (2005) *Handling Qualitative Data: A Practical Guide*. London: SAGE.

Seale, C. (1999) *The Quality of Qualitative Research*. London: SAGE.

Silverman, D. (2015) *Interpreting Qualitative Data*, 5th edn. London: SAGE.

Strauss, A.L. and Corbin, J. (eds) (1997) *Grounded Theory in Practice*. Thousand Oaks, CA: Sage.

Strauss, A.L. and Corbin, J. (2015) *Basics of Qualitative Research: Techniques and Procedures for Developing Grounded Theory*. Thousand Oaks, CA: SAGE.

SECTION 2

KEY THEMES

INEQUALITY AND HEALTH

MAIN POINTS

- A relationship exists between income inequality and health inequality.

- The more equal a society is the better the health and some other issues of that society.

- The more unequal a society the worse the health of that society.

- Inequality does not only affect those in lower socio-economic groups, but affects everyone in a gradient.

- Inequality has increased both in individual nations and globally.

- Inequality leads to health problems by creating a fragmented, less cohesive society where those at the bottom are vilified and disempowered from being able to make the kind of changes that would make their lives healthier.

INTRODUCTION

Inequality is now accepted as a serious global issue not just by academics, but by politicians and even multi-billionaires such as Bill Gates and Warren Buffet. They are concerned that inequality, whether between different countries or between different social classes in the same country, is having an adverse and deeply damaging effect on many aspects of society. The main thrust of this concern is that inequality makes a society less cohesive, less functional, less democratic, less successful economically and, given what we are about to discuss here, less healthy.

The differences in life expectancy between social classes in highly unequal societies can be stark. In high-income countries, such as Scotland in the United Kingdom, the city of Glasgow provides one of the biggest gaps of all. In one of the poorest and most deprived areas, a place called Calton near the city centre and not far from the Clyde River (which used to be home to one of the world's largest ship-building industries), average life expectancy for men is a low 54 years – a life expectancy that is below the average male life expectancy of countries such as Nigeria or Bangladesh. If you were, however, to take a twenty-minute car ride to the outskirts of the city and arrive in a place called Lenzie, the life expectancy there is considerably greater at 84 years. We will return to the reasons why this disparity exists later in the chapter, but for now just note that it is not because of access to health care as Calton is closer than Lenzie to Glasgow's major hospitals, nor is it down to air pollution, as Glasgow's days as a major heavy industrial centre are long gone.

It is not just in high-income nations such as Scotland that health inequalities exist between groups of people in the same society. In the middle-income nation of South Africa, health differences by socio-economic group are also evident. The extent of major diseases and disability is greater among the lower socio-economic groups than in the higher socio-economic groups. Now, some of that may be explainable as the outcome of poverty. A sizeable section of South Africa's population remains in some form of poverty. In 2011, 45.5% of the population were living in moderate poverty and 20.2% were living in extreme poverty (Statistics SA 2014). Certainly many of the diseases that are found among the poorer sections are often associated with poverty (for example, AIDS/HIV, influenza and TB). What is notable, however, as Ataguba et al. (2011) point out, is that non-communicable disease, the types of disease such as diabetes and hypertension, which are more commonly associated with the challenges of living in a demanding, unequal society, are evident and higher among lower-income groups as well.

The difference between countries is equally stark too. The world's highest life expectancy, according to the WHO (2015), can be found in Japan, with an average life expectancy of 84, while Norway and Sweden have average life expectancies of 82. By contrast, the world's lowest life expectancy belongs to Sierra Leone at 46, while average life expectancy in South Africa and Malawi is 60. Now, some of those reasons can be explained by reference to under-development, war and chronic poverty, with their roots in historical processes such as colonialism. There are, though, some interesting counterintuitive examples. Life expectancy on the small Caribbean island of Cuba is 78, while the Central American country of Costa Rica is 79. Both countries are not particularly wealthy but exhibit life expectancies that are either the same or very close to the global superpower of the United States, where average life expectancy is 79. So, not everything is explained by war or poverty; other processes are at work too.

In this chapter the relationships between poor health and inequality are explored. Two main points emerge. The first is that the greater the inequality in a society is, then the worse the health of that society is. The second is that inequality affects everybody. It is not just those at the bottom of society who are the only ones whose health is damaged, lives are shortened and overall wellbeing is compromised. Inequality creates a gradient where your health and wellbeing relates to where you are in the social hierarchy.

The chapter begins by charting the rise and extent of global inequality. Here we survey the main trends in global inequality and the emergence of the super-rich, a trend that begins in the late 1970s. The reasons why inequality has increased are tackled next. What is made clear here is that inequality is not an inevitable process, nor is fantastic wealth necessarily related to talent or hard work; increasingly those who own the greatest wealth, especially in the United States, have inherited rather than earned that wealth. Once the parameters of inequality of have been established, the connections between health and inequality are sketched out by drawing on the work of Wilkinson and Pickett, and Marmot. The chapter concludes by considering what policies could be undertaken to reduce inequality.

On the companion website: Chris Yuill talks through the issues of inequality and health.

HOW DO WE MEASURE INEQUALITY?

The standard measure of inequality is the **Gini coefficient**, as developed by Italian sociologist and economist Corrado Gini. The actual statistical method of computing a particular country's level of inequality is not relevant here, but rather what the final figure means. One advantage of the Gini coefficient is that it is quite simple. It operates between two points. The first point is 0, which is absolute equality (where everyone possesses the same level of income), and the second point is 1 (where a very small minority have everything and the rest none). Since no country is either completely equal or unequal most countries fall somewhere in between. So, what you have is a continuum where if a nation's Gini coefficient is, let us say, 0.25, it is fairly equal, and if another country's Gini coefficient is 0.65, then it is fairly unequal. To add readability, sometimes the coefficient is expressed as a percentage, so the 0.25 becomes 25% and the 0.65 becomes 65%. Table 5.1 displays the Gini coefficients of a variety of countries.

Table 5.1 Gini coefficients in various countries

Country	Gini coefficient
Norway	25.9
Sweden	27.3
Denmark	29.1
United Kingdom	32.6
France	33.1
United States	41.1
Costa Rica	49.2
South Africa	63.4

Source: The World Bank available at: http://data.worldbank.org/indicator/SI.POV.GINI

WHAT IS THE EXTENT OF GLOBAL INEQUALITY?

At the 2014 gathering of the World Economic Forum in Davos, where leading politicians and business leaders gather annually in order to discuss economic and social matters, the charity Oxfam released a report on the extent of global inequality. The headline points from that report are quoted below:

- Almost half of the world's wealth is now owned by just one percent of the population.
- The wealth of the one percent richest people in the world amounts to $110 trillion. That's 65 times the total wealth of the bottom half of the world's population.
- The bottom half of the world's population owns the same as the richest 85 people in the world.
- Seven out of ten people live in countries where economic inequality has increased in the last 30 years.
- The richest one percent increased their share of income in 24 out of 26 countries for which we have data between 1980 and 2012.
- In the US, the wealthiest one percent captured 95 percent of post-financial crisis growth since 2009, while the bottom 90 percent became poorer. (Oxfam 2014: 2–3)

QUESTIONS

What is your reaction to the above statistics? Do you feel that the disparities in wealth are morally acceptable or morally unacceptable?

What is important to understand here is that when reference is made to the rich and to the wealthy it is not well-paid, white-collar workers nor middle-class professionals, such as doctors or lawyers, as the wealthy once were, but a small elite group whose wealth and income is vastly disproportionate by comparison. As Sayer (2015) notes, exactly who the individuals are who populate the stratospheric levels of wealth are often unknown to the general public. There may be some wealthy celebrities that are familiar, but often their wealth will pale in comparison. So, for example, people may be familiar with the British celebrity couple Victoria Beckham and David Beckham, who are reputed to be worth £470 million. For most people £470 million is a considerable amount of money, but in comparison with Britain's richest man, Leonard Blavatnik, who is estimated to have a personal wealth of £11,000 million (eleven thousand million), it is not quite as much. If we then place those two examples in a global context, we find that the Beckhams' wealth is not as much as someone like Warren Buffet who has a personal wealth of $58.2 billion.

QUESTIONS

Try to work out what you think a reasonable level of income is for someone living in the same society as yourself. How much would they have to earn to be able to live somewhere that meets the basics of being dry and warm, being able to feed and clothe themselves and to be able to engage in some form of social activities with others? Once you have worked out that level of income, compare it what you expect to be earning. Where does your potential salary stand in relation to the minimum income you identified at the beginning of this task?

Sometimes this group is referred to as the '1%', which may provide a useful shorthand when discussing inequality but obscures where the real wealthy are actually located. For example, in the United Kingdom the Institute for Fiscal Studies (IFS) (2015: 29) noted that even those in the top 99th percentile of income (somewhere just under £2,500 per week) 'are arguably a long way short of what would usually be considered the "super rich"'. Dorling (2014) also makes the same point in his research on inequality: when trying to understand who the super-rich are we must explore the fractions within the top 1% – just as much of a jump exists between those at the bottom to the top of the 1% group as does between the bottom of the normal income distribution and the top 1%.

HOW DOES INEQUALITY COME ABOUT?

Inequality is not a natural phenomenon. The reasons why some countries exhibit higher levels of inequality are to be found in how those nations organise themselves and what social and economic policies they decide to enact. So, analysing why countries such as Norway, Sweden and Iceland regularly appear at the top of various global indexes for happiness, equality or wellbeing, we discover that their social policies are orientated to maximising the overall welfare of their citizens and to creating a society that allows individuals to flourish to the best of their abilities by creating a steady and secure basis on which they can build and realise themselves as individuals. Swedish academic Lars Trägårdh (1997) has dubbed this distinctive mixture of individualism and the strong presence of the state as 'statist individualism'. The Nordic countries should not, according to Trägårdh, therefore be mistaken as an example of socialism, despite the emphasis on equality. We should instead understand these highly equal Nordic countries as another way of doing capitalism, where an emphasis is applied to the wellbeing of the citizens, just as much as it is to making a profit.

However, in countries such as the United Kingdom almost the reverse is true. Policies enacted by both Labour and Conservative administrations have sought to bring about a less equal society. One of the main areas where this has been visible is taxation, where the top tax rate has been reduced from 83% in the mid-1970s to 45% in 2014 (IFS 2015). There are some other specific reasons for the rise in inequality in the United Kingdom.

- Decline in traditional, skilled blue-collar work. Back in the 1950s and 1960s people, typically men, who did not leave school with academic qualifications could find reasonably well-paid stable industrial work in engineering, ship building or in factories. Those jobs relied on manual skills and crafts that could be acquired through apprenticeships or on-the-job training. That kind of work is disappearing now. The reason why that has happened can be found in several interweaving reasons, such as globalisation and the move in the 1980s to re-orient the British economy away from manufacture and towards finance.
- Decline in trade union power. There has been a sharp fall in the number of workers in the United Kingdom who belong to a trade union. In 1979 13,212,000 workers belonged to a trade union. In 2012–13 that figure was down to 7,086,000 (Department for Business, Innovation and Skills 2014: 6). What the trade unions provided was a source of power to act, in effect, as a counter-weight to the power of big business and the state. In practice, that power means the capacity to protect the wages and working conditions of union members.
- In countries where inequality is lower than in Britain, such as the Nordic countries and in Germany, trade union membership in much higher. In fact, in Germany trade unions still yield considerable power, and by law (the *Mitbistimmung* legislation) companies that employ over 500 people are required to have trade union representation on the management boards. In terms of health, research by Navarro et al. (2006) has found that countries where trade union membership is high and organised tend to exhibit better health.

In addition to these reasons for the growth in inequality, which are nation-specific, a number of more general global trends are responsible for increasing inequality. French economist Thomas Piketty (2014) has charted the growth of what he calls 'patrimonial capitalism'. His work points to how the concentration of wealth in a small layer of families is akin to a return of the massive inequalities that provided the narrative context of the novels of early nineteenth-century English writer Jane Austen, where large landholding families possessed a wealth far in excess of the rest of society at that time. The reason for the rapid growth in inequality since the mid-1970s has been brought about by the increasing returns that profit, interest and rent now supply for the small, elite 1% of society. What is notable about where the wealth and income of the global elite 1% comes from is that it is not through working hard or through creating industries that employ vast amounts of labour, but is income derived through finance. In turn, that wealth and money is being contained in certain families where the children of the richest 1% become the new richest 1%, purely by the brute luck of being born into a rich family rather than by any outstanding talent or abilities.

WHAT IS THE RELATIONSHIP BETWEEN HEALTH AND INEQUALITY?

There are many pathways by which inequality can exert a negative effect on health and wellbeing and we shall explore several in this section. Before we begin to do that it is worth highlighting that the focus here on social inequalities and health does not imply that the reason for health inequalities are all explicable by social processes. Marmot (2005) provides a rough ratio of about one-third of our health being due to what we think of as traditional risk factors when it comes to health (smoking, poor diet and drinking), but the remaining two-thirds of what causes health inequality are influenced by social processes. He is quick to point out that we have to take care in assuming that smoking, drinking and poor diet are purely down to choice or personal decision making. For a start, if smoking was purely a personal matter, then the pattern would be random, but it is not: patterns of smoking follow a social gradient, so something else must be going on. There are two points being made here. The first is that focusing on risk factors is only part of the overall explanation. Smoking is definitely bad for your health and cutting down levels of smoking is in itself a worthy pursuit, but in itself it is not enough to reduce all health inequality. The second point is that what may seem like a bad choice in terms of one's health is also conditioned by social reasons. Marmot (2005) cites the work of Hilary Graham on understanding why lone mothers smoked and spent money on smoking. The end reason was that for the lone mothers it was the only part of their budget that was spent on themselves, where everything else was spent on someone else. It was the one luxury they could have that made life bearable.

QUESTION

Discuss your reaction to the point that Marmot makes concerning choice. In what other ways may circumstances inhibit the choices that people can make about their health?

A good place to begin in understanding the relationship between health and inequality is with the research of Marmot (2015) and Wilkinson and Pickett (2010), who make the point that inequality not only affects those at the bottom of society but it affects *everyone*. A gradient exists where different levels of advantages and disadvantages are distributed across society according to your position in that society. What the gradient means is that people, let us say, in the middle will have on average better health than those below them, but not as good health as those above them. To make that point a little easier to understand, Figure 5.1 sets out the early mortality rates by social class for the United Kingdom. What can be clearly observed is the existence of a gradient. You should notice that people

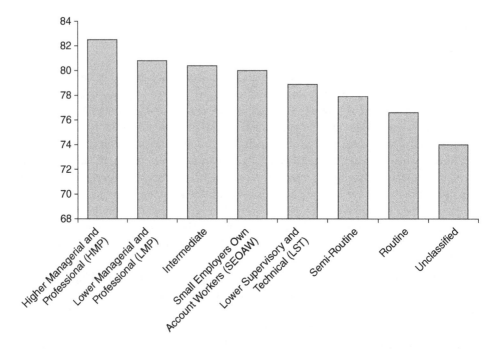

Figure 5.1 Male life expectancy at birth by NS-SEC class, 2007–11, England and Wales, using National Statistics Socio-Economic Classification 7 analytic class schema (ONS 2015)

Source: National Statistics website: www.ons.gov.uk/ © Crown copyright

in the highest social class – the higher managerial and professional class – exhibit a longer life expectancy than the lower managerial and professional group just below them, but in turn the lower managerial and professional group exhibit a lower level of early morbidity than those below them.

If we shift our focus to somewhere else in the world, that gradient also becomes evident. Returning to Ataguba et al.'s (2011) analysis of health inequalities in South Africa, a relationship between cumulative shares of illness, levels of disability and socio-economic group is also evident. Both the United Kingdom and South Africa exhibit distinct differences by socio-economic group. Though the measures are different in each case, what is important is the overall picture of a health gap between socio-economic groups. The health differences by socio-economic group in Sweden provide a further interesting contrast. What is evident here is that a gradient does exist between social groups (Eriksson et al. 2014) but all people, regardless of class, live longer than in either South Africa or the United Kingdom. Overall, if you were to choose which country to be poor in, then you would probably choose the United Kingdom and Sweden over South Africa, but best of all is Sweden, where being in the lowest socio-economic group gives you the longest life of all three.

INEQUALITY AND THE SPIRIT LEVEL

The gradient is important as it draws attention to patterns that exist in society and the fact that health and wellbeing are ordered along social lines. How that gradient is shaped can be traced to income inequalities in a society. *The Spirit Level*, by Wilkinson and Pickett (2010), advances a serious, well-constructed and evidenced understanding and explanation of health inequalities and other social maladies in contemporary high-income ('rich') societies such as the United Kingdom or the United States. Their central message is that once a society has gone beyond a certain material threshold (usually somewhere about an average per capita income of $10,000), then it is not the *absolute* levels of income that animate social problems but rather *relative* income. Critically, the larger the income inequality existing between the richest and poorest sections of a society, the greater certain social problems facing that society.

A substantial array of data drawn from a variety of sources is marshalled into a series of thought-provoking graphs (see Figure 5.2 below) to support and outline Wilkinson and Pickett's (2010) thesis. Each graph in turn consistently plots the same relationship between inequality and a number of social problems, such as health inequality, drug misuse, high rates of teenage pregnancy and increases in the number of people experiencing some form of mental distress. The United Kingdom and the United States prominently figure as the worst examples of the relationship between high inequality and social problems. In contrast, the Nordic countries and Japan

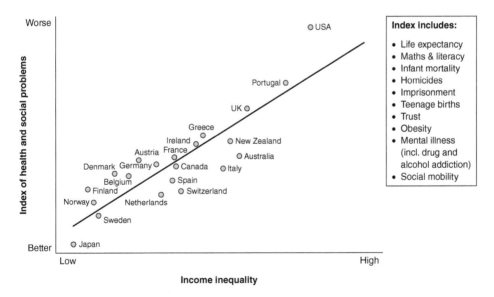

Figure 5.2 Health and social problems are worse in more unequal countries

Source: Equality Trust, available at: www.equalitytrust.org.uk/spirit-level

consistently do well, exhibiting both high levels of equality and low levels of the examples of problems just listed.

Wilkinson and Pickett's (2010) emphasis on relative income differences and inequality may, at first, seem counterintuitive. A wealthy society should, after all, be more than able to meet the basics of the good life that its members require. It should be in a position to provide sound housing, an adequate diet and reasonable education – the accepted building blocks of 'wellbeing'. The evidence Wilkinson and Pickett present strongly overturns such an otherwise reasonable observation. Wealthy societies can be quite incapable of eradicating health inequalities if they exhibit high levels of inequality. The United States, the world's richest nation-state, for example, demonstrates some of the worst health differences between the richest and the poorest sections of its society despite its substantial wealth. That is possibly one reason that explains the observation made earlier that the wealthy United States has roughly the same life expectancy as less wealthy Cuba and Chile.

How that inequality translates into health inequality is explained by reference to **psycho-social perspectives** and how they translate into a variety of biological systems within the human body. In an earlier work, Wilkinson (2005) neatly sums up why it is important to focus on psycho-social processes as opposed to purely psychological or sociological processes:

> Psychological literature, concentrating as it does on the individual, too often ignores our susceptibility to the powerful sociological processes that drive social differentiation and discrimination against those lower down the social hierarchy. On the other hand, the sociological literature that addresses issues of social class stratification usually ignores its interaction with individual psychology. (2005: 33)

A focus on psycho-social factors allows Wilkinson and Pickett (2010) to go beyond (but not necessarily completely dismiss) material factors, such as poor housing or bad diet, and to explain how people's experiences of inequality can have such a devastating effect on their health and on wider society. In part, the reasons for health inequality are to do with stress (albeit stress of a chronic and persistent nature), which is connected to having low control over one's life, for example. The reasons for health inequality are, however, as Wilkinson and Pickett (2010) argue, more to do with what we have inherited from our evolutionary past. Humans have evolved to be aware of status and rank, and are sensitised to experiencing and perceiving hierarchy. The experience and perception of status and rank trigger various internal biological systems that, in turn, create a variety of harmful states that negatively impact on our health.

Wilkinson rallies a variety of non-human primate studies to provide empirical proof for the relationship between psycho-social factors and biology. In *Unhealthy Societies: The Afflictions of Inequality* (1996), he draws on the work of primatologist Sapolsky. Researching wild baboons in the Serengeti, Sapolsky (1992) identified how social hierarchies and social dominance within those hierarchies lead to deleterious physiological effects on these primates. Key to harm occurring is the release of glucocorticoids triggered by social stressors. The long-term presence of these biochemicals increases the chances of cardiovascular disease and high blood pressure.

Other researchers working with humans have similarly noted the negative effects of certain physiological systems being 'switched on' for too long. McEwen's (2000) work on stress in humans, for example, identifies the highly damaging effects of having one's stress system permanently active. A variety of biochemicals, in particular the corticoids, which are adaptive for short-term stressors, become highly maladaptive when produced over extended periods, especially when one's body permanently adjusts to being chronically stressed.

QUESTIONS

Can you identify times when stress has had an effect on your life or on the lives of other people you know? What was the cause of that stress? What does that suggest about the relationships between certain aspects of our biology and ourselves as social beings?

INSECURE EGOS AND NARCISSISM

In addition to the biological reactions outlined above, Wilkinson and Pickett (2010) claim that highly unequal societies generate particular forms of harmful social interactions, divisive cultures and damaged individual subjectivities. Chief among damaged subjectivities, for example, is the increase of a self-promoting, insecure egotism. Easily mistaken for having high self-esteem, those with insecure egos who exhibit self-promoting behaviours (think of the time people spend on Facebook and what they say about themselves) can experience high evaluation anxiety and increased cortisol levels when others perceive them as failures.

Though citing other factors, such as the unintended consequences of promoting self-esteem, psychologists Twenge and Campbell (2010) indicate that inequality is one of the reasons why American culture is currently gripped by what they term a 'narcissistic epidemic'. What their research, and others' research, has found is that personality traits that are normally associated with people who have a Narcissistic Personality Disorder are appearing in the general population. These traits include an overestimation of how good, attractive and competent an individual believes themself to be.

The downside of this epidemic is that if reality does not match self-perception, then a variety of negative consequences follow. As Twenge and Campbell (2010: 259) note: 'Narcissism is the fast food of the soul. It tastes great in the short term, has negative, even dire consequences in the long run ...' Those dire consequences include problems for the narcissistic individual, such as poor mental and physical health, but also for others. Their behaviour can impact on the quality of life of their friends and family, as their wellbeing is ignored in order for the narcissist to reach his or her goals.

Inequality also exerts negative pressures on society in terms of corroding bonds of trust between people, ultimately leading to a retreat from the community into more private, but more troubled, spheres of life. As a result of this more inward lifestyle, people look to protect themselves and create cultures that place symbolic and actual barriers between themselves and others.

QUESTIONS

Do you accept Twenge and Campbell's assertion that we are living in a narcissism epidemic? Are people self-obsessed in a negative way?

ROSETO: A CASE STUDY OF HOW EQUALITY IS GOOD FOR HEALTH

An interesting historical example is provided by Bruhn and Wolf's (1998) classic work on the small town of Roseto in Pennsylvannia in the United States. Roseto was not an affluent community; in fact in many respects it was a poor community like so many others nearby. Unlike the neighbouring towns with which they shared much in common, Roseto from the 1930s to the 1950s exhibited a higher level of good health, especially in relation to heart disease. This health advantage intrigued many health researchers, who at first thought it might be due to a better diet, or increased exercise or a low levels of smoking, or perhaps moderation in drinking alcohol. Each of those explanations was rejected as the evidence indicated that there was nothing special about Roseto with regard to those risk behaviours. Ultimately, the health advantage experienced by the Rosetans came down to one explanation: high levels of social cohesion. Rosetan culture at the time was built around strong civic engagement, with residents being members of various clubs and societies. There was also a strong culture of equality. So if you owned more than your neighbours, it was frowned upon to display that advantage. What all this cohesion and equality meant for health was that the stresses and strains of living in the poorer reaches of society were avoided. People could rely on each other for support.

From the 1960s onwards, however, the community gradually became increasingly immersed into US culture and the individualism of US culture. Parents wanted their children to do well, that is to become wealthier and to become outwardly more successful. That may sound laudable but it came at a cost: the old, tight community bonds and collective nature of Roseto began to disappear. As the collective culture began to erode so did their health advantage and instances of heart disease increased.

Urban researcher Anna Minton (2009) highlights a similar dynamic in her work. She notes the increasing privatisation of formerly public space and the parcelling up of the urban landscape into supposedly secure, but ultimately isolated, gated communities. Fear of an imagined other, then, appears to be part and parcel of an unequal society. Inequality also breeds harsh disrespect for those lower in the social hierarchy and obsequiousness towards those above. A bicycling metaphor is employed by Wilkinson and Pickett (2010) to illustrate this situation. This metaphor projects the image of someone holding the handlebars of their bike as if bowing to someone above them, while at the same time kicking down on those below as they pedal away.

More recently, Marmot (2015) highlights the damaging effects that *disempowerment* exerts on health. His basic point is that the lower down someone is within the social hierarchy and the steeper that hierarchy is, the more disempowered that person will be. Disempowerment is not just individual disempowerment but the social disempowerment of whole groups of people within a society. Disempowerment creates barriers and denies access to resources that can make a positive change in people's lives that will result in better health, or, as Marmot (2006: 2086) put it, '… they do not have the opportunity to lead lives they have reason to value'.

The steepness of the social hierarchy is critical when it comes to disempowerment. All countries exhibit a social hierarchy, although in some countries that hierarchy is not as steep as in others. A social hierarchy exists in the Nordic countries, which are consistently held up as exemplars of equality, but the social hierarchy there is not like the social hierarchy to be found in the United States or in the United Kingdom – drawing attention to the importance of national contexts was a point made earlier.

According to Marmot (2015), disempowerment can be conceptualised in three forms:

Material disempowerment exists where the money or the resources are simply not there to provide adequate nutrition, shelter or clothing. This form of disempowerment can have a relative or absolute dimension. So, in the context in a low- or middle-income country it can mean having no or little food, while in high-income nations it can be relative, where citizens may have access to the fundamentals of life but that are of a level far below what could be reasonably accepted. At the end of the day, what matters is that it is difficult to make effective choices if food, housing and clothing are problematic.

Psycho-social disempowerment exists where people do not have the control over their lives to make the kind of decisions that would be beneficial for their overall health and wellbeing. Marmot illustrates the psycho-social form of disempowerment by reference to the Scottish city of Glasgow. Substantial health disadvantages exist there, as indicated in the introduction to this chapter. Underlining those health problems is a deep-seated sense of lack of control. Some of this lack of control can be explained by the particular history of Glasgow. Collins and Levitt (2016) have noted that Glasgow has been subject to a series of historical events (mainly related to the management of industrial decline) that have deprived many communities of the sense of purpose and identity they once had. The end effect of this historical process is that loss of control.

Political disempowerment exists where a collective voice is absent either in civil society or within political institutions to create the social policies that would allocate the necessary resources to improve the social fabric of a particular country. As we noted earlier, how a society is shaped and what levels of equality and inequality it exhibits are very much shaped by the kind of social policies that it enacts.

QUESTION

Can you identify examples of each of the three forms of disempowerment beyond the examples given elsewhere in this chapter or book?

Marmot (2015) points to disempowerment as being social in cause and tied into the structures of a society, where society is organised in such a way that those iniquities are continually produced and reproduced. It is necessary, he argues, to provide education in health behaviours so that people can make informed choices but also, if not more so, to create the social bedrock that allows people to enact those choices to experience a healthy, meaningful life.

THE NEO-MATERIALIST CRITICS

Other sociologists have criticised the inequality arguments outlined in the previous sections. The majority of objections to what Pickett and Wilkinson (2010) claim in their work on inequality is voiced by a group of scholars commonly referred to as the 'neo-materialists'. Their points of criticism can be briefly summarised as follows. Wilkinson and Pickett provide no insights into how inequalities arise in the first place, nor do they provide an analysis of the processes and social forces that maintain and perpetuate income inequalities. The main reason for that, as Scambler (2001) suggests, is that Wilkinson and Pickett call off their search for causes too soon. The journey to discover the causes of health inequality is signposted but not fully travelled. More needs to be done to tease out the full depth and causality of inequality. Such a move would require getting to grips with deeper structural forces and, in particular, the role of social class. One can, however, sense that Wilkinson (2002) is not disposed to engage in such an activity. The reason, as Yuill (2010) suspects, is that he is keen, if not impatient, to get on and do something about health inequalities in a more direct way. Wilkinson's frustration with those who chide him for not plumbing deeper into society is evident in this response to neo-materialists Muntaner and Lynch:

> In an attempt to lay down boundaries and avoid an infinite regress into causes of causes, I simply stopped at saying that wider income differences carry health costs. Others could wrestle with the extremely complicated, but crucial, issues of how income distribution can be influenced. (Wilkinson 2002: 361)

Overall, the criticisms are very useful, but do not detract from the main observation that Wilkinson advances, namely that inequality needs to be addressed – a point even his most trenchant critics also note (for example, Lynch et al. 2000). It is how any reduction in levels of inequality is effected that is important.

CONCLUSION

What we can conclude from this chapter is that health inequalities are a pervasive element of modern-day health. It does not really matter where you are in the world to a large extent: wherever you are in the social hierarchy has a relationship with your health. The lower down that hierarchy you are the worse your health will be, whether mentally or physically. Where overall income inequality is higher, the health of those in that society will be worse than in countries that are more equal overall.

SUMMARY POINTS

- Inequalities in health exist due to inequalities in society.

- Health inequalities do not just affect the health of those at the bottom of society but everyone. In more equal societies everybody's health from the bottom to the middle to the top is better than their counterparts in a more unequal society.

- Global income inequalities are increasing, with the top of the top 1% increasingly leaving the other 99% further behind.

- Inequality affects health through a variety of mechanisms: increase in narcissism, disempowerment, and a the creation of a toxic competitive and unforgiving society.

CASE STUDY

LAURA'S STORY

Shopping is the worst part of the week for Laura. It isn't because she cannot afford – well most of the time – to feed her two children (Amy and Pete, 3 and 2 years old respectively), but the food that she fills her basket with is all from the supermarket's Basics range, the packaging of which is a radiant bright orange that just proclaims low budget. All those aisles neatly packed out with the tempting ranges of food in the carefully designed and interesting packets were not for her. She wants to try them, to experience new flavours, and to have her children be able to run around the supermarket and pull something off the shelf that they might want to try, but no. Shopping is a strict, disciplined exercise where preference is very much a secondary consideration to necessity.

The trip to the supermarket is a chore too. It requires two bus trips as the local corner shop is way too expensive, plus it only stocks canned goods – and there are only so many baked beans a girl can eat! The bus journey itself is not that unpleasant, the estate where she lives is by-and-large OK, but just a bit run down in places. Built in the 1960s it is a bit past its best. It was once a showpiece of urban redevelopment and a model of how social housing could be – all clean and spacious in comparison with the old Victorian housing that used to exist in this part of the city. There is always some affection in Laura's mother's recollections of the estate in those days. Perhaps not street parties every weekend, but people would at least know who their neighbours were, and that meant pretty much all the people in the whole street, not just the people living on either side of Laura, who are the only neighbours Laura knows.

In fact, there are fewer people on the estate of late. There's the occasional boarded-up property now, where the tenants have left and no one else has moved in. The windows and doors have been sealed up using flame-retardant metal grilles, just in case there's another spate of fire-raising, usually by bored kids (and not so young adults, too) dropping lit rags through letter boxes or a box of matches into a litter bin. That doesn't cause too much damage, though it can get serious. Last year one of the empty properties, an empty three-storey low-rise, was almost burned down. The local authority has also stopped spending so much on keeping the various common areas neat and tidy. The grass on the roadside verges needs cutting; it's becoming overgrown and messy, and just makes the whole estate look less of a nice place in which to live.

Her estate, though, is quite different from the one just three stops away on the second bus she has to take to the supermarket. It is a stop where nobody gets on or off. This estate is all single houses, with two cars or more in the driveways, and finished off with perfect gardens boasting neat green lawns. She would like to live there. It just looks so much nicer.

Laura's health is fine; it could be better, but she can't complain and she is definitely better than other people on the bus. There is always someone coughing (too many cigarettes, or perhaps something else?) but mainly people look worn down or, as they say around here, 'done in'. What always surprises her is just how much some of her friends have aged of late. They look a good ten years older than they should, even the ones who eat OK, don't smoke and keep themselves active. Laura puts her mind back on the shopping she's about to do, and the same routine of tightly focusing on what she can pick off the shelves and what she simply must ignore.

QUESTIONS

1. Read Laura's story and think about the ideas and theories we have discussed above. What helps to explain both her health and general situation?
2. Can you identify any examples of what Marmot terms disempowerment in Laura's story?
3. What social policies could be enacted that would improve the health of Laura and the people who live on her estate?

TAKING YOUR STUDIES FURTHER

This chapter will have helped you understand many of the key terms, concepts, theories and debates relating to health inequalities. Listed below are books that will provide deeper and more detailed discussions of the points raised in this chapter. You will also find additional resources on the companion website, including downloads of relevant material, links to useful websites, videos and other features. Please visit the companion website at https://study.sagepub.com/barryandyuill4e

RECOMMENDED READING

Marmot, M. (2015) *The Health Gap: The Challenge of an Unequal World*. London: Bloomsbury.

Wilkinson, R. and Pickett, K. (2010) *The Spirit Level: Why Equality is Better for Everyone*. London: Penguin.

6

GENDER AND HEALTH

MAIN POINTS

- Gender is not a fixed biological state, but rather the outcome of myriad social and cultural processes.

- We should also be wary of making simple binary distinctions of there being men and women and think instead of different forms of masculinities and femininities.

- The various health and wellbeing issues that affect men and women can be traced to the prevailing gender order: how it is to be a man or a women shapes and conditions behaviours and attitudes and in turn health and wellbeing.

- Care must be taken to trace which particular gender process affects and influences which particular aspect of health and wellbeing.

- There are two approaches to policy in relation to gender and health. The first is to adapt and work with existing constructs. The second is to challenge prevailing gender orders and to rethink how we construct masculinities and femininities.

INTRODUCTION

One theme throughout this book is that social processes play very powerful roles in influencing and shaping – if not determining, at times – core aspects of our lives and our health. Gender is no exception. Though we often think in terms of gender being located in very distinct biological terrain, gender is just as much an outcome of social processes as the other social structures discussed in this section: class, sexuality and ethnicity. What we explore in this chapter is why understanding the social construction of gender is vital in understanding the implications that has for health and wellbeing. That perspective allows us to understand and explain why across the globe women are more likely to develop HIV/AIDS, be subject to physical and emotional violence, or report greater levels of lung disease than men, and also why some men's health can be compromised by certain expectations placed on them to be a 'real' man.

The chapter begins by teasing out one central issue: what is gender? What we find is that gender is incredibly fluid, morphing and transforming over time, with no real settled and consistent form. Power is also central to any consideration of gender. The headline message here is that men dominate many aspects of life, whether that is economically, culturally, symbolically or physically. There have been considerable shifts in the balance of power, especially since the 1960s and 1970s with the emergence of strong women's movements, but many instances of inequality still persist and endure in contemporary society. Some countries are further ahead on this road to equality than others, but overall some distance still remains to be travelled. The theories of Judith Butler and Raewyn Connell are then called on to assist in thinking through the various dimensions of gender, what gender is and how gender is produced and reproduced in society.

After discussing how gender can be theorised we move on to consider how the social construction of gender relates to health. Much of what is presented here is guided by Connell's observation that we must seek to identify specific gender practices and how they relate to health. What she means by that is that we cannot simply say it is all down to gender, as if it is one undifferentiated entity that presses down on people like a cookie-cutter, but rather what is it about certain gender practices that can exert a negative or positive bearing on health and wellbeing?

Finally, how gendered health inequalities could be overcome is considered. Two broad approaches are sketched out. The first approach discusses how aspects of masculinities and femininities can be called on and adapted in order to promote health. The second approach outlines a deeper approach that calls for fundamental changes to the gender order, seeking to tackle the root causes of gender inequality in society. Before we set about these issues, a brief overview is undertaken of how sociological approaches to gender and health have changed over time.

> On the companion website: Chris Yuill talks through the main points of this chapter, focusing on the importance of understanding how social constructions of gender influence health.

Changing approaches to gender and health

A shift has occurred in medical sociology over the last twenty or so years. Older studies on gender and health were not really about gender in the widest sense, but rather focused more on women and their health (Hankivsky 2012). There were many good reasons for that exclusive focus on women, as women's health and women's bodies had been historically subordinated and marginalised within medicine. In early Victorian medicine, for example, women's bodies were depicted as being inferior to men's bodies and were presented as a pale copy of the male body. From the late 1990s onwards, however, greater emphasis was given to men and their health (Courtenay 2000). Research on men's health has identified some interesting and counterintuitive findings. It was commonly assumed that men's dominant position in society would result in a health advantage over women. What we do find – albeit a little nuanced – is that the demands of certain male gender practices can be harmful to men's health. Attention now within medical sociology has moved on even further, going beyond just thinking about men's health and women's health. Instead, attention now falls on how gender as a whole is constructed within a society and how the various power relations inherent within those relations affect the health of both men and women.

What is gender?

Gender may seem fairly unproblematic. We are either male or female, and that sense of being male or female is derived from our biology and the outward appearance of our bodies. What sociology and other social science disciplines argue is that gender is a great deal more complex than what we might first think. What it is that makes us identify as being male or female lies, however, outside biology, and can be found in the social and historical context in which we live. If biology was dominant in deciding and creating our gender identities, then what you would expect to find is that all men and all women would be the same the world over and exactly the same across time. What you actually find is that this consistency is simply not there, that there is instead considerable variability in what it means to be a man or woman depending where in the world you live or where in historical time you are.

Focusing on the historical aspects first, let us take the case of what happened in the United States and the United Kingdom before, during and after the Second World War (1939–45). Prior to the war women in those countries occupied what we would call traditional domestic roles, typically focused on the private sphere of the home where women were responsible for running the home and acting as primary carers of children. If women did work, then working-class women typically worked as domestic workers, servants or cooks, and middle-class women did secretarial work. Any type of work that was more physical or technical was considered not just inappropriate as work for women, but also beyond what women were deemed capable of. During the war, with many men in the armed services, there was a shortfall of key workers (engineers, industrial and assembly line workers) to keep the economy running. Women were called upon to fill these positions. That, however, clashed with the traditional gender role just outlined. What we witnessed over the war years was a change in that gender role, with what we would now consider a more progressive or liberated role for women. A useful example of this is the character of Rosie the Riveter, as depicted in Figure 6.1. She was an imaginary propaganda figure devised by the United States government, but thousands of real-life Rosies existed. In the image Rosie is depicted wearing a headscarf, a traditional sign of femininity in 1940s America, but she is

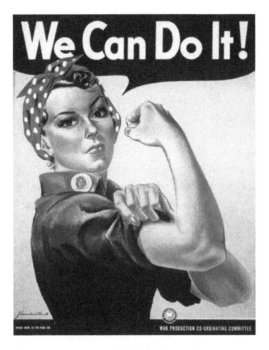

Figure 6.1   Rosie the Riveter (US National Archives)

Image courtesy of US National Archives

also wearing a blue boiler suit and flexing her muscles, which are both traditional signs of masculinity. The slogan of the poster is 'We Can Do It!', an empowering and progressive message that was adopted by later feminist movements in the 1960s and 1970s.

In that short space of time, what it was to be a women changed markedly from being a passive homemaker to an active, skilled factory worker. In Britain, the first ever example of pay parity between men and women was found in the Air Transport Auxiliary where women pilots were paid the same as male pilots. At the end of the war, however, the gender role for many women was almost reversed back to what it had been before the war, and there was a cultural and social move to effectively re-domesticate women into the private sphere of the home.

QUESTION

What other examples can you find where gender roles and constructs of gender have changed and altered over time?

The colour pink provides one other historical example of the fluidity of gender and how it is constructed at different points in time. We think of pink as being exclusively a colour for young girls and women generally, and, more importantly, a colour that is somehow naturally associated with women, that there is some quality of pink that is innately feminine. On closer inspection that assertion does not hold up. In Victorian Britain, pink was perceived to be a boy's colour, regarded as a juvenile tone of what was then accepted as the very masculine colour red.

What both the examples above indicate is that ideas around gender change frequently over time. It is not a stable entity. Looking at different societies we can again identify distinctly different ways in which gender is understood. The main lesson so far is that gender is very fluid across time and space as to what it is to be a man or a woman. Further challenges to notions of gender being static are provided by the experiences of trans-gendered people, where the biological body and the sense of gender identity are not congruent.

Gender inequality

One notable feature of the gender landscape is that considerable inequalities have existed and continue to exist between men and women. The extent of inequality is dependent on where you are in the world, but inequality exists in many different guises and forms across the globe. In high-income nations such as those found in Europe, like the United Kingdom, many of the gaps between men and women are narrowing, though there is still much distance to be travelled before full equality is reached; while in low-income and middle-income countries in South America and in Africa the position of women remains highly unequal.

Taking the United Kingdom first, we can observe that over time the pay gap between men and women has narrowed, though it still persists. In 1975, 16- and 17-year-old men and women could earn roughly the same amount of money, but thereafter men started to out-earn women. By the age of 38, the pay difference was 61%. Wind that forward nearly 40 years and the position is different. Women and men through their teens, twenties and into their early thirties earn comparable wages, and it is not until the mid-thirties that a gap opens. By the age of 49, men are earning 45% more than women (ONS 2014). The general trend, then, has been towards equalising pay, but sizeable inequalities still persist.

In other global regions women often face barriers that prevent them accessing and completing education, are restricted in what types of work they can enter, and face difficulties in having financial independence. Data gathered by the World Bank (2015) indicates some of the following global gender inequalities (all figures are rounded up where necessary):

- In low-income nations the completion rates for primary-level education are 70% for men and 63% for women.

- The global workforce participation rate is 50% for women and 77% for men.
- Women can lack access to their own bank accounts which could allow them financial independence and to avoid being reliant on men. In middle-income nations 62% of men have access to financial accounts in comparison to 52% of women.
- Globally, in 2013, women held only 23% of all ministerial seats in national governments.
- In low- and middle-income nations women are more likely than men to work for nothing in family-run businesses.

There are many reasons why gender pay differences endure in the United Kingdom and in other places too despite the existence of anti-discriminatory legislation or policy commitments that espouse gender equality. Women can be trapped between 'sticky floors' and 'glass ceilings', where because of discrimination and a lack of resources it can be difficult to gain promotion or to find alternatives to low-paid work. In South Africa, for example, despite a very progressive post-apartheid constitution which extols gender equality, the daily reality for many women is quite different. Patriarchy is deep within the country's culture and traditions, which can make it difficult for women to gain access to well-paid employment or promotions when they are in work.

Inequality and male advantage are much wider than pay. As Walby (1990) noted in her classic work on how patriarchy functions in society, male dominance permeates all spheres of society and not just in the workplace. In particular, she highlights that the presence and power of patriarchy can also be observed in areas such as culture, politics, sexuality and in domestic violence.

QUESTIONS

Try to identify and discuss examples of how patriarchy structures and shapes the areas of society to which Walby draws our attention. Are there are any other areas of life where men dominate? Try to think of those examples too.

As Penny (2013) has argued more recently, sexism morphs and adapts the form it takes and the spheres of society in which it operates. She is critical of how the internet has provided a platform for new forms of sexism to emerge. The anonymity the internet provides in social media can allow men to degrade, threaten and abuse women, with minimal chance of their identities becoming known. When Caroline Criado-Perez campaigned in 2013 for the greater inclusion of famous and significant women on bank notes issued by the Bank of England she met with a storm of violent misogynistic abuse on Twitter. The threats made against her included killing her and raping her.

Theorising gender

The discussion so far has raised questions about gender, by challenging commonplace assumptions. So, then, what is gender? How can we adequately understand gender and avoid lapsing into misleading stereotypes? We must turn to theory to answer these questions.

Within the sociology of health and illness, how we theorise gender has shifted away from out-and-out feminist theories, which concentrated on how women are dominated by men, to theories that focus on gender relations and gender order. These theories explain how interactions between men and women are affected by the ideas of masculinity and femininity that pervade society (Annandale and Hunt 2000). This is not to claim that we should drop all the insights that feminist theories gave us – or to suggest, for one moment, that we have moved away from a society where gender ceases to act as an arbiter of power and privilege, particularly in favour of men. For instance, feminist theories, which provided a rich analysis of patriarchy (male domination), allowed us to understand how society privileges men on a variety of fronts. This, though, does not take into account the experiences of men and implies that all men are part of a 'unified' bloc, who all share similar dispositions and access to power and economic resources, for example. Current theoretical thinking on gender acknowledges that there exist many varieties of 'maleness' and masculinity in society, as well as 'femaleness' and femininity, which should also be acknowledged and theorised.

Two in particular are detailed next. The first are the ideas and theories of Judith Butler. One key point that Butler makes in her work is that gender is not an innate state of affairs, where our gendered identities are pre-set in our genes or biology – a point that was raised earlier. Gender, for her, is a property which emerges as we perform our gender according to how gender is scripted by the society in which we live.

Connell provides another useful theory, which, this time, brings out the power relationships inherent in gender. Figure 6.2 captures the basic tenets of her theory. What is evident is that instead of one single form of masculinity and femininity there are different forms of masculinity and femininity. It is more accurate to refer to masculinities and femininities. What we find here is a move to escape categorical thinking about gender that gender can be reduced to two simple categories of men and women.

At the top, and the most powerful element, of this gender order is **hegemonic masculinity**, to which all other forms of masculinity and femininity are subordinate. The concept refers to how one form of masculinity (in this case one which is healthy, heterosexual, wealthy, assertive, aggressive and white) is associated with power, being successful and being the form of masculinity that should be aspired to in western societies. By being the 'top dog', so to speak, this form of masculinity is hegemonic, which means it controls everything else. Some good examples of men who epitomise hegemonic masculinity are the car-show presenter Jeremy Clarkson, and in America the former actor and governor

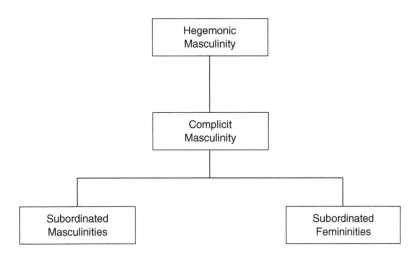

Figure 6.2 Connell's gender hierarchy

of California, Arnold Schwarzenegger. Next in the gender order is *complicit masculinity*. This is a form of masculinity that may not live up to the full expectations of hegemonic masculinity, but still affords a reasonable amount of power. We then see subordinated masculinities and femininities, which are beneath both hegemonic and complicit masculinity in terms of power and status. *Subordinated masculinities* include gay men and, in terms of health, men whose masculinity is challenged or undermined by physical or mental illness. *Subordinated femininities* include *emphasised femininity*, which refers to women who comply with hegemonic masculinity; this involves matching up to hegemonic male expectations of attractiveness and femininity. In terms of health, this can mean, especially for older women, taking on care duties for children, disabled people or older relatives in the home. There also exists *resistant femininity*, where women reject the demands and norms of emphasised femininity. This tends to be a less visible group of women (for example, lesbians and spinsters) in society, given the prevalence and profile of emphasised femininity.

One final point that Connell puts forward is that you do not have to be male to comply with the characteristics of hegemonic masculinity. She, like Butler, also denies an essentialist position of gender that gender is fixed by our biological self. Rather, she sees that these are socially created roles and women are not barred from adopting the trappings and practices of hegemonic masculinity. Examples of women who fit the hegemonic masculinity category include former British Prime Minister Margaret Thatcher, German Chancellor Angela Merkel or Winnie Mandela, former wife of South African President Nelson Mandela.

QUESTION

Reflect on a society with which you are familiar: how does Connell's theory of patriarchy help to analyse the connections between gender and health?

Perhaps we have it the wrong way round? We see what appear to be naturally occurring bodies. Men with muscles and petite women, and therefore assume that is how men and women naturally are. However, these bodies are the outcome of a variety of social processes that begin in infancy and continue throughout life. Taking physicality as an example, if we think about the types of sport that boys and girls are encouraged to play, they produce certain forms of bodies. Young (1980) takes this issue up in her classic work 'Throwing like a girl'. Women are not only channelled into sports that do not develop a physically muscular body, but are also encouraged, by informal norms and sanctions, to act in a non-physical manner, to be weak and passive in sport, and in everyday life.

QUESTION

Reflect on your own life. Can you think of times when you were directed toward certain activities, whether in the home, at school or in other spheres of life that shaped your body in a particular way?

The point just made about physicality also encourages some reflection on the old notion of nature versus nurture. That binary distinction was once a popular way of discussing issues of gender, contrasting the social with the biological as if the two are completely separate and divorced from each other. It is more fruitful instead to think through the interplay of social processes and human bodies, and how we are as people emerges out of that interaction. Connell provides the example of pregnancy. She argues that childbirth may seem the most natural state in which for women to be, where biological process must surely be the dominate force. Applying the sociological imagination, what is revealed is that pregnancy is mediated and structured by a variety of social and cultural processes. One useful example is provided by the age of the woman when she first becomes pregnant. In the United Kingdom the age of first pregnancy has increased from x in 1950 to y in 2010. The reasons why that has occurred are down to how the position of women in British society have changed in that period with the rise of the Women's Movement and the availability of oral contraception. Both of those events have allowed women to take control over reproduction. If we also consider that for some women in the United Kingdom the choice to put career first and delay motherhood until reaching their forties or fifties also illustrates the place of the social in pregnancy.

Gender and health

So, how do these theories explain how gender affects health? As Connell noted we must search out how particular gendered practices (the way we do gender in our society) shapes and conditions health. There are some clear examples where gender practices influence men and women in a way that is detrimental to health. As Connell claims, trying to live up to the demands of hegemonic masculinity requires men to act in ways that are not necessarily conducive to good health. One element of hegemonic masculinity is demonstrating that you are brave and risk-averse. That could explain why we find that young men are over-represented in statistics relating to accidents. In Scotland, for example, the number of young men who reported to accident and emergency wards was x because of accidents, while for young women it was x.

Pietilä and Rytkönen (2012) found that for Russian men, trying to accord with how masculinity is constructed in Russia was potentially damaging to their health. The researchers found that gender roles were constructed along very traditional lines. Men were cast as the breadwinners and were expected to behave and act in a very hegemonic masculine way. Having to act like that may explain why, when they cannot achieve that role because they cannot work, for instance, due to changes in the Russian economy, they resort to heavy drinking as a means of attaining a masculinity they cannot perform elsewhere.

Apprehension of appearing less than masculine can also deter men from openly communicating their health needs (O'Brien et al. 2005, 2007). This is especially so when it comes to minor illness. Admitting to not being able to cope with an illness that is not life-threatening could be interpreted as failing the requirements of hegemonic masculinity. Any man doing so runs the risk of slipping down the hierarchy of masculinity and heading towards a subordinated masculinity.

Some subtlety and complexity does exist, and we must be careful not to make blanket statements. O'Brien et al. (2005) found in their research that men who were employed in jobs such as a fire-fighting found it relatively easy to talk about their health as their job strongly accorded with a very masculine identity. It is dangerous and risky work that embodies many traditional stereotypes of being a man. Therefore, no one was going to challenge a fireman as being a weak and subordinate male if he starts to share his health or his feelings. The opposite applied to men whose work did not have access to that resource, men who worked in offices for example. Admitting to what they perceived as a weakness could undermine their complicit position in the gender hierarchy. One other subtlety the research found was that if an illness threatened to overwhelm them altogether and thereby fundamentally challenge any claims to masculinity, then that would prompt health-seeking behaviour.

More recent research in Canada by Johnson et al. (2011), this time focused on men and depression, also highlighted some of the subtleties that are at play. They found that men interpreted their experiences of depression in different ways but which still referred to some ideal of masculinity. So, for example, some men would seek treatment, but the preferred treatment was cognitive behavioural therapy (CBT) rather than approaches that relied on talking and expressing emotions. The men in this study preferred CBT because it provided them with a clear rationale of steps to help their mood. In some respects this active approach is similar to other aspects of masculinity, such as following the instructions to repair a car or fix something round the house, hence its appeal. Even the men who reported that they sought help framed doing so in a masculine way, interpreting their actions as being active partners in a process as opposed to passive patients.

In the middle-income nation of Ghana in Africa the unhealthy intersection of gender and poverty is evident in the high levels of lung disease, such as chronic obstruction pulmonary disease (COPD) among women. The condition accounts for 2% of the disease burden in the country. Constructions of gender in Ghana assign women a place in the home in charge of cooking and the provision of domestic nutrition. It is in the home, especially in the more rural and northern areas, that one of the consequences of poverty is experienced. Poor Ghanaians can typically only afford to cook using biomass fuel (mainly charcoal or wood), which, when combusted, emits noxious and harmful substances. So, in this instance, poorer women in Ghana are required to be in the home where they are in turn placed at a higher risk of lung disease than men.

MacPherson et al. (2012) provide another example of how gender and power interact. They sought to find the social processes that lay behind why women in Southern Malawi are more likely to contract HIV than men. Interviewing men and women in a fishing community, they identified the interplay of poverty and gendered power dynamics. Among the men three levels of power were evident. At the top were boat owners, the wealthiest men in the community; next were the boat captains, who were responsible for the day-to-day running of the vessels; and finally the boat crews, the men at the bottom of the hierarchy who lacked any power and were poorly paid. The women in the community worked as fish traders, taking the catch to market, where they would attempt to support their families with the money they earned. This was a highly precarious economic position to be in as it was not always certain how much they could earn. A steady income was never guaranteed and there were times when they did not have enough money to buy fish from the fishing boats. At this point, gender dynamics were at their most telling. For the women, transactional sex became an option open to them to acquire the fish to sell at market, the transactional sex occurring typically with the boat captains or the crew. Since the women were in the least powerful position they could not negotiate the use of condoms or other safe sex procedures. It was not that the men or the women did not have the requisite knowledge concerning the transmission of HIV, it was that the women lacked the power to practise that knowledge and to challenge the dominant economic and gender power of the men in this situation.

Policy – working with or challenging the gender order?

The discussion in this chapter has hopefully highlighted that the demands and expectations of gender roles are the deciding issues that influence the health and wellbeing of men and women. Emphasising the primacy of gender roles in shaping the health of men and women raises some interesting policy issues on how to reduce gendered health inequalities. After all, gender being a social construction rather than an innate characteristic means that it can be changed, challenged or engaged with. Two broad forms of policy that seek to reduce gender health inequalities can be put forward.

The first approach works with an understanding of what it is to be a man in a particular society, and to craft health policy accordingly. Earlier we discussed how men can be reticent to communicate and share concerns that they may have about physical health or feelings of emotional distress. Men's Sheds provide one approach to overcome this problem. Originating in Australia, the Men's Sheds concept seeks to create a space for typically older men where they can participate in activities such as carpentry. The health and wellbeing benefit is not just the activity, but rather the opportunity to be able to meet with other men in an environment that feels familiar and safe enough to share problems and issues.

A similar policy initiative that also works by appealing to aspects of masculinity can be found in Scotland. Sport and the physically strong body are fundamental elements of masculinity, particularly in a Scottish context. The programme seeks to assist men to exercise more and eat healthier by locating those activities in the local football club. The men involved in the programme attend their local football club, where they are coached by the training staff of that team, who provide exercise and nutritional advice. At some clubs, such as Hibernian in Edinburgh, men who have attended the programme have the opportunity to participate in a goal shoot-out at half time when their team is playing at home. The opportunity to do so acts as an incentive to adhere to the programme and allows for a performance of masculinity. By creating a health programme that relates to constructions of masculinity, men are attracted to it because it does not threaten their masculinity but it can achieve a positive change in health and wellbeing.

The second approach is dealing with how gender is constructed in a society in the first place. This approach requires going deeper into the social structures of a society and transforming the power relationships that underpin gender. Mane and Aggleton (2001) call for a rethink and transformation of gender relations in society. They highlight that even though constructions of masculinity are the root problem, it is not men themselves who are the problem. Blaming individual men ignores the fact that constructions of masculinity require men to act in certain ways. It also glosses over the differences that exist between men, and that there are men who want to see a new gender order that breaks away from older models of hegemonic masculinity.

Trying to establish actual programmes of intervention is hard, but not impossible. Mane and Aggleton (2001) suggest intervention programmes that orientate boys towards different forms of behaviour that are more positive and progressive than traditional ideals of masculinity. They also advocate, following work in the informal settlements, or favelas, of Brazil, working with young men who have experienced the damage that men have impacted on both women and men, but who feel trapped by the constructions of masculinity they are supposed to follow. By offering alternative models of masculinity then, perhaps the problems of the past can be countered. In terms of reducing levels of HIV in South Africa, Meyer and Struthers (2012) endorse a similar approach by challenging conventional modes of masculinity, as they act as a barrier for men to seek help when they require help and prevent them from engaging in healthier and more responsible behaviours.

> This suggests breaking away from stereotypes and, instead, treating men as complex individuals whose behaviour is informed not only by their own notions of what it means to be a man but also by their communities, their families, their culture ... (Meyer and Struthers 2012: 8)

Finally, referring back to MacPherson et al. and their research in Malawi, the main factor that they identified that could lead to a reduction in levels of HIV infection in the fishing community would be to increase the economic power of the women. That would allow the women not to have to rely upon transactional sex in order to feed themselves and their families.

QUESTIONS

Which of the above approaches do you favour? Why? What policies can you put forward that may bring around a positive change in the area of gender and health?

CONCLUSION

Gender emerges in this chapter not as a fixed and stable biological destiny, but as a restless, changing social and historical construction. In that flux, power dynamics are at play and inequalities exist that allow differential access to economic, symbolic, cultural and physical resources not just between men and women, but between men and men and women and women. As embodied humans we live in that flux of change and gendered inequality and it is that which affects our health. So, rather than looking for reasons within, at the levels of genetics and biology, our attention must be focused externally on how the gender order in the society in which we live constructs gender and the conditions of how we perform gender.

That emphasis on the social also provides hope and optimism that issues related to health can be changed. If a social phenomenon such as gender is constructed, then we can perhaps construct it in different ways, where the negative and damaging aspects of gender can be changed and transformed.

SUMMARY POINTS

- Gender is not a fixed immutable entity. What constitutes being a woman or a man is contingent on the society and the historical time in which you live.

- Sociologists understand gender as being a performance of roles but a performance that takes place with a hierarchy of power. They are also different ways to be masculine and different ways to be feminine.

- It is the meeting of the expectations of gendered practices that impacts on health. Specific demands can lead to specific health outcomes.

- Improvements in health can be made through adapting or challenging the prevailing gender order.

CASE STUDY

Shaun is in his fifties now, living in a deprived area of town. Life has been tough for him both economically and just getting through the daily round of life in his neighbourhood. He is not one of the hard men who live locally, but he has made himself pretty tough over time. If someone insults him he has no problem in stepping up to defend his reputation. Most of that time it just involves puffing his chest and trying to outstare someone else. There have been a few occasions when he has resorted to using his fists, though not that often. He actually doesn't like fighting.

Lately he has been experiencing pains in his chest and he seems to be coughing almost constantly. Usually a cough clears up pretty soon, but this time it has dragged on for weeks. He is beginning to think that there might be something wrong. But he's had problems before and always got through them, working out his own solutions. It'll be the same this time, no doubt. Besides, he doesn't want to take any time off work.

QUESTIONS

1. Using Connell's concept of hegemonic masculinity, why do you think Shaun behaves the way he does?
2. Pretend you are devising a local neighbourhood policy that is targeted at men like Shaun. Outline what form that policy could take and discuss your thinking behind that policy.

TAKING YOUR STUDIES FURTHER

This chapter will have helped you understand many of the key terms, concepts, theories and debates relating to gender and health. Listed below are journal articles and a book that will provide deeper and more detailed discussions of the points raised in this chapter. You will also find additional resources on the companion website, including downloads of relevant material, links to useful websites, videos and other features. Please visit the companion website at https://study.sagepub.com/barryandyuill4e

RECOMMENDED READING

Connell, R. (2012). 'Gender, health and theory: Conceptualizing the issue, in local and world perspective', *Social Science & Medicine*, 74(11): 1675–83.

Hankivsky, O. (2012) 'Women's health, men's health and gender and health: the implications of intersectionality', *Social Science & Medicine*, 74(11): 1712–20.

Meyer, M. and Struthers, H. (eds) (2012) *(Un)covering Men: Rewriting Masculinity and Health in South Africa*. Chicago, IL: Jacana Media (Pty).

ETHNICITY, MIGRATION AND HEALTH

MAIN POINTS

- We live in a global world with multiple flows of migration.

- Global migration requires us to rethink and reconsider how we understand the relations between ethnicity and health.

- Ethnic minority groups often have worse health than ethnic majority groups.

- Care must be taken when using concepts such as race and ethnicity as each can be easily misused.

- Any health inequalities experienced by ethnic groups are not explicable by reference to either cultural or genetic causes.

- Racism appears to be the main cause of those health inequalities.

- Context is important: experiences of racism vary by ethnic group and by location.

INTRODUCTION

One feature of globalisation is the increase in flows of people moving around the world. There were just over 231 million migrants globally in 2013 according to the United Nations (2013). That movement of people takes many different forms: from people moving from the global south to the global north or people migrating to other countries in the same global region.

There are multiple reasons why people make the challenging and difficult decision to migrate. Leaving one's country of birth is not an easy option for most people to make, but one that is often the result of circumstances beyond their control. War, societal breakdown, famine and economic downturns are the main triggers for migration, where the life one had known or would like to live has been taken away. Castles and colleagues (2013: 16) have termed the various transformations that occurred in migration in recent years as the '**new migration**', which they claim comprises six identifiable trends:

1. *The globalisation of migration*: immigration begins to be experienced by more and more countries around the globe, with those global migrants possessing highly diverse backgrounds in terms of skills, qualifications and experiences.
2. *The changing direction of dominant flows of migration*: where people migrate from and to is changing. Patterns vary across time. Countries that were once sites of emigration (where people would leave from) become destinations of immigration (where people travel to). Countries that have not experienced much immigration before, such as the Gulf States, can increasingly become a destination of choice for many migrants.
3. *The differentiation of migration*: migration now occurs for many different reasons. In the past, the reason for migration tended to be restricted to labour migration (or what is sometimes termed economic migration), but the reasons now are multiple and complex, including reasons such as family ties, education or seeking refuge.
4. *The proliferation of migration transition:* refers to the point in time when countries switch and begin a transition from being places of emigration to places of immigration.
5. *The feminisation of migrant labour*: the traditional migrant was a male seeking employment elsewhere and after establishing himself in a new country he would be joined by his wife and family. However, that form of labour migration is largely historical, with women now making up a considerable percentage of the numbers of global migrants.
6. *The growing politicisation of migration*: migration is often the subject of international treaties and agreements. An example of this is the freedom of movement open to citizens of nation states that are members of the European Union.

The new migration refers to multiple changes in global migration. In the past, migration typically involved male migrants from the colonial territories of the European nations and the motivation was mainly for economic reasons. In present-day society the patterns, destinations, starting points and reasons for migration are complex and varied.

The new migration challenges how we must think about and understand the health of what are termed ethnic-minority groups. Since most countries now experience a diversity of migrant groups arriving from different countries, older modes of understanding ethnicity and health require updating and challenging. Earlier editions of this book, for example, tended to discuss ethnicity and health in terms of a narrow Anglocentric perspective that focused on how ethnicity was framed in the United Kingdom by immigration from territories within the British Commonwealth from the 1950s onwards. That line of discussion focusing on the experiences of one nation state (such as the United Kingdom) becomes increasingly unsustainable given the variety of migrant and ethnic groups now living within the United Kingdom.

QUESTION

Why does migration need to be considered as a global phenomenon as opposed to focusing on one nation state?

That Anglocentric perspective also ignored how countries outside the United Kingdom have their own distinct historical and contemporary experiences of migration and ethnic relations. Those distinct historical experiences have in turn a particular effect on the health of what are deemed ethnic minority groups in those countries. So, for example, racism in South Africa was embedded in many state and private institutions in the form of apartheid, which witnessed the segregation of people on the grounds of skin colour and ethnicity. Apartheid as a legal and social system was dismantled by the mid-1990s but its effects still persist today, as is discussed later in this chapter. In Australia, the current ethnic profile of the nation was influenced by a series of policies enacted from the 1850s to 1901, commonly referred to as the 'White Settler' policy. The purpose of those policies was to establish the primacy of white European, if not British, values and to act, as Moran (2005) notes, as a justification of the taking of Aboriginal lands, which ultimately displaced the indigenous inhabitants of the continent. The White Settler polices were slowly dismantled from the Second World War onwards. However, even though Australia is now a multicultural country, the legacy of those years is still felt today and is evident in the exclusion and discrimination experienced by a variety of ethnic minority groups.

By stepping back from focusing on one nation state and adopting a more global view, we can perhaps obtain more insights into the various social processes that are at play and that influence and condition the relations between ethnicity and health. What emerges during the discussion of ethnicity and health in this chapter is the fundamental importance of society and of the social. One key point is that it is how a *society* is organised that exerts the main influence on ethnicity and health rather than anything intrinsic to the culture or biology of ethnic minority groups. Or put another way, as Nazroo (2012) invites us to do, we must ask 'what is it about a particular society that influences the health of ethnic minorities?'. His question is quite intriguing as it shifts the perspective away from considering what is it about an ethnic minority (its culture and customs or even its genetics) on to how a wider society understands, categorises and regards certain groups of people. Our focus is therefore on the wider social processes that shape the lives and lived experiences of people from ethnic groups and *not* the supposed innate characteristics of particular groups.

QUESTIONS

Nazroo invites us to explore 'what is it about a particular society that influences the health of ethnic minorities?' Why is that question phrased the way it is? And why is it more sociological than asking 'what is it about particular ethnic minorities that influences their health in society?'?

What emerges from the discussion on ethnicity and health in this chapter is that one social process acts as a prime mechanism in deciding the health of ethnic minority groups: racism. How that racism is manifested and experienced depends on where and in which society it occurs.

In many countries around the world if one is a member of an ethnic minority group, then the chances of ill-health, poor wellbeing and early mortality are much higher than for ethnic majority groups. The inequalities between ethnic groups is further troubling given that ethnic minority groups tend to exhibit a younger age profile and encounter health problems sooner in life than would be expected.

Before moving on to discuss specific health issues it is essential to clarify and outline key terms. While that is a useful task to undertake in any piece of sociology, it is perhaps especially useful, if not critical, here because if concepts such as race and ethnicity are not handled with care and subtlety one can lapse into stereotyping and an analysis that glosses over important nuances and subtleties.

RACE, RACISM AND ETHNICITY: DEFINITIONS, DEBATES AND ISSUES

Race refers to supposed biological differences between people based on skin colour and other physical features, though the actual differences between them genetically are extremely small.

Ethnicity refers to the cultural heritage and identity of a group of people.

Racism refers to the supposed racial superiority of one group over another.

Issues of **race** and **ethnicity** are complex and challenging to explore in any field of sociology. The complexity is due to the contentious and sometimes political nature of how we define and perceive supposed differences between people. In this section we shall explore how perceiving the world as composed of different and distinct races is highly problematic and ultimately false. We also explore how **racism** develops out of specific historical and social influences. Finally, we question what can appear to be the relatively neutral concept of ethnicity, and point out how it too can be problematic as both a sociological concept and a neat and easily bounded category that can be applied to groups of people.

Race

One aspect of modern life is that skin colour is often accepted or regarded as being a major way of defining differences between people. The focus on skin colour follows on from the idea that humanity consists of different and distinct races, in which there exist discernible and enduring genetic and cultural patterns that clearly separate one group of humans from another. Adopting such a perspective of fixed and immutable characteristics can be referred to as *essentialism*, where certain traits are seen as naturally given and outside social and historical influence. Essentialism implies that a range of characteristics are fixed and that people are born in a certain way that is with them for life. From a sociological perspective, however, this particular view can be challenged and shown to be false. We can also identify how such a view is heavily influenced by racist prejudice and stereotyping.

First, can classifying humans into separate races be scientifically justified? The concept of race implies that there are different species of people, just as there are different species of animal. The scientific evidence indicates that there exist virtually no major differences between groups of humans. Biologist Steven Rose (2005: 37) usefully summarises the genetic science thus:

> The definition of race is essentially a social one, as in reference to Blacks or Jews. While there are differences in gene frequencies (that is, differences in the proportions in which particular genetic variants occur) between population groups, these do not map onto the social criteria used to define race. For instance, Polish Jews resemble genetically their fellow Polish nationals, non-Jews, more closely than they do Jews from Spain. Gene frequencies in Black Americans differ from those in Black South Africans. And for that matter, gene frequencies differ between people in North and South Wales, yet no one would think of classifying those two populations as two different races. This typological thinking has not disappeared: it characterizes, of course, the poisonous propaganda of racist political groups, and has not entirely vanished from popular scientific writing.

What Rose is saying here is that people, regardless of exterior markers such as skin colour, are almost identical. Humans, as a life form, are fairly genetically homogeneous; one is likely to find more differences between people who are seen or see themselves as, let us say, Asian than between Asian people and people who are seen or see themselves as, let us say, white. This is not surprising as in evolutionary time *Homo sapiens* is comparatively recent, emerging out of Africa only *c.* 200,000 years ago. That is simply not enough time to evolve into different groups, species or races!

Rather than seeing differences between humans as being essential or natural, we must look to how differences are *socially* constructed over time and in different societies. The whole tradition of thinking in terms of race has a distinct history that is mired in prejudice and oppression. It also emerges out of particular historical and social circumstances. Using skin colour, or race, as a delimiter, or way of distinguishing one group of people from another, is historically recent. The first attempt to 'scientifically' classify people did not happen until the mid-1800s and is associated with the work of de Gobineau, and was, at best, based on flimsy pseudo-science and carries no validity today.

The roots of thinking in terms of race require us to step a little further back in time to the rise and expansion of European colonialism and the development of the slave trade from the mid-1600s to the early 1800s. As Blackburn (1998) has discussed, the need for cheap mass labour to work the new plantations in the Americas and the Caribbean led to the enslavement of millions of black Africans. The sheer brutal and bloody exploitation required some form of justification both on the plantations and in Britain, with many white working-class movements in Britain, such as Chartism, being opposed to slavery. So, starting as an oral tradition on the plantations, before becoming part of mainstream European thought, the racist idea that black people were of a lower order, perhaps even subhuman, and therefore not allowed full human rights, spread and developed as part of this process of justifying the slave trade.

Prior to that period, the main ways of seeing differences between people have varied considerably over time. In the ancient world of Rome, Greece and Egypt, race and skin colour were not seen as important: instead the world was divided into civilised people

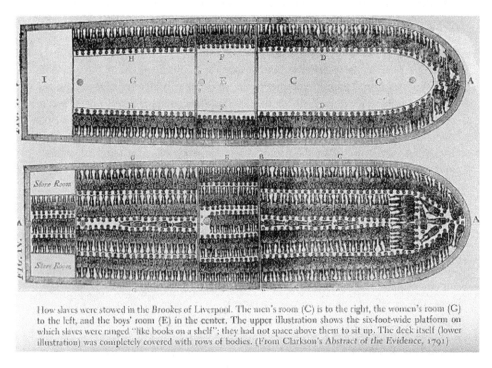

How slaves were stowed in the *Brookes* of Liverpool. The men's room (C) is to the right, the women's room (G) to the left, and the boys' room (E) in the center. The upper illustration shows the six-foot-wide platform on which slaves were ranged "like books on a shelf"; they had not space above them to sit up. The deck itself (lower illustration) was completely covered with rows of bodies. (From Clarkson's *Abstract of the Evidence*, 1791)

Figure 7.1   Anti-slavery leaflet from 1789

and barbarians. Notably, what constituted being civilised was independent of skin colour, with barbarians including white Northern European people and civilised people including black North Africans. Some key historical figures, such as the Roman emperor Septimus Severius, were what we would now regard as black. Indeed, much of the culture of the ancient world to varying degrees was, as Bernal (1991, 2001) has argued, a fusion of European, North African and Asian influences.

Figure 7.1 is taken from an abolitionist anti-slavery leaflet from 1789. It illustrates the brutal and inhumane way in which enslaved Africans were transported from Africa to the Americas. People were chained to platforms for weeks on end with no access to toilets or fresh air. Millions of Africans died on this transatlantic journey. British ports such as Bristol, Liverpool and Glasgow both directly and indirectly benefited from this trade.

Eamonn (Figure 7.2) belongs to one of the UK's fastest expanding ethnic minority groups. Born in Scotland, he is of mixed heritage with a white Irish mother and a black African father. In future years he will have an array of ethnic identities to adopt. He could choose, for example, to call himself Scottish or black Scottish or maybe black or black British. Or perhaps he might prefer Irish or African. In fact, he has a large number of ethnic identities he could choose and then discard throughout his life. Any ethnic identity he may select will be alongside other aspects of his identity too. For example, he'll be someone's son, someone's partner and so on.

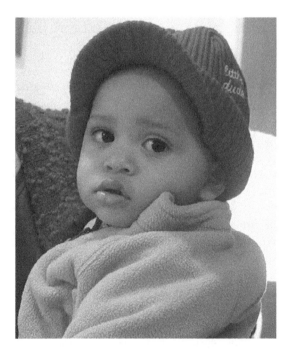

Figure 7.2 Eamonn

Ethnicity

Given the problems associated with race, as identified in the previous section, the concept of ethnicity is frequently favoured today in many different contexts. With ethnicity there is no essential basis; reference is not to supposed biological or genetic traits, but rather to purely *social* phenomena. Ethnicity refers to a common cultural heritage that is socially learned and constructed; this means that as we grow up we take up and internalise what we see happening about us. So, one sees certain ways of dressing and eating, for example, as being normal and adopts them as one's own.

In many respects the concept of ethnicity is a useful advance on, and correction to, the problems of race, with its emphasis on the social as opposed to the biological. Ethnicity too can be problematic. We shall now discuss how this is so, considering two main problems in the way that it can sometimes be (mis)used.

QUESTIONS

To which ethnic group, if any, do you regard yourself as belonging? What are the features (for example, dress, language, food, religion, etc.) of your ethnic group? How much of a role, if any, does your ethnicity play in how you see yourself?

Static or fluid?

Ethnicity can be misused in a way that reduces culture to a static list of attributes, with the assumption that everyone who is identified as being in a particular ethnic group shares the same characteristics with regard to, for example, family, life, culture, food, and attitudes to illness and health services. Ethnicity is therefore seen as being like a shopping list or a 'cookie cutter', where everyone turns out the same. Ethnicity is far more complex than that. One of its complexities is that, like other forms of identity, it is dynamic, evolving and changing over time (Carter and Fenton 2009). Another one of its complexities is that people who are, let us say, seen as being South Asian in one context are not the same as people who are seen as being South Asian in another context.

For example, people with a Pakistani heritage who have grown up and live in Glasgow in Scotland can be quite different from people with a similar heritage who have grown up in Bradford in England. As Virdee et al. (2006) note, people with a Pakistani heritage living in Glasgow report that their ethnic identity is shaped both by being Scottish (in particular, speaking with a Scottish accent is an important signifier of being accepted as being Scottish in Scotland) and by their Pakistani heritage (in this case being Muslim). While for Bradfordian Asians, their sense of identity is shaped by a complex and contradictory relationship with being English and British, that differs by generation too (Bagguley and Hussain 2008). If we expand the example a little further, we can go on to say that

116

both Glaswegian and Bradfordian South Asians would in turn be quite different in many respects from South Asian people who have lived and grown up in South Africa.

It is useful here to mention that in the wider sociological literature on identity the idea of a fixed static identity is clearly rejected (Jenkins 2004). What is emphasised is that identity is fluid. By claiming that identity is fluid we mean that we can switch between different identities (for example, being British or English, student or therapist, member of a youth subculture or churchgoer) depending on the *context* in which we find ourselves and in what ways we wish to present ourselves in that context.

In relation to disability, we can find how these complexities of identity and how other forms of identity, in addition to an ethnic identity, can be important in deciding how people perceive themselves in society. Researching how South Asian deaf people negotiate their identity, Islam (2008) found that the people in their study did not see themselves in a singular way. Rather, they subscribed to a variety of identities depending on context. These multiple identities ranged from seeing their identity as part of a wider deaf community, to religious identities, and to a fusion of British and Asian identities. Focusing on the experiences of disabled Muslim women who have migrated to Canada, Dossa (2009) points again to the complexities of identity. The women in her research contested and struggled with different identities of disability, their ethnicity and, in some cases, their disputed identity as legitimate citizens of Canada.

Another useful example, this time concerning ethnic identity generally, is how Caribbean migrants thought of their identity in the late 1940s and how it has changed over time. Many early migrants, regardless of which Caribbean island they were originally from, saw themselves not as African-Caribbean (the currently preferred term) but as British. The following quote is from someone who arrived on the *Empire Windrush* in 1948 as part of the initial phase of migration from the Caribbean into Britain:

> I wouldn't say that we had our own identity. We were always British. In Jamaica I can remember, when it was the Queen's birthday or the King's birthday or the Coronation, everything was done the way Britain wanted us to. (Phillips and Phillips 1999: 12)

A unified and distinct African-Caribbean identity developed in Britain in response to the sometimes less than welcoming reception that early migrants encountered.

QUESTIONS

The above discussion talks a lot about fluidity, change and fusion. Identify ways in which both mainstream culture and your own personal life display elements of that fluidity and fusion. You may wish to think about TV programmes, dress, food, and so on. Also, why is it important to be aware and knowledgeable about other cultures and ethnicities?

Ethnicity as too general

There is another distinct problem with ethnicity as a concept and how it can be used. The terms used in the United Kingdom are very loose and wide-ranging in their coverage. 'South Asian', for instance, covers a huge geographic range with a population of millions, including India, Sri Lanka, Bangladesh and Pakistan. It also includes a variety of major languages (Punjabi, Gujarati, Pashto, Bengali, Urdu and English) and major religions (Hindu, Islam, Sikh and Christian). Such terms lack any real specificity and can miss out many important and telling differences within an ethnic group. A warning on simplifying ethnic groups into large undifferentiated units was raised by Nazroo (1998) after breaking down the ethnic identity of 'Indian' into religious groups. He found that there were some differences in the reporting of fair or poor health. Indian Hindus, on average, reported similar levels, and Indian Christians slightly better, than the majority white population, while Indian Muslims reported, on average, worse health than all the previously mentioned groups.

In the United States, Zsembik and Fennell (2005) have drawn attention to the difficulties associated with the concept of a Latino category. Here, again, a variety of people, also from a large and varied land mass, are brought together under one overarching heading. Zsembik and Fennell identify considerable and notable differences in culture, perceptions of health, social class and acculturation for different Latino people. So, instead of this one overarching title of Latino, it would be more effective to break that particular category down into smaller and more representative categories to identify Mexicans, Puerto Ricans, Dominicans and Cubans as separate groups.

Racism

Even though we have rejected the validity of race on the grounds that the concept is not soundly based in any real science, this does not mean that we can reject racism as a force in society (Bradby 2012). Racism is a defining experience for many ethnic groups in the United Kingdom, the United States and elsewhere. As a concept, it refers to one group holding itself to be inferior or superior to another group. Earlier we saw that ideas of race and racial superiority developed out of slavery and European colonial expansion. Even though the plantation system, which prompted the emergence of thinking in terms of white superiority over other groups of people, has disappeared, racism and all its problems still continue today. The climate of the 'War on Terror', and wider conflicts in the Middle East, have also increased tensions concerning Muslims in western countries.

Levels of reported prejudice in the United Kingdom reveal a complex and highly differentiated picture. A recent survey by the British Social Attitudes Survey (2013) indicated that the levels of people reporting being either very or a little prejudiced have been generally increasing since 2002. Before that date the number of people reporting being very or a little prejudiced was declining. Overall, somewhere in the region of three in ten people in the United Kingdom report being very (3%) or a little prejudiced (27%). Such a figure does not mean, however, that levels of prejudice are evenly spread across the United Kingdom. Not all social or age groups report that level of prejudice. Younger people, especially those born after 1980, and people with a degree-level education tend to report higher levels of no prejudice, as do people working at a professional level and people who live in inner London. However, older people, born either before 1939 or in the baby boomer years of 1940–59, are more likely to report higher levels of prejudice, as do those with a CSE or equivalent educational qualification or those with no qualification and those who work in unskilled occupations. One possible explanation for these differences is that people whose lives are precarious and lack security are more likely to see migrants and people with what are perceived to be different cultural heritages as a threat to what they have (particularly jobs and housing).

The actual manifestation of racism and the form it takes in society have changed over time, though arguably the result is the same: the systematic disadvantaging of specific minority groups. In the early days of the slave trade, racism centred on the supposed subhuman nature of enslaved African people, with claims that they were a lesser species of humans than white Europeans, and inferior to them in just about any conceivable way. At the high point of the British Empire in the late 1800s racism took on a paternalistic form, with notions that colonised peoples required the guidance and help of supposedly more advanced and enlightened Europeans. During the 1980s racism became more disguised and subtle, with the emphasis being on how the survival of indigenous British culture could be overwhelmed by the cultures of migrant ethnic groups. Prime Minister Margaret Thatcher, at the time, went as far as saying that British culture would be 'swamped' by the new groups arriving in the UK. In the wake of the attack on New York on 11 September 2001 and the ensuing 'War on Terror', 'Islamophobia' has been on the rise, with Muslims often being portrayed as a potential threat, or having to justify aspects of Islamic culture in a way that other minority ethnic groups are not required to do.

Racism consists of three dimensions. First, there is **prejudice**, which relates to negative attitudes about someone from another race or ethnic group. In a day-to-day context this would mean name-calling on the street and putting forward opinions that denigrate an ethnic group. Next, there is **discrimination**, which relates to actions that treat people from another race or ethnic group unequally based on prejudice. This could mean, for example, preventing someone of an ethnic group from getting a job. Research by Wood (2012), for example, found that employers were less likely to employ someone with a typically Asian name than someone with a typically British name. Finally, in recent years in the UK one of the most highlighted and debated forms of racism has been **institutional racism**. The main focus on institutional racism has been in the wake of the Macpherson Report (1999) looking at the failures of the Metropolitan Police in investigating the murder of black student Stephen Lawrence. It is in this report that a very useful definition of institutional racism can be found:

The collective failure of an organisation to provide an appropriate and professional service to people because of their colour, culture or ethnic origin. It can be seen in processes, attitudes and behaviour which amount to discrimination through unwitting prejudice, ignorance, thoughtlessness and racist stereotyping which disadvantage minority ethnic people. (Macpherson 1999)

It is not just in the police force that institutional racism is evident. In the next section we will look at how prejudice and racist stereotyping within health and medical services adversely affect the health of ethnic minority people. Health professionals within the NHS also face institutional racism, with a variety of reports suggesting that health professionals from ethnic minority groups are worse off than white health professionals with equivalent training and expertise (Kline 2014).

QUESTIONS

What are your views on the levels of racism today in the society in which you live? What do you think are the main issues and problems that we face in trying to bring about a more tolerant society?

ETHNICITY AND HEALTH

So how do ethnicity and health interact? Older perspectives on ethnicity and health tended to focus on the genetic make-up or cultural practices of particular groups. An indicative example of this older approach can be noted in research on South Asians and coronary heart disease (CHD) (Nazroo 1998). Work by Gupta et al. (1995) inferred that the predisposition of South Asians to CHD was either to be found in their genetic make-up, or in their cultural practices such as cooking with ghee, not exercising or not making the best use of medical services. Part of the reason why this 'victim blaming' came about was the research method used. Drawing on certain statistical and quantitative approaches, ethnicity here was treated in a stereotypical manner, casting all South Asians as genetically and culturally identical. Such approaches also ignored the socio-economic context in which South Asian people found themselves, for example class and the effects of poorly paid jobs.

Sociological perspectives have developed and become more refined since then. Explanations that focus on genetic factors have been discarded for the reasons outlined above in the section on race – that humans are basically so similar that seeking out genetic explanations can lapse into the biological racism of previous generations. We can also be wary of pointing to explanations that stress that the ethnic and cultural traditions of a group of people are responsible for any health inequalities.

Sickle Cell Disease (SCD) provides an interesting example of both the problems in uncritically using the concept of ethnicity and also of seeking out genetic or biological reasons to explain ethnic health inequalities. The blood disorder of SCD emerges from a genetic mutation that historically developed as a protection against malaria. One symptom of SCD is extreme pain, which occurs during a sickle cell crisis when abnormal sickle-shaped cells can block blood vessels, which in turn can damage bodily tissue or organs. Other symptoms include tiredness and fatigue.

SCD is often solely associated with people whose ethnic identity is assumed to be African or African-Caribbean. While higher incidence rates of the disease are found in those groups, it is not exclusive to African and African-Caribbean people. It can affect white people from southern Europe, Hispanic people and people from the Middle East, or, to put it another way, people who have an ancestry in a country where malaria was common at some historical point. The exclusive association of SCD with one or two particular ethnic groups raises an interesting sociological point.

As Carter and Dyson (2011, 2015) point out, SCD has been involved in a process of **ethnoization** of a disease. What they mean by ethnoization is that a disease becomes associated with one particular ethnicity and becomes in the popular imagination a disease that *only affects that group* of people: in this instance, people who are African-Caribbean or African. The ethnoization of SCD indicates how ethnicity can be misused as a sociological concept and as a method of categorising people. As Carter and Dyson note, the assumption made is that ethnicity refers to a discrete and distinct group of people, who are sealed off from other ethnic groups. SCD reveals that that is simply not the case and that the boundary lines between ethnic groups are at best blurry, and can fall down altogether on closer inspection. Dyson (2005) also draws attention to how focusing on ethnicity as a sole risk factor in developing the disorder may miss out people who are at risk, but because their presumed ethnicity does not match the risk profile, they may not be identified as being at risk. For example, someone who is assumed to be ethnically white British may develop SCD because they have an ancestor who, by dint of coming from an area where malaria was a risk, developed the disorder. However, because SCD is commonly presented as being a disorder associated with people with an African-Caribbean heritage, someone who is from that white ethnicity may not be perceived as being at risk.

> Ethnoization refers to a process where a particular condition, disease or disorder is popularly and often falsely attributed to a particular ethnic group or sometimes groups. Doing so can create a false understanding of that condition, disease or disorder and can contribute to stereotyping and misinformation.

If we can dismiss – or at least heavily critique – appeals to biological or cultural explanations, then what is left as a possible explanation? Contemporary sociology of health turns to the social processes that shape, form and interact with how ethnic groups are defined, how people define their ethnic identity and how ethnic hierarchies in specific contexts impact negatively on health. We consider those social processes in greater depth next.

RACISM AND HEALTH

The prime social process to consider is racism. We discussed racism and the various forms that it can take earlier in this chapter. What we need to do now is understand how and why racism affects health. The relationship between racism and poor health has been noted for some time. Karlsen and Nazroo (2002a, 2004) in the United Kingdom, Krieger et al. (2005) in the United States and Harris et al. (2006) in New Zealand, for example, have all come to similar conclusions that we have to take the lived experience of racism seriously if we are to have a full and rounded understanding of what contributes to ethnic health inequalities. More recently, research by Brondolo et al. (2011) and Braveman (2012) have also strongly supported the linkage between racism and poor health outcomes. This racism can come in a variety of forms: the day-to-day racism of name-calling and prejudice; actual physical abuse and assault; and institutional racism. It is also important to note that it is not just the *direct* but also the *indirect* experience of racism that has an effect. This means that someone does not have to be name-called in the street or attacked; they simply need to have a perception or expectation that racism exists and that it could happen to them – in short, a fear of racism, and the worry and stress this creates (Karlsen and Nazroo 2004). In many ways indirect experiences of racism share an affinity with the stress-related psycho-social pathways of health that we explored in Chapter 5 on inequality and health.

Priest et al. (2013) have undertaken a systematic review of the research literature that seeks to understand the impact that racism can have on the health and wellbeing of young people. Their review of 153 published papers relating to 121 separate pieces of research carried out across six geographic regions (Australia/New Zealand, South America, Canada, Europe/UK, Israel and the USA) indicated that racism could affect health in ways similar to the pathways outlined above but in other ways too:

1. restricted access to social resources
2. negative emotional reactions
3. patho-physiological processes
4. reduction in uptake of healthy behaviours
5. direct physical injury.

They found that an array of mental health and emotional distress issues were prevalent for young people who had experienced racism and racist discrimination. Experiences of anxiety, depression and distress were common, while feelings of good or high self-worth and self-esteem were less likely. Notably, physical health problems returned lower levels of association, which means that young people's physical health was less likely to be affected by racist discrimination.

Priest et al. (2013) also noted one new observation in their review: the relationship between racism and behavioural issues such as alcohol and illicit drug use. The use of alcohol and drugs possibly developed as a response to the racism that young people can encounter, and which may in turn further exacerbate any mental health or emotional health problems they are experiencing. Paradies (2006) also found similar relationships in a review of the research on racism and health. Again, a relationship between emotional distress and racism was evident.

What is notable in the relationship between wellbeing and racism is that it is mental health that appears to be most affected and physical health much less so. One possible reason to explain why emotional and mental health is affected is that some form of time lag exists between the appearance of mental health issues and those issues translating into physical symptoms. As we have discussed in other chapters in this book, our emotional health and physical health are not separate spheres, and stressful emotional issues that we experience in everyday life can become physical problems too. There is no strong evidence to support this explanation at the moment, but it indicates one direction for further research into how racism affects health and wellbeing in its widest sense.

The discussion so far has focused on the relationship between racism and health. Earlier in this chapter we discussed how care must be taken when exploring issues of ethnicity and racism. Just as ethnicity varies across different countries and across history, so does how racism is expressed and experienced. How racism is structured and experienced is not the same the world over.

We are now drawing attention to the role played by the social context in which racism is both manifested and experienced. By doing so we are returning to Nazroo's point that the focus should be on what it is about a particular society that creates health problems for ethnic groups. What emerges from other research is that it is not so much where you are from that is important, but where you are in the world, and how you are perceived there goes a long way in explaining health inequalities for ethnic groups.

A study by Nazroo et al. (2007) helps to explain the points just made, that context is important and that racism varies by social context. In their analysis of survey data of health and ethnicity that compared the United States with the United Kingdom, they compared the health of five different ethnic groups:

- black Americans
- Caribbean Americans
- white Americans
- white English
- Caribbean English.

It might be a reasonable assumption to make, given what we have been discussing so far, that the health of the black ethnic groups listed above would be uniformly worse that the health of the white groups. That, though, does not turn out to be the case. Instead, different health outcomes both by ethnic groups and by country were evident in this research. Caribbean Americans have better health than black Americans and Caribbean English and are on a par with white Americans. If we begin by comparing the Caribbean

English with the Caribbean Americans we can bring to the fore the importance of context. In England, Caribbean people are perceived in a more negative light than Caribbean people are in America. As Bécares et al. (2012) discussed in a study similar to that of Nazroo et al. (2007), Caribbean Americans are positively stereotyped as being hard working, while the reverse applies to Caribbean English, who can be negatively stereotyped as lazy and drug users.

A historical dimension also exists. In the discussion on the fluidity of ethnic identity earlier in this chapter, we highlighted how a distinctive, unified and *British* African-Caribbean identity emerged after migration to England from the 1950s onwards and that experiences of life in England were often marked by racism and discrimination. English Caribbeans therefore have had a longer exposure to a particular form of racism than American Caribbeans.

QUESTION

The discussion above emphasises the importance of the context in which people live. Why is context important and what does it tell us about the formation of ethnic identities in a specific society?

Other research also points to supposedly the same ethnic groups but in different locations experiencing different health outcomes. Comparing whites, South Asian Indians and African-Caribbeans in the Netherlands and in England in a study on metabolic syndrome, Agyemang et al. (2012) found that the Dutch ethnic groups exhibited higher prevalence rates of metabolic syndrome than their English counterparts. The difference between the Dutch and English ethnic groups, they felt, was explicable by reference to the context in which the ethnic groups lived.

The key message to highlight again is that it is not just being black or Caribbean that affects health in the cases just discussed, but what it means to be black or Caribbean in a particular context and how those ethnic identifiers are interpreted, stereotyped and understood within that context.

So, if we are claiming that context is important, what about societies where racism has historically been a central organising principle of that society, where racism was built into the fabric of social institutions and actively promoted by the government? South Africa provides an example of one country where racial discrimination was embedded deeply into society. Racial and ethnic segregation and discrimination have long been a feature of South African society, the roots of which can be found in the country's colonial past when the various parts of what would become South Africa were under Dutch and British rule. After independence from the British in 1948, racial segregation became institutionalised in the brutal system of apartheid. The word 'apartheid' comes from the Afrikaans language, meaning 'to separate'.

124

The various peoples living in South Africa were subjected to a strict form of racial hierarchy that institutionalised and entrenched white supremacy and was often based on arbitrary criteria, especially for people classified as Coloured (those of mixed heritage), where different members of the same family could be deemed to belong to different racial groups. The four different racial groups – blacks, whites, Indians and Coloured – were then segregated into different areas.

Apartheid came to an end in the period between 1991 and 1994, when legislation that enforced apartheid was repealed and the African National Congress (ANC), led by Nelson Mandela, was elected to power. That point in time may be stretching into the past now, but the legacy of the past exerts a strong influence on the present. Williams et al. (2008) and Atwoli et al. (2013) have carried out research in post-apartheid South Africa. They used the same categories that were enforced in the apartheid era and what they found was that the black, Indian and Coloured groups had worse mental health, especially in terms of distress, than the white ethnic group. Again, discrimination, whether racially or non-racially motivated, played a part in explaining the higher levels of mental health problems. The researchers also noted that some form of historical trauma may also exert an influence on current generations of black South Africans. Historical trauma refers to the pain and suffering caused by discrimination and racist acts of inhumanity in the past whose effects have been so damaging on a group of people that it requires generations to heal.

INTERSECTIONALITY

One final aspect of ethnicity that needs to be considered is how other social structural processes operate in relation to ethnicity. Is it purely down to ethnicity or do other social structures, such as class and gender, make a difference too? If we say no, or keep the focus on ethnicity and the various issues that entails, then the social structures on class and gender have no bearing. However, research indicates otherwise and points to what sociologists call *intersectionality*. The roots of intersectionality emerge out of the writings of black US feminists from the 1960s onwards (hooks 1987). As a concept, intersectionality speaks to the need to consider that people's lives are not just defined by one process. People are not simply understood by reference to, or are reducible to, their ethnicity, but rather are simultaneously shaped by their social class and by their gender. These different processes therefore intersect, cut across, fuse together and influence each other. As Higginbottom (2006: 585) usefully summarises, variations in ethnicity and health and ill health 'arise from the coalescence of complex factors such as migration, cultural adaptation, racism, reception by the host community, socio-economic influences and prevailing societal ideologies'. Research from around the world indicates that other forms of inequality, concerned with class and gender, also affect many ethnic minority groups.

CONCLUSION

We have explored in this chapter one form of health inequality that, given current trends and globalisation, is increasing in importance. The key message is that it is not the fault of ethnic minority groups that they experience worse health than ethnic majority groups, whether one points to culture or genetics. Rather, it is how groups of people are categorised into distinct ethnic groups and perceived within a particular society. How that categorisation and perception takes place in turn exposes that group to various forms of racism that can be direct (name-calling or physical violence) or indirect (discrimination and an expectation of discrimination) in having an effect on health. The evidence so far points to mental health and emotional distress being the prime health and wellbeing consequences of racism, but further research could establish how those psychological issues translate into physical health problems.

Overall, what we find is that much of what makes our health and wellbeing good or bad depends very much on our place and location in the society in which we live.

SUMMARY POINTS

- We live in a globalised world with increasing levels of mobility, with people moving to and from various regions of the globe.

- Race and ethnicity are contested terms in sociology. Great care must be taken in how those terms are understood and used.

- It is racism that is the prime cause of ethnic health inequalities, rather than biology or culture.

- It is how the ethnic identity of a particular group of people is constructed that indicates what levels and what forms of racism they might encounter.

CASE STUDY

Mike remembers what his dad told him about what he had to endure at work back in the 1970s. Being the first African-Caribbean person to work in the local council housing department, he had to deal with all sorts of abuse and disrespect. Sometimes this was out-and-out racism. A small group of people in the office often verbally abused him. On several occasions they left bananas or literature from far-right racist parties on his desk. What Mike's dad found worse, though, were the attitudes of other office workers, who, even though not openly hostile to him, always seemed a little suspicious. Mike's dad constantly had to make jokes about his skin colour in order to be accepted in any way. He hated having to act in that way as he found it demeaning. This added an extra layer of stress to an already stressful job. It was having to deal with all these issues that, Mike believes, led to his dad developing a heart condition in his late fifties. In fact, his dad had to take early retirement as a result of his poor health. To this day he still claims to feel quite poorly most of the time and is not as healthy as he would like to be.

For Mike, many of these problems are firmly in the past. The office in which he works is like the rest of the city, with a mixed, cosmopolitan and diverse workforce. He works alongside people who are white, Asian or African-Caribbean and who, like him, see themselves as British born and bred. He gets on well with just about everyone in his section and he faces none of the outward racism that his dad had to face. However, more subtle forms of racism persist. Despite the diversity of the workforce, the managers are uniformly white. Mike has put in for promotion several times but each time he has been rejected, despite working hard, putting in the hours and being respected by many of his colleagues as a good worker. Other people with a less strong profile than his have advanced up the ranks much quicker than him. He now suspects that it is something to do with his ethnicity. Regardless of how much he works, it just never seems to be enough. This is starting to get to him. Lately, he has found himself becoming more stressed and feels generally down.

QUESTIONS

1.   What elements of the case study reflect some of the wider social changes that were discussed in this chapter?
2.   Discuss the ways in which racism has had an effect on the health of both Mike today and his father in the past.
3.   Besides issues to do with ethnicity, what other social factors could be exerting an influence on Mike's health?

TAKING YOUR STUDIES FURTHER

This chapter will have helped you understand many of the key terms, concepts, theories and debates relating to race, ethnicity and health. Listed below are journal articles and a book that will provide deeper and more detailed discussions of the points raised in this chapter. You will also find additional resources on the companion website, including downloads of relevant material, links to useful websites, videos and other features. Please visit the companion website at https://study.sagepub.com/barryandyuill4e

RECOMMENDED READING

Bécares, L., Nazroo, J., Jackson, J. and Heuvelman, H. (2012) 'Ethnic density effects on health and experienced racism among Caribbean people in the US and England: a cross-national comparison', *Social Science & Medicine*, 75(12): 2107–15.

Carter, B. and Dyson, S.M. (2011) 'Territory, ancestry and descent: the politics of sickle cell disease', *Sociology*, 45(6): 963–76.

Nazroo, J.Y. (2006) *Health and Social Research in Multiethnic Societies*. Abingdon: Routledge.

Priest, N., Paradies, Y., Trenerry, B., Truong, M., Karlsen, S. and Kelly, Y. (2013) 'A systematic review of studies examining the relationship between reported racism and health and well-being for children and young people', *Social Science & Medicine*, 95: 115–27.

MENTAL HEALTH AND EMOTIONAL DISTRESS

MAIN POINTS

- Many more people in contemporary society are reporting and experiencing distress and depression.

- Sociology helps us understand how mental health is framed in and by society.

- The attitudes of others and wider society greatly affect the wellbeing of those experiencing distress.

- Wider social inequalities are also visible in the distribution of diagnosed and reported mental health problems.

INTRODUCTION

Mental health issues and emotional distress is of worldwide concern, becoming one of the leading causes of disability. The World Health Organisation (WHO) (2015) identify that 350 million people globally are affected by depression. They also note that depression can lead to suicide, with suicide being the second most common cause of death for 15–29 year-olds. Despite being so common and prevalent in society, mental health has been regarded with suspicion and sometimes fear within society, and has been seen as a lower-status field in which to practise by the medical profession. Much of this is to do with how social attitudes negatively frame mental illness. In previous centuries, for example, mental illness was seen as possession by demons, a curse by God. Even in more enlightened times it was the ultimate transgression against reason and rationality. As a result, mental illness became stigmatised, the badge of the outsider and the deviant, and associated with danger and violence.

Sociology has an important role to play in trying to understand the full intricacies of mental illness, especially when it comes to the ways in which society *influences* and *frames* both how we see mental health and illness and how society creates situations that can negatively impact on individuals' mental health. Busfield (2000: 554) neatly summarises what sociology can offer the study of mental health and illness, and how sociology tells us about

> the importance of social processes in a range of areas: in the definition, boundaries and categories of mental disorder; in any adequate understanding of the factors that give rise to mental disorder; and in the understanding of the character of mental health practice and the professionals and others who shape that practice together with the ideas that underpin it.

This chapter will explore many of the issues associated with mental health and illness. Much of the focus, as suggested above, will be on how mental health and illness are framed by society. A great deal of the research indicates that this framing (attitudes held by the general public, how people's behaviour is interpreted by others, and the influence of medical classifications and categories) can affect the lives of people with mental health problems much more than the symptoms of their particular condition. We will look at some of the debates that exist in relation to defining and identifying what is seen to be mental illness. Attention will also be given to the effect that social attitudes, whether expressed by official bodies or by the lay general public, have on people who are experiencing some form of distress. This will lead us to the theory of stigma, which helps us understand how people with certain traits and characteristics are made to feel unwelcome and excluded by society. We will also look at depression in some depth. This will allow us to consider some of the particular circumstances and issues that affect people who experience this condition. Finally, consideration will be given to sociological perspectives on suicide.

WHAT CAUSES MENTAL ILLNESS?

Giving a clear and concise answer to the question 'What causes mental illness?' is highly problematic. Part of the reason for this is the complexities and uncertainties that surround the whole process of diagnosis and identifying mental illness in the first place. Unlike physical illnesses, there is often no clear-cut objective sign that someone is experiencing a mental illness. One cannot, for example, find a broken bone or a cell that has become cancerous. Instead, doctors and psychiatrists have to rely on what people tell them – which is, in itself, highly problematic, as we shall see. McPherson and Armstrong (2006: 50) summarise these concerns well, when they say:

> What is pneumonia or appendicitis or cancer can be agreed internationally with reference to the presence or absence of certain clearly defined physical characteristics. In psychiatry, however, there is no such external biological referent to act as an anchor for diagnosis. Essentially, psychiatry classifies on the basis of a patient's patterns of symptoms which might vary according to how they are elicited and interpreted.

Because, then, we cannot always clearly identify what mental illness is, this makes the search for a cause all the harder. Lack of certainty means that no single authoritative answer can be put forward, and over the years we have seen many competing explanations come and go. Broadly speaking, explanations for mental illness fall into one of two camps: biological explanations and social explanations. These look in very different directions and see quite different reasons for the existence of mental illness, as outlined below.

Even though there are often no apparent organic signs, biological explanations (typically favoured by mainstream medicine) still privilege a focus on faulty genes or imbalances in the chemistry of the brain. There is, for instance, an association between low levels of serotonin and depression. This way of thinking, of looking for a biological cause, is increasingly reinforced by the proliferation of pharmaceutical interventions, such as SSRIs (selective serotonin reuptake inhibitors) for treating depression, which suggest that if an illness can be treated by chemicals, then it must have a biological, organic basis.

Social explanations, on the other hand, fall into two general categories: social causation and social constructionist. The social causation perspective refers to how the various inequalities in society (mainly to do with ethnicity, gender and class) produce toxic levels of stress for some people. As a result of this stress, people may be 'tipped' into mental illness, whether it is a woman expected to bring up children on her own and keep down a job; or the experience of someone from an ethnic minority group of being racially abused by a neighbour; or the constant soul-destroying grind of poverty and not being able to lead the life that others enjoy. We shall look at some of these issues later in this chapter.

The other main social explanation is social constructionist. Mental illness, from this viewpoint, does not exist as a 'fact' or as 'real' and it has absolutely no organic basis. This sociological view is influenced by the work of Foucault (1967), who has argued that there is no single incontestable truth that can be discovered and agreed on by everyone. Rather, society is constructed by the ideas and conceptualisations of both individual people and also, more importantly, certain powerful groups. Some groups, such as psychiatrists, are able to construct a discourse that privileges a certain viewpoint above others, which allows them to effectively rule out and rule in ways of conceptualising, for example, what constitutes mental illness. Constructing such discourses allows such groups to become dominant in

LINK

See Chapter 1 for more information about Foucault and discourse.

society and allows them to regulate and control the activities of others. Such a perspective allows us to question the factual basis of what is deemed to constitute mental illness, which is useful given the lack of solid evidence by which psychiatry sometimes proceeds. It also points to the way in which, as with other aspects, medicine can discipline and gain control over our lives.

Both biological and social explanations can definitely tell us something about mental illness. We have, however, to be careful here of not falling into the trap that either explanation on its own is sufficient to address the complexity of mental health and illness. What is certain is that mental illness does not fit into simple 'A-leads-to-B-leads-to-C' explanations. Rather, there is a complex interweaving of both society and biology, where both have to be understood as often working together in complex and dynamic ways.

Some of this complexity and dynamism is captured by Rose (2005) in his discussion of the causes of mental illness and how biology and society interact. He points out that just because a change in the chemistry of the brain takes place does not mean that the chemical change caused the illness. He urges that we must be careful in thinking about the processes which cause changes to happen. The example he uses to illustrate this point is that if someone has a headache, they take an aspirin. If we were then to check the chemicals in the person's brain in order to discover the chemical basis of a headache, we would find aspirin. Thus, according to the biological explanation, we would claim that aspirin causes headaches, because people who do not have headaches do not have the chemical aspirin present in their brains. Now, obviously, we know this not to be the case. What Rose is saying here is that, yes, chemical changes do occur, but they could equally be the *result* of other (in this case *social*) factors.

This takes us to an explanation put forward by Pilgrim and Rogers (2014), which acknowledges and develops that last point. They put forward a critical realist perspective on mental health and illness. This approach is useful in that it does not fall for the either/or impasse outlined above. Rather, it brings in the consideration that to fully understand what causes misery and suffering in the world we have to be aware of one of the complexities of human life: that humans are simultaneously organic biological *and* social beings. This perspective allows us to see that both aspects of being human are important and that humans are not entirely reducible to either. What this means is that a critical realist perspective fully acknowledges the strong and influential role of culture, but does not say that it is all down to society; it also accepts the importance of medical information

LINK

Chapter 1 provides an overview of sociological theories and perspectives.

and research. However, crucially, it questions how diagnoses are framed by the social influences on the medical profession (this is explored further in the next section). Finally, a critical realist perspective accepts that biological processes are at work but, like Rose (2005), as outlined above, attempts to place those processes in a wider context where social factors may be the cause of biological changes.

ATTITUDES TO AND CONSTRUCTIONS OF MENTAL HEALTH AND ILLNESS

We usually accept medical terminology and classifications as given, that is, as being fact, value-free and scientific. Various sociologists and other writers, however, have challenged these notions. This is because medicine (like every other aspect of human activity) takes place within a social context. This social context influences how people think, in all sorts of subtle and not so subtle ways. Those who work in medicine, such as doctors and psychiatrists, can also be quite easily influenced by, and in turn play an important role in, prevailing social attitudes. It is useful to remember this when thinking about mental illness and the way it is framed in and by society, especially when someone is judged to be acting in an 'unusual' and 'problematic' manner; for those judgements, made by doctors and psychiatrists, may be based not on purely neutral 'scientific' criteria but on social values and cultural norms (Foster 1995).

One useful example is the way in which both psychiatry and society have changed their perception of homosexuality. Until relatively recently, being gay was considered and framed as a form of mental illness. Gay men, for example, could find themselves on the receiving end of quite draconian interventions, such as incarceration. During the 1960s, however, social attitudes towards homosexuality changed, partly due to the activities of campaign groups such as the Gay Liberation Front and events such as Stonewall, when gay people fought back against police harassment. As the stigma and stereotyping diminished, so did the view that homosexuality was an illness rather than just one of the many forms of human sexuality.

Many myths and unhelpful images surround people deemed mentally ill. One common misconception is that people diagnosed with schizophrenia have a 'Jekyll and Hyde' personality, whereby they are sane and rational at one moment and violent and deranged the next (Angermeyer and Matschinger 1999). Unfortunately, these negative images appear to be widespread and persistent. Early research by Star (1955) identified negative stereotypes in the United States, while similar work by Hall et al. (1993) in England found people possessing similar attitudes nearly forty years later. Wider representations of mental illness also conflate and confuse mental illness and danger. Jorm (2000), researching in Australia, has found that many members of the public have a very limited knowledge of mental illness. Using vignettes of someone with depression or schizophrenia, Jorm found that few people could identify the depicted mental illness according to medical classifications: only 39% correctly identified depression, and even fewer, 27%, correctly identified schizophrenia.

'Mental imbalance' often characterises many a movie or soap series villain. These are not just neutral images, however, that are contained within the safety of the cinema or the TV screen; they form beliefs and constructs held by people in everyday contexts. In turn, these social stigmas increase the stress of those with mental illness and exacerbate feelings of social exclusion and social distance.

The *Counting the Cost* survey by Baker and MacPherson (2000) for MIND highlighted the extent of stigmatising images and the effects they had had on people with mental illness. For many respondents to the survey, the social stigma was harder to deal with than the symptoms of their particular condition. Some key results from this survey are summarised below:

- 73% of respondents felt that the media had been unfair, unbalanced or very negative over the previous three years
- 12% felt that the media had been fair, balanced or very positive
- 50% claimed that poor media coverage had a negative impact on their mental health
- 24% experienced some hostility from neighbours and their local communities as a result of media reports. (2000: 5)

QUESTION

Why you think mental illness attracts such negative imagery?

Negative views of mental illness and mentally ill people are also evident among young people. The *Tomorrow's Minds* survey reached a similar conclusion on stereotyping and prejudice (Baker and MacPherson 2000). Sixty per cent of young people in the survey admitted to using abusive terms such as 'psycho', 'schizo', 'nutter' or 'loony' to describe mentally ill people.

Historically, these images of mental illness have their roots in ideas of demonic possession (Scheff 1966) or the loss of rationality (Foucault 1967). Currently, negative images of mental illness are presented in newspaper articles, films, documentaries and popular dramas. Again, we see a dominance of stereotypes and misleading images. Philo (1996) noted that the majority of images were associated with violence, particularly violence towards other people, though also to self. The dominance of so many negative images in the media is not necessarily to do with the prejudiced attitudes of programme makers; rather, it is to do with the restraints imposed by the format of television shows, especially soaps. Programmes are restricted to half-hour slots, have multiple plotlines and need to provide dramatic entertainment that unfolds over a relatively short period. Realistic portrayals of mental illness, with all the various subtleties and intricacies that distressed individuals experience, are therefore ignored or glossed over. In addition, the need for storylines to develop, peak and pass quite quickly may result in a very unrealistic portrayal of an illness, how it develops over time and how it can affect someone's life.

Stigma

Goffman is probably one of the best-known sociologists to have studied and theorised how certain groups of people attract **stigma**. His humanistic and sympathetic work focuses on why certain attributes of an individual or a group deny them full acceptance in given situations and lead them either to be excluded or to be left with a feeling of not 'fitting in'. Goffman (1968) classifies stigma into three broad groups:

- *physical stigma* – mainly to do with aspects visible 'on the surface' of people, for example facial scarring, a physical impairment or an amputation
- *personal/character stigma* – mainly to do with aspects 'below the surface', for example drug use, sexuality or mental health
- *social stigma* – belonging to a particular group or ethnic minority.

> Stigma refers to an attribute that 'discredits', or prevents, someone's full acceptance in a particular situation.

QUESTION

Can you identify conditions, mental or physical, that could be potentially stigmatising? Try to figure out why they could be stigmatising.

Like other symbolic interactionists, Goffman seeks to explore the subtleties and intricacies of how people present themselves to the outside world, especially if their identity is in some way 'spoiled' or stigmatised. How that identity can be spoiled or stigmatised varies greatly. Sometimes it is highly visible, in the case of facial scarring for example, or it can be highly invisible, such as a history of depressive episodes. Whatever it is, it may completely alter social identity. In some respects we all have something in our lives that we wish to keep hidden, or pieces of personal information that we manage in certain ways so as to maintain a particular 'face' to those about us.

Another aspect of Goffman's notion of stigma is that it is highly relational, depending on the situation in which we find ourselves. The previous section outlined how people experiencing mental health problems are portrayed in a negative light, and, if their status is known, in certain situations the effects can be quite damaging. If, let us say, a person was with others who shared similar mental health problems, then the stigma would be reduced or non-existent. Notions of what is normal, or what stigma is, are thus highly contextual; each of these labels is socially constructed and has no inherent or natural basis.

> Passing refers to attempts to conceal a potential stigma and prevent its disclosure.

People respond in a variety of ways to a potentially stigmatising condition or situation, although, as Goffman argues, this can depend on how concealed or 'displayed' the stigma is. For those with a concealed or concealable stigma, an attribute that Goffman terms 'a discreditable stigma', there is the possibility of managing, manipulating or presenting information so as to avoid revealing the stigma. This is termed **passing** and entails devising a routine. This routine may involve being careful about what one talks about, where one goes, what one wears, and so on – basically managing daily life so as to keep potentially stigmatising information secret.

Goffman points out that trying to maintain this round of secrecy can come at a terrible cost and be quite emotionally draining and demanding. There is always the chance of letting information slip or it being discovered, and the consequences, real or imagined, would then have to be endured.

As persuasive and elaborate as Goffman's ideas are, he has been criticised for not acknowledging the material basis of stigmas and for overly reflecting on the individual. His ideas do, however, provide a challenge to health professionals as he stresses the importance of constructing identity. As the work by Baker and MacPherson (2000) illustrates, the social stigma of a condition can at times be more of an issue for someone with a mental illness than the condition itself. We need to be aware of how the social framing of mental health and illness affects the lives of people who are experiencing distress.

CASE STUDY

Mary provides an example of stigma and passing. She encountered severe mental health problems shortly after leaving university with a degree in plant science. Feeling very depressed, she found herself unable to leave her flat and even to attend to her personal hygiene. After several years of drug therapy and counselling she became more socially confident and able to deal with aspects of her mental health. She soon reached the point where she wanted to start working and perhaps catch up with old friends again. However, she did not want them to find out about her mental health problems and was worried that they might find her strange or dangerous. The potential problem was made worse by having a gap of several years in her life when she was ill and did not start a career like so many of her old university friends. Fortunately, she managed to find a job working in the greenhouses of the local botanical gardens. Her job involved routine repair and cleaning activities, even though she was qualified to take on more complex and demanding work. The job, though, gave Mary the cover of saying that she was working in the botanical gardens, making it sound as if she was currently in work of an appropriate level for a graduate with several years' work experience, even though it was not. This made it easier for her to catch up with old friends as she could pass herself as 'normal' and hide aspects of her biography that she did not want revealed.

PATTERNS OF MENTAL HEALTH AND ILLNESS

As mentioned in the introduction to this chapter, mental illness affects a wide cross-section of people of different ages, sexes and ethnicities. Nevertheless, certain conditions tend to be found in some groups more than in others and certain people, for a variety of reasons, are more at risk. Overall, mental illnesses are fairly common. The most widespread form of mental illness is depression.

There is a tendency for mental illness to be distributed unevenly across the class scale, and in particular, among women. In the research, this association between social class and mental illness has long been noticeable. Early researchers such as Faris and Dunham (1939), in their study of the various residential zones of Chicago, observed that schizophrenia was more frequent among working-class people. Slightly later US work by Hollingshead and Redlich (1953) also identified class factors in relation to mental disorder. The now classic work by Brown and Harris (1978) similarly noted class differences: they came across higher rates of depression among working-class women with children than among their middle-class counterparts.

ETHNICITY AND MENTAL HEALTH

There are a number of explanations for why people from black and other ethnic backgrounds appear to have higher rates of mental illness and a different, often coercive, relationship with services. These explanations include:

- racist and prejudiced attitudes on the part of service providers and agencies of the state, such as the police
- lack of cultural sensitivity
- more frequent exposure to stressors in the form of, for example, unemployment
- adjusting to a new society if recently arrived
- racism generally.

These explanations are useful when trying to understand the situation of people from ethnic minorities in relation to mental illness. However, Pilgrim and Rogers (2014) point to another, related concept that may help us in this context. They draw on Foucault's concept of seeing madness as part of the 'other', that is, groups of people who are regarded as being outside the norms of society and as constituting a threat to the order of society. In previous times people with mental illnesses were excluded from society, banished to the Ships of Fools that traversed European waterways in the Middle Ages, or to the asylums of the Victorian age. Here we see, they argue, a relationship between new racism and psychiatric discourse.

LINK

These issues are discussed in greater depth in Chapter 7 on ethnicity and health.

The new racism also deals with this supposed threat to social and cultural identity by using exclusion, this time by excluding black and Asian people from full social acceptance into British society on grounds of non-Christian religions, diets, involvement in terrorism, or other 'non-western/white' aspects of identity behaviour. Thus, psychiatric practice reflects, in its treatment of black and Asian people, wider aspects of racism within society by further excluding these groups from full social participation by identifying their behaviour and activities as pathological and insane.

GENDER AND MENTAL HEALTH

Every review of the literature concerning sociology and mental health reaches the same conclusion when discussing **gender**: women always display higher rates of certain mental illnesses than men (Bebbington 1996; Foster 1995; WHO 2015). Much research has attempted to explain this particular phenomenon, with various results. Some explanations point to measurement artefact effects and to men seeking alternative outlets, such as drink, that mask depressive disorders; others point to role strain and conflict; while yet others indicate that social factors, such as poor housing or social class, are the cause. Other explanations point to the pressure on women to conform to prevailing norms of femininity and attractiveness. For example, the British Medical Association (BMA 2000) warned that media images of very thin models and celebrities could have very damaging and negative effects on young women's perceptions of their body image and their self-esteem, which could lead to feelings of distress and anxiety.

Gender refers to the cultural differences between men and women, while sex refers to physical differences.

Measurement artefact means that women exhibit higher rates of mental illness than men because the design of questionnaires and the way data are collected produce a 'statistical mirage', which artificially generates a problem where there is not one. Earlier work by Gove (1984), among others, indicated that faults with the way in which data were collected meant that women appeared to exhibit higher rates of depression.

LINK

See Chapter 6 for more information on gender and health.

In a substantial review of the literature relating to women and depression, however, Bebbington (1996) and Nazroo et al. (1998) argued that there was little evidence of measurement artefact being responsible for the high levels of recorded depression in women. In their carefully constructed study, Nazroo et al. (1998) demonstrated that women did report more depressive episodes – whether distant, mild or exaggerated episodes. There was little evidence for men masking their depression by turning to alcohol or substance abuse, as had been suggested by other studies.

What Nazroo et al.'s research pointed to was the effect that gender roles and life events had on men and women. Looking at a range of crises that related to children, reproduction, housing, finance, work, marital issues, crime and health, the researchers concluded that women were more likely to develop depression if a crisis involved children, housing or reproduction. The chance of depression was increased if a woman's role identity meant that she attached greater importance to those areas. So if, for example, a woman feels a particularly close attachment to and sense of responsibility for children because of her role identity, then the chance of depression is much greater if there is a child-related problem, such as difficulties at school or drug misuse. For crises involving finance or work, marital issues, crime or health, there appeared to be no gender role difference.

One of the best-known pieces of sociological research on women and mental health was carried out by Brown and Harris (1978), who sought to analyse the relationship between social factors and mental health in the Camberwell area of London. From their research they developed a multifactorial model (Figure 8.1) which attempted to explain the intricacies and subtleties of why some women develop clinical depression while others, living in similar conditions, do not. The model contains the idea that the onset of depression (the dependent variable) will occur if other factors are present (the independent variables). Key components of the model are:

- *Current vulnerability factors*. These factors relate to events that have happened in a woman's past and indicate whether or not she may be more susceptible to depression. Brown and Harris identified four vulnerability factors:
  - losing their mother before the age of 11
  - presence at home of three or more children under the age of 15 years
  - absence of any confiding relationships, particularly with the husband
  - lack of full- or part-time job.

- *Provoking agents*. Here Brown and Harris identified various events that could occur in a woman's life, which could then trigger a depressive episode. The events mainly relate to loss and disappointment, for example death, losing a job or discovering a partner's unfaithfulness. Ongoing difficulties were also noted as being contributory; they included dealing with a variety of 'background' problems ranging from housing problems to headaches.
- *Symptom-formation factors*. Women over 50 years of age and women with low self-esteem were at greatest risk of developing depression.

One way of thinking about this approach is to imagine someone on a tightrope. The chances of falling are increased if there are any existing vulnerabilities, which means that the tightrope begins to sway, making it harder to maintain a sure footing. There is an even greater chance of falling if a provoking agent, such as an adverse life event, comes along and impacts on the person, making it likely that they will be knocked off. Finally, any possibility of staying on the rope may be diminished if balance is poor due to low self-esteem.

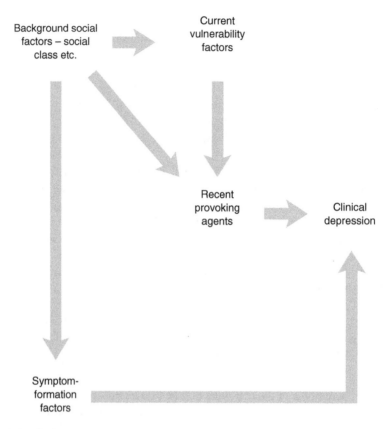

Figure 8.1 Schematic representation of Brown and Harris' model of depression (Brown and Harris 1978: 265)

FOCUS ON DEPRESSION

Depression is becoming an increasingly common condition not just in industrial capitalist societies such as the United Kingdom, but across the globe. As Ferrari et al. (2013) note, YLD (Years Living with Disability) rates per 100,000 for depression indicate that Australia, Nigeria and the United Kingdom experience similar levels of depression, while South Africa is similar to France. Psychologist Oliver James (1998) makes the point that even though we are now, in many ways, richer economically, we are definitely poorer emotionally. This, he argues, is due to the tendency of contemporary society (mainly through hyped-up media images) to heighten our expectations of what life should be about – expectations which are ultimately impossible to fulfil. This leads to a depressing 'gap' between where we think we should be in life and where we actually are, or, as James puts it, we think we are losers even though we are winners. As referred to in the discussions on inequality in Chapter 5 and on health policy in Chapter 13, depression due to the problems of modern living and the health challenges they create are not just restricted to high-income European and North American countries.

One problem when discussing 'depression' is the term itself. In lay usage we use the word to describe and refer to a vast variety of states and feelings in everyday life. So, for example, you could claim to be feeling depressed after your football team loses yet again on a Saturday afternoon, or when the essay you feverishly worked on receives a lower grade than you had hoped. The emotional states indicated in these two examples will be highly unpleasant and perhaps lead to some, albeit temporary, change in behaviour, for example having a cry or wanting to be on your own. This is quite different from what is meant by experiencing depression as a mental illness. Through confusion between the state of everyday blues and the illness of depression, many of the subtleties and issues which face people with clinical depression are lost. The severity of the condition and the experiences that people with depression go through may be unfairly diminished and not taken as seriously as they would be if the person was, for instance, experiencing a severe physical illness instead.

Depression is, therefore, considerably more than feeling just a little down or blue. People with clinical depression experience a highly distressing and debilitating combination of mental *and* physical symptoms that can last over a period of months or even years. In terms of mental states and emotions, people with depression experience a substantial reordering of how they think, see themselves and perceive others. Their thinking changes in that they interpret the world very negatively and see everything in the worst possible and most despairing way. Frequently, people with depression are acutely sensitive to the smallest of things. So, for example, if a friend does not sit next to them in a lecture, this can be taken as a sign that nobody likes them and that life is terrible. What is important here is that this change in thinking cannot be 'snapped out of', as is sometimes popularly thought. Such changes in thinking often seem beyond the control of the person with depression. They wish they could stop thinking in such a negative and horrible way but find it almost impossible to do so. The following quote from someone with depression illustrates this point:

> It is so total ... There is no reason to wake up in the morning. I just let the blinds stay down ... Sometimes I wonder what life will be like, where I can find a fixed point, a hold to my life. (Kangas 2001: 86)

At worst, changes in thinking can take the direction of suicidal thoughts, where taking one's life begins to appear as a 'suitable' way of dealing with life's problems. These thoughts are deeply despairing. We examine sociological perspectives on suicide later in this chapter.

As well as all the changes in thinking, there are considerable physical changes. Among the more common changes that affect the body are exhaustion, difficulties in sleeping, loss of appetite, loss of weight and loss of interest in sex. These physical changes indicate how the differences between physical and mental illness are not so clear-cut. Just because something is mainly seen as a mental illness does not mean that it is only experienced as a set of feelings. The same also goes for physical illnesses, which often have an emotional side to them too.

Throughout this chapter, there has been reference to how society views or frames mental illness. Depression is no exception, and there are considerable cultural differences in how people from a particular society frame this mental illness. In a US study, Karasz (2005) found that there were differences between European Americans and South Asian immigrants in how they viewed depression. Two key differences emerged. The European Americans were more likely to see depression as a disease and a medical condition, not related to any social context, while the South Asians had the opposite viewpoint: they saw depression more as an emotional response to what was going on in someone's life and tied very closely to social context. Other social and cultural differences have been noted elsewhere. Fenton and Sadiq-Sangster (1996) found that South Asian women expressed depression in physical terminology, for example saying that they had a pain in their heart with little or no allusion to feelings or thoughts. What should be noted here is that just because different cultures frame depression in different ways does not mean that one is more accurate and correct than the other. All that this demonstrates is how social influences affect our ways of expressing our moments of suffering and anguish.

SUICIDE

We saw earlier the high suicide rates for young people aged between 15 and 29 (WHO 2015), with suicide becoming the second leading cause of death for that age group. Suicide often appears to be an unfathomable act, impervious to analysis or systematic understanding. After all, how can any research be carried out on an action that takes place in isolated and lonely circumstances, where the subject is someone whose life has reached the place where ending it appears a valid choice?

There has been much (perhaps too much, some would say) sociological work on suicide, mainly because of early work by functionalist Emile Durkheim. Durkheim used suicide as an example of how the most apparently individual of acts can be opened up to sociological investigation. First published in 1897, *Suicide: A Study in Sociology* was the first sociological attempt to systematically understand suicide (Durkheim 1970). Without denying that individual circumstances could affect a person's decision to take his or her own life, Durkheim noticed patterns in suicide rates between countries and between different groups in the same society. Protestant countries had higher rates than Catholic countries, while Jewish societies had the lowest suicide rates of all. What was also notable was the constancy of relative suicide rates between countries. After further analysis Durkheim identified four different types of suicide:

- *Egoistic suicide.* If an individual was not sufficiently integrated into society then they were at a higher risk of suicide. This explains why Protestants were at greater risk than Catholics. The Protestant faith emphasises individualism, while Catholicism emphasises community, with greater integration for a community's members. In addition, people who were unmarried or childless were more likely to commit suicide than those who were married and had children, because of the former's lack of integration with a family unit.
- *Anomic suicide.* The opposite of egoistic suicide, this occurs where a society fails to regulate the individual, for example when a society collapses and all the usual norms and patterns of life fall apart, leaving people bewildered and unsure of what is happening. The classic example of this is the 1928 stock market crash that just about devastated American life, with people losing security, savings and their homes. Here the loss of all that was considered normal led to an increase in suicide rates.
- *Altruistic suicide.* Here a sense of duty, linked to a high level of integration into a particular society, leads someone to take their own life. There are numerous examples around the world: the Japanese kamikaze pilots who flew their planes directly into American battleships in an attempt to sink them during the Second World War; the Hindu practice of suttee, where a wife kills herself at her husband's funeral; and the Irish Republican hunger strikers, such as Bobby Sands, who starved themselves to death in pursuit of their political beliefs.
- *Fatalistic suicide.* This form of suicide refers to the despair of living in a highly regulated society with no opportunity for personal freedom and control. It is very rare in contemporary society and Durkheim only included it for historical interest. Mainly applying to highly restrictive societies, this type of suicide could be seen among slaves in ancient slave societies.

As with any other ground-breaking and important piece of sociology, Durkheim's theory of suicide has attracted much debate, with many proponents and opponents. Some critics point out that suicide statistics are notoriously unreliable. Coroners or doctors may record a death as due to some cause other than suicide, in an attempt to avoid problems for surviving family members. Other critics point out that his observations could not always be proved or researched properly.

LINK

Chapter 1 discusses functionalism in more depth.

The strongest critique, however, came from interpretive sociologists such as J.D. Douglas (1967). He put forward two points:

1. All suicide statistics should be treated with caution, as there may have been collusion between officials who record and categorise deaths and family and friends. The degree of integration here may affect the decision. The more integrated the suicide in a social group, the greater the possibility of a cover-up taking place.

2. Durkheim failed to take into account the motive for and meaning of the suicide. Suicide can be a way of communicating revenge, eliciting sympathy or dealing with guilt, or a way of meeting cultural obligations. This information could be elicited by studying diaries and suicide notes.

LINK

Chapter 1 discusses interpretive perspectives in greater depth.

More recent sociologists have criticised theories of the interpretive approach of sociologists such as Douglas, and sought to construct more elegant and sophisticated theories of suicide. Taylor (1989, 1990) also agreed that statistics are unreliable, and noted, in a study of deaths on the London Underground, a number of contributory factors that could lead to a death being recorded as a suicide or not. These included whether or not the person had a history of mental illness, or the views and opinions of people who knew the deceased. If the coroner asked a close friend or family member then suicide would often be denied, while if the coroner asked a casual acquaintance then a verdict of suicide was more likely.

Taylor then went on to identify four different types of suicide. The categorisation is similar to Durkheim's, but Taylor's emphasis is less on social factors and more on what people think of themselves and their relationships with others – and the certainty or uncertainty of these feelings is important. These suicides divide into two main categories: ectopic, which relates to a person's view of him/herself, and symphisic, which concerns the person's relationship with others.

Ectopic suicides (self)

- *Submissive suicide*. This occurs when someone has decided that there is no point in going on and that their life is at an end. This may be because of the death of a loved one or because of terminal illness. Any attempt at suicide is carried out with the full intention of taking one's life and may take place in an isolated place so as to avoid the chance of discovery.
- *Thanatation suicide*. This relates to feelings of uncertainty, and the attempt at suicide is not as earnest as a submissive suicide, the person leaving it to chance as to whether they actually die or not.

Symphisic suicide (relationships)

- *Sacrifice suicides*. Here the person takes their own life in order to make others, such as partners or former lovers, feel guilty or incur censure from friends and family. Any suicide note will indicate on whom the blame for the suicide rests.
- *Appeal suicide*. This occurs when someone is uncertain how others feel about them. The person who attempts suicide is not necessarily trying to end their life, but is testing the reactions of others. The suicide attempt may be staged in such a way, in front

of others for example, as to enable the person who is making the attempt to see how much someone else cares about them.

QUESTION

Which of the above theories do you find the most satisfactory in attempting to explain suicide? Provide justification for your answer.

The above three sociological theories of suicide present interesting and different perspectives on why people decide to take their own lives. Each has a particular strength or weakness, and in many ways a combination of all three provides some useful insights into why people attempt suicide. Durkheim offers useful ideas on how social pressures and wider aspects of a society affect suicidal behaviour, while Douglas cautions against accepting suicide statistics at face value and urges us to look at meaning. In Taylor's work we find explanations of why some people leave notes, or attempt suicide in a variety of locations with different levels of secrecy or openness.

CONCLUSION

A theme running through this chapter has been how distress, suffering and mental health issues are framed and very much influenced by society. This extends from trying to define what is meant by mental illness and the ways in which wider attitudes (and prejudices) impinge on official discourses and perspectives, to the difficult experiences of people with mental health problems and the ways in which they can be stigmatised by wider society. Indeed, for many people who feel depressed or experience other issues with their mental and emotional wellbeing, it is the reactions of others that can cause them more problems in their day-to-day lives.

We have seen once more that, as with other aspects of health, great social inequalities exist. Women, working-class people and people from minority ethnic groups all appear to report higher levels of distress. Again, social influences are at play here. We can see the pressures created by expectations of socially constructed femininities, the experiences of stress and poverty, or the results of racism all having potential negative consequences. This chapter has highlighted that mental health has to be understood in its widest context, with sociology providing insights into the social processes that influence and define the misery and suffering of many people in society today.

Given the higher profile of mental health issues and wellbeing in contemporary society, it appears that interventions in improving and maintaining good mental health have to take place at a social level just as much as, if not more than, at a personal level.

SUMMARY POINTS

- Mental illness, particularly depression, is common in contemporary society.

- Many people hold negative images of mental illness. These negative images often associate mental illness with danger, whether to others or to the mentally ill person. Media portrayals of mental illness are often similarly negative. The stigma created by negative images can have an adverse impact on people with mental illness.

- Ethnic minorities have a different experience of mental health care than do white people. African-Caribbean young men are more likely to be perceived as difficult or violent and more likely to enter mental health care via the police. Cultural stereotyping and racist attitudes affect the care of people from ethnic backgrounds. This also includes white ethnic groups, such as Irish people.

- Women have a different experience of mental health care and mental illness from men. Women tend to have higher rates of depression than men. Stress created by attachment to gender roles is likely to be the cause of those higher rates.

- Overall suicide rates are decreasing, but suicide rates for young people aged 15–29 are increasing. Various sociological theories point to a variety of reasons as to why people take their own lives. Durkheim stresses social and cultural factors; Douglas warns against accepting statistics at face value and emphasises the need to understand individual meaning; while Taylor looks at feelings of uncertainty and certainty with self and others.

CASE STUDY

John has recently been relocated into a community hostel that helps those with a variety of mild and non-violent mental illnesses to reintegrate into society. The hostel is situated in a reasonably affluent suburb near a sizeable public park.

It was during his fourth year at university that John first came into contact with the psychiatric services. Until then John was a fairly standard student, competent but not especially noteworthy. This was probably due to his participation in a rather hectic social life, in which he appeared to be one of the prime movers. This particular group of friends clubbed quite extensively at the weekends and some of the group took drugs. As he himself remarked to a case worker: 'Yeah, drugs were part of what we did at the weekends but it was nothing serious – dope mainly and speed. Well, speed most Fridays and Saturdays just to help us get that extra energy boost.'

In his third year, one of this group was killed in a random accident. They had been out on a Friday night and John had encouraged everyone to try to drink and smoke as much dope as possible. After the club closed they headed down to the nearby beach to watch the sun come up. It was there that John's friend slipped on a rock and fell to his death. Strong feelings of guilt overcame John as he felt he was to blame for the accident. He gradually became more withdrawn from his friends, and his use of alcohol and soft drugs increased. At the start of his fourth year a relationship with another student fell apart. She found his increasingly pessimistic moods difficult to handle. In addition, his overall behaviour was becoming more compulsive: he constantly analysed what lay behind her words and actions. Invariably, all his conclusions were negative and he firmly believed that she was bored with him. After she left, he ceased attending classes and his coursework suffered. He spent most of his time in his flat, unable to sleep and constantly fixating on what he had done wrong in his life. One night in an attempt to sleep he drank half a bottle of whisky and took some sleeping tablets. A flatmate found him unconscious on the living-room floor and rushed him to hospital.

In the following weeks he was advised to see a counsellor and was referred to cognitive therapy. He made some progress, but as the year went on his university friends finished their courses and moved out of the area. This left John feeling alone and isolated. Consequently, his problems returned, and this time he was placed in the local psychiatric hospital. The seven months that he spent there seem to have made some difference to him. During his stay he responded well to medication and to the various therapies, and hints of his former self appeared. At various social events the charismatic aspects of his personality, which had been quite strong during his university days, surfaced. However, the outside world still seemed problematic to him and he found it difficult to be among large groups of people on his own. In addition, he had nowhere to stay, as he was no longer entitled to student accommodation.

It was decided that the hostel was the best place for him as his family might find it difficult to care for him. His father had left home to set up a new life for himself and his new partner, a former office colleague, and his parents divorced. As a result of the separation John's mother developed severe long-term depression and found life generally difficult to cope with. Recently, she had been experiencing some ill effects from a course of Fluoxetine prescribed by her doctor. This led to her taking several days off from the department store where she worked. Her managers were reasonably supportive but a proposed restructuring of the department was causing her some anxiety because of the possible loss of a part-time assistant, which would increase her workload. It was proposed that John's father might help to care for him, but John did not feel that he was ready to re-establish such a relationship with his father as he still felt some ambivalence towards him for leaving the family home.

Life at the hostel had until recently been going reasonably well. John was managing to socialise again and felt confident about interacting with the world at large. In fact, he had managed to get to know some local people his own age. They knew he was at the hostel but he claimed that he was a worker there, and with his quick wit and outward appearance of calm there was no reason to doubt this. However, one day in the nearby supermarket John suddenly felt quite anxious and rushed out of the store, discarding his shopping as he left. This was witnessed by one of his new friends who started to have doubts about John's true identity.

QUESTIONS

1. Discuss how John's sense of identity has been affected by his mental illness. How important is maintaining a sense of identity for John?
2. What has happened in his mother's life that has led her to feel depressed? Which theory could help us understand her situation?
3. What passing technique does John employ?
4. If you are a health professional student, what type of involvement would you have with someone like John?
5. The assumption is that John is white, but how might his treatment and subsequent care and recovery have been different if he was a young African-Caribbean male?

TAKING YOUR STUDIES FURTHER

This chapter will have helped you understand many of the key terms, concepts, theories and debates relating to mental health. Listed below are books that will provide deeper and more detailed discussions of the points raised in this chapter. You will also find additional resources on the companion website, including downloads of relevant material, links to useful websites, videos and other features. Please visit the companion website at https://study.sagepub.com/barryandyuill4e

RECOMMENDED READING

Busfield, J. (ed.) (2001) *Rethinking the Sociology of Mental Health*. London: Blackwell.

Goffman, E. (1968) *Stigma: Notes on the Management of a Spoiled Identity.* Harmondsworth: Penguin.

Pilgrim, D. (2014) *Key Concepts in Mental Health*, 3rd edn. London: SAGE.

Pilgrim, D. and Rogers, A. (2014) *A Sociology of Mental Health and Illness*, 5th edn. Buckingham: Open University Press.

SEXUALITIES AND HEALTH

WITH MEGAN TODD

MAIN POINTS

- Sexuality is socially constructed.

- The hierarchical social ordering of sexuality gives rise to a number of social divisions and inequalities.

- Structural inequalities lead to differential experiences, and treatment, of service users along lines of sexuality.

INTRODUCTION

The topic of sexuality in relation to health and inequality remains relatively neglected, and perhaps even taboo. Arguably, sexuality has often been secondary to other important issues, such as class, gender and ethnicity. As we shall see, this can have potentially serious consequences for the wellbeing of many service users. This chapter aims to introduce readers to the topic of sexuality by considering the diversity of sexuality in order to provide a deeper understanding of the implications for workers in the field of health and social care, thus enabling them to work better with a range of service users. Although this chapter will focus mainly on lesbian, gay and bisexual lives, there is not an assumption that heterosexuality is the norm; all sexualities, including heterosexuality, need explanation.

Sexuality is often presented as the most natural and private aspect of identity. Social constructionists would argue that sexuality is shaped by social structures. What is considered normal changes over time and between cultures (Weeks 2003).

One reason why it is problematic to write about sexuality is that the available terminology can be difficult to negotiate, is often inadequate and can so easily offend. Before we begin the chapter proper, therefore, it may be useful to have a brief discussion about terminology. *Sexuality* in this chapter refers to sexual identity or orientation, rather than simply sexual activity. Where possible, the term 'homosexual' has not been used; this is because it is derived from nineteenth-century sexology and exhibits many negative connotations associated with medicalisation. Instead, where possible the terms 'LGBT' (lesbian, gay, bisexual and transgender) or 'lesbian' and 'gay man' are used because these are the terms more usually used by the lesbian and gay communities. Also used often is the phrase 'coming out' to refer to those (LGBT) people who acknowledge their sexuality openly, and the related 'closeted' for someone who has not come out of the closet. It is also important to recognise that coming out is not a one-off event: decisions about when and where to disclose one's sexuality can be a daily experience. Partly because a chapter of this length cannot do the topic justice, and partly because it is not necessarily about sexual identity, no specific discussion about transgender and transsexual health issues is included. Readers seeking to find out more about this area are advised to look at the burgeoning literature elsewhere (Hines and Sanger 2010; Stryker and Whittle 2006).

We also need to proceed with caution when using statistics. First, we do not know how many lesbians and gay men live in the United Kingdom; current statistics – which suggest roughly 5–7% of the population are gay – are likely to be underestimates. Despite a recent raft of policies aimed at moving towards equality, we still live in a *heteronormative* society where gay men and lesbians are relatively marginalised and often hard to reach. Thus many people are not 'out' and may not label, or indeed recognise, themselves as gay or lesbian.

Heteronormative refers to the assumption that heterosexuality is the norm, is natural and superior. Consequently, anything else is rendered marginal or abnormal. In order to think usefully about sexuality, we first need to consider the ways in which gender, sex and sexuality are inextricably linked. Gender is often understood as a system which divides society into two categories – masculine and feminine – and is relational, in that one cannot understand what is meant by 'masculinity' without having some notion of what it is to be 'feminine' and vice versa. Gender is something which organises virtually every aspect of our lives without us thinking about it. Sometimes it is difficult for us to see it in operation precisely because it is everywhere: we declare our gender when we walk into public toilets or changing rooms, and it's stated on our birth certificate, driving licence and passport. Because of this, gender can seem natural. However, much research (for example, Margaret Mead's (1930) observations in Papua New Guinea) highlights the fact that gender is not expressed in the same way across the globe or over time. We can therefore argue that gender is *socially constructed*. It is often conceptualised as the social and cultural expression of sex. The binary system, crucially for feminist thinkers, operates as a set of hierarchies, in that we tend to privilege the masculine over the feminine. It is therefore a system of power and not just about observable differences and similarities. Understanding that gender is socially constructed, however, means that there is potential for change: the system has not always operated in this way and need not continue to do so.

When gender is used in feminist analysis, it is defined in relation to **sex**. Feminist thinkers were the first to separate gender from sex. In our society, we recognise only two sexes – male and female – but it is important to state that this is not a universal approach to sex. Sex is often conceptualised as the natural, or biological, differences between men and women. This binary system may not be as stable as we might think:

LINK

More information on gender can be found in Chapter 6.

if you were to take a cross-sample of society and test people's chromosomes, hormones, genes, physiology and so on, very few would fit into the 'ideal' male or female categories. Many sociologists would argue that how we categorise sex is also influenced by culture.

Ideas about *sexuality* are intimately tied up with gender and sex. Heterosexuality is viewed, in contemporary western society, as the appropriate or proper expression of gender. A truly 'masculine' man is heterosexual. Within western society, it is argued, we privilege men; male sexuality is acceptable in itself. By contrast, appropriate female sexuality is passive and is synonymous with the reproductive role; motherhood is the only acceptable expression of female sexuality. Heterosexual sex (penetration of a vagina by a penis) in our society is deemed to be real sex or natural sex. This is reflected in our legal codes. It is only recently, for example, that UK law has broadened the definition of rape to include the penetration of an anus (so men can now be legitimate victims of rape). To date, women cannot be guilty of perpetrating rape, as only forced use of a penis constitutes rape; use of fists, bottles or other instruments only qualifies as sexual assault. Heterosexuality is a powerful conceptual tool in society. Adrienne Rich (1980) refers to 'compulsory heterosexuality'. This is the idea that heterosexuality is the default or obligatory sexuality and is something which further subjugates women. Like sex and gender, sexuality is often thought to be an innate or natural essence of our identity. Social constructionists would argue that in fact sexuality is also shaped through social process. Heterosexuality and homosexuality are relatively recent concepts (1902 and 1897 respectively), being inventions of the Victorian sexologists. Early 'scientists' understood 'the homosexual' as a woman trapped in a male body, and they labelled this person as an 'invert' – in other words, someone who was not correctly gendered. This stereotyped view of gay men as effeminate and lesbians as masculine persists in dominant discourses, reflecting the fact that we can only conceptualise society along heterosexual lines. The new labels created categories which regulated our behaviours and created, for the first time, sexual identities. Before the invention of the homosexual and the heterosexual, we had a variety of acts which didn't necessarily define the individual. Foucault (1979b) has argued, therefore, that sexuality is historically and culturally constructed, rather than biologically derived. Our current system also, crucially, positions some sexualities as 'good' and others as 'bad'; heterosexuality is desirable and 'normal', whereas same-sex attraction has historically been read as symptomatic of sickness or sinfulness. One could say that society has rigid, and arbitrary, rules about what we can do and with whom. Having given some thought to terminology, we will now move on to consider some of the ways in which sexuality bears an important relation to health and social care.

DOMESTIC AND OTHER ABUSES

An important consequence of living in a heteronormative world is that LGBT people are framed by their sexuality, unlike heterosexuals. Despite the fact that someone who has a lesbian identity may never actually have sex with another woman, she is seen, by the rest of society, as being overtly sexual. More attention is paid to lesbian and gay lifestyles than to heterosexual lifestyles. This means that more focus is given to the potentially harmful effects of a 'homosexual' lifestyle. Issues related to heterosexual lifestyles tend be discussed purely in terms of gender (Wilton 2000). In relation to this, we know that married men fare better than single men in terms of general health, for example, whereas single women live longer than married heterosexual women.

Sylvia Walby describes patriarchy as 'a system of social structures and practices in which men dominate, oppress, and exploit women' (1989: 214).

Years of feminist research have revealed that heterosexuality can place women in great danger. Studies consistently show domestic violence to be a significant social problem, with UK figures suggesting that one in four women will experience this form of abuse at the hands of a man (Walby and Allen 2004). From feminist perspectives, male violence against women is persistent and severe, and both reflects and maintains their unequal positions within society. **Patriarchy**, it was argued, could be explained as a consistent pattern of ideological and structural practices that serve to justify and perpetuate men's oppression of women. Patriarchy (and heteronormativity) also, it is argued, establishes hierarchies not only between women and men, but also between men and men and between women and women (Connell 2002). It has been argued that, consciously or not, all women are aware of their vulnerability to becoming victims. Even in the absence of a specific threat, awareness of vulnerability governs many women's lives and choices. Kelly, for instance, suggested that 'while not all women live in constant fear, many of women's routine decisions and behaviour are almost automatic measures taken to protect themselves from potential violence' (1988: 32). Legislation in relation to violence against women has arguably reflected patriarchal heterosexuality. Rape in marriage, for example, was not recognised as a crime in Scotland until 1989 and in the rest of the United Kingdom in 1991; the assumption was that a woman was the property of her husband, and so marriage gave conjugal rights which could be forcibly taken if not freely given. Across the globe, women's subordinate status means that their physical and mental wellbeing is constrained. Women and girls are forced or coerced into having their genitals mutilated, or herbs inserted into their vaginas to tighten them in order to increase their male partner's pleasure. Most forms of contraception also carry health risks for those women engaging in heterosex. Indeed, so prolific are the abuses inflicted upon women that many have suggested that gender-based violence should be classified as a hate crime.

It took many decades of campaigning on the part of feminists to get the abuse of heterosexual women recognised as a crime. However, there are suggestions that this produced a dominant discourse about domestic abuse which rendered other groups invisible. We are only just beginning to acknowledge, for example, that men can be victims of abuse by their female partners. We are also just beginning to address the fact that domestic abuse is a significant problem within LGBT communities (Ristock 2002), although given that this is a stigmatised and hidden population, we must be cautious about statistics. For some, much feminist analysis of violence based on male privilege and power may seem irrelevant or inapplicable to same-sex relationships. This is one reason why there has been relatively little research in this area to date. Yet while neither partner in a lesbian relationship, for example, enjoys male privilege and power, lesbians have other identity/power positions while living in a society that promotes hierarchy, power differentials, inequality and violence. These are endemic to patriarchy and can occur in all relationships lived in this cultural milieu. Additionally, same-sex relationships are directly influenced by other societal power inequalities that impact on all citizens – including sexism and those based in class, racial, ethnic and economic inequalities – as well as on interpersonal differences in power. Evidence points to the fact, however, that those services which provide help and support for victims of domestic violence do not have the awareness, training and provisions to cope with male victims or instances of same-sex abuse.

Another harm that occurs as a direct result of sexual orientation (either real or perceived) is anti-gay hate crime. Recent reports in Scotland have indicated a rise in homophobic hate crime, although it is difficult to assess whether this reflects an actual rise in offences or changes in reporting (Archibald 2011). What is clear is that it is a significant problem and one which can have additional impacts depending on ethnicity, disability and gender.

Drug and alcohol abuse

Use and misuse of tobacco, alcohol and other drugs appears to be higher among LGBT people (Drabble et al. 2005; Hughes and Jacobson 2003). One explanation may be related to the stress linked to living with prejudice and homophobia. Another reason may be that it is difficult for gay men and lesbians to enjoy taking part in the leisure activities that many heterosexuals take for granted. Recent studies, for example, have pointed to the difficulties and anxieties related to a gay man or lesbian becoming part of a (unquestionably heterosexual) sports team, with individuals being reliant on the goodwill and tolerance of heterosexual team members. As a result, in many towns and cities, gay areas have developed which offer a degree of safety and security. Such gay spaces tend to be heavily commercialised and revolve around pubs, bars and clubs, where it becomes difficult to avoid alcohol. This might also be an issue related to recruitment. The LGBT population, despite recent social and legal shifts, is stigmatised and thus is a relatively marginalised and hidden group. Many studies into LGBT lifestyles, therefore, recruit from 'gay villages'; thus a study into alcohol consumption is likely to encounter some heavy drinkers if the sample is taken largely from bars and clubs.

HEALTH

Mental health

For decades homosexuality itself was considered a mental illness. Despite the fact that research findings have effectively collapsed any evidence for this belief, a significant number of psychiatrists and clinicians still maintain that homosexuality is an illness *per se*, or symptomatic of mental ill health. Research findings do suggest that LGBT men and women have a higher instance of mental health problems than the wider population (King and McKeowan 2003) – anxiety, depression, self-harm and suicidal behaviour being the main expressions of this ill health. Arguably it is homophobia, rather than being gay, which is the cause of such anxiety – with rejection, discrimination, exclusion and victimisation being identified as primary reasons for the ill health (Musingarimi 2008). A lack of appropriate social spaces, as discussed above, has also been cited as an additional source of stress for young LGBT people, particularly in rural areas. Studies into sexuality and mental health have shown consistently that the majority of those interviewed do not have faith in current healthcare providers and state they would prefer to see an LGBT-specific counsellor (Chakraborty et al. 2011).

QUESTIONS

Should LGBT people have separate provisions for health and social care? What might be the benefits of this and what might be negative consequences? What might an alternative be?

Breast and other cancers

One health issue which appears to be a particular problem in the lesbian community is breast cancer (Breast Cancer Care 2011). 'Over 1 in 12 lesbian and bisexual women aged between 50 [and] 79 have been diagnosed with breast cancer, compared with 1 in 20 of women in general' (Hunt and Fish 2008). It is important, however, to unpick the problem here. Lesbians are not at higher risk of breast cancer because they are lesbians. Rather, it is because there are certain characteristics associated with lesbian communities and lifestyles which place lesbian women at greater risk. These include childlessness (thus, crucially, not breast feeding), obesity and excess consumption of alcohol. Figures are extrapolated from small-scale studies, and, as discussed above, populations may well be drawn mainly from bars and clubs, given the relatively 'hard-to-reach' nature of the population. We do not know how many lesbians have breast cancer as the NHS does not routinely make a note of sexual identity. Neither do we know how many lesbians have children. Much research (e.g. Hunt et al. 2007) has found that lesbians continue to have negative experiences in health services despite anti-discriminatory legislation. Thus there is a very real chance that lesbians suffering ill health do not seek medical advice or, if they do, do not wish to add to the stress by coming out (Fish 2010).

There is also a suggestion that lesbians are falling off the radar when it comes to cervical cancer. Many lesbians either believe, or have been told by medical practitioners, that they do not need to have smear tests. Certainly, it would appear that women who have never had sex with a man are at less risk of developing cervical cancer. First, however, many lesbians have had sex with men, either before they came out or after (despite neat labels, many people do not conform to rigid boundaries of 'gay' or 'straight'). New evidence also suggests that human papillomavirus (HPV), a cause of cervical cancer passed by sexual contact, can be transmitted by female-to-female sexual contact. In addition, smoking is a risk, and it is thought that lesbians are more likely to smoke or have smoked than heterosexual women.

STIs, HIV and AIDS

Certain groups in society are particularly at risk of contracting sexually transmitted infections (STIs). Often, these groups are at risk because of misleading dominant discourses. For example, figures suggest that STIs and HIV are rising among older people. Age Concern England (ACE 2002a) has shown that more than 10% of those men who are HIV positive are over 50 years old. Partly, this is because they are less likely to use condoms as they do not perceive themselves to be at risk. In addition, post-menopausal women have thinner vaginal tissue and less natural lubrication, which means their skin is more likely to tear. This is particularly worrying given that we know older people take longer to access services than younger people.

Much writing and research into gay sexuality and health has been concerned with HIV/AIDS. Similarly, much writing on HIV and AIDS has focused on gay men – thus, in part, perpetuating the myth that this is an issue that pertains only to the gay community. Certainly, many of the earliest cases involved young gay men and, as a result, many assumed that it

HIV stands for human immuno-deficiency virus, a retrovirus which infects and destroys the immune system. Thus someone with HIV has reduced protection against infections and cancer. The infection can be transmitted in a variety of ways, but the greatest risk is when semen is deposited in an anus or a vagina.

AIDS, or acquired immune deficiency syndrome, refers to the infection(s) which attack someone with an immune system weakened by HIV. Recent drug treatments used in the west have meant that HIV is now seen as a chronic rather than an acute condition.

was a disease which affected the gay community only. Some doctors called it gay-related immune deficiency (GRID) and the tabloid press in Britain, for example, referred to it as the 'gay plague'. Given that this was a time of more general homophobia, this assumption was generally accepted, and led to the stigmatisation of the disease. This is another example of how 'homosexuality', the subject of many powerful sanctions, is contaminating by association (Plummer 1981). As Watney (2000) argued, the ongoing misinformation that HIV transmission is related to sexual orientation, rather than sexual behaviour, places the heterosexual community at risk. World Health Organisation (WHO) studies consistently show that, globally, HIV is spreading as a result of unprotected hetero-sex. Other groups who have recently been identified as at risk include asylum seekers and prisoners. Society's conceptualisation of 'real' sex as penile penetration and anything else as 'not real sex' has placed other groups at risk. For example, sex between women carries a low risk of transmitting HIV but it is not always safe.

QUESTIONS

Collect from the internet the annual reports of as many health and social care service providers as you can. Do they make reference to heterosexual, lesbian, gay or bisexual service users? What are the possible consequences for your own profession?

AGEING

Ageing in general is increasingly becoming an issue of importance, partly because we are an ageing population. In addition, with the recent Coalition government in the UK, pressures on *older* people have increased and are likely to continue to do so. We know that older people are disadvantaged in the labour market, partly because they are perceived as being unable to learn new skills. Older people are more likely to live in poverty. It is also important to remember that older people are not a heterogeneous group with similar needs; they are a diverse group reflecting different social divisions. In other words, structural inequalities persist into old age. So, for example, issues of gender and class impact in older age: older women are more likely than older men to live in poverty, and older working-class people are more likely to live in poverty than older middle-class people. In a youth-oriented society, older people become marginalised and invisible. Recent stories about the representation of older women on television show how this is something which arguably impacts on women especially, where older women are deemed to be less attractive and less acceptable than older men (Cochrane 2011). Stereotypes about older people abound in our society. We tend to perceive older people as vulnerable, incapable and asexual (Gott 2005). These dominant discourses about sexuality in later life can have serious consequences for older people's quality of life. Positioning sexuality in later life as unnatural, shameful or disgusting can have the effect of rendering it invisible. This, of course, not only affects older people's sense of self, but also excludes them from the services and resources available to them.

There is not always agreement about what constitutes *older* in research. For some this includes those individuals who are 65 and above. For others, including many who research into older LGBT people, the term refers to 50 plus. Until recently, little effort had been made to explore the lives of older lesbians and gay men, and the area has remained relatively unexplored in health and social care work. There is, however, a small but growing body of research which allows us to look at the LGBT experience of growing older in relation to the heterosexual experience. Older LGBT individuals are, for instance, more likely to live alone, to age as a single person and not to have children. This means that compared to their heterosexual counterparts, many lack key social support networks. Research has shown that many younger LGBT people rely on friendships forged in the LGBT community, these friendships forming 'families of choice'. Such communities, however, are increasingly commercialised and youth oriented, meaning that older LGBT people may not be welcome. They are also, arguably, more in need, therefore, of formal services. Although the twenty-first century marks, in many ways, an unprecedented age of positive legislative and social change for gay men and lesbians (e.g. the Civil Partnership Act 2004; the Equality Act (Sexual Orientation) Regulations 2007), it is important to acknowledge that many older lesbians and gay men have lived through less liberal times. They will have experienced not only informal discrimination, but also formal discrimination – and this will impact on their use and experience of health services. The defection of Burgess and Maclean in 1951, for example, directly and indirectly impacted on the lives of many gay men and lesbians. The central scandal was the fact that these were two upper-class English men defecting to the Soviet Union – but the revelation that they were gay was used to cement the outrage, and perhaps even to explain it (Vargo 2002: 83). The combined fear of communism and homosexuality was a pervasive one in the 1950s. In England and Wales, the arrest of gay men rose by 50% between 1950 and 1955 – in part as a result of deliberate 'sting' operations, with homosexuality frequently being linked to general subversiveness and threats to the nation (2002: 103). Awareness of the fact that a homosexual identity was a stigmatised one, as far as much of society was concerned, may well have impacted on the ability of lesbians and gay men to access services. Older lesbians, gay men and bisexuals are five times less likely to access services for older people than is the older population in general, because they fear discrimination, homophobia and ignorance and believe that they will have to hide their sexuality. Older lesbians and gay men experience an unfortunate paradox. They live in a time of increasing sexuality, and at a time when, arguably, it is easier to be gay, yet they also live in a society where they are told older sexuality is distasteful. In addition, as older members of the LGBT community – a commercialised, youth-oriented population – many older LGBT people feel marginalised. This sense of isolation, marginalisation and invisibility impacts on many aspects of older LGBT lives.

Domestic abuse

As we have already seen, domestic abuse among LGBT people is a significant problem. Older same-sex couples suffer both direct and indirect discrimination in relation to this (ACE 2002a). If the image of the older lesbian and gay man as depressed, isolated, desperate and sexless is prevalent (Ginn and Arber 1995), if risks are associated with an 'out' identity in certain circumstances, and if there is little sense of support from LGBT communities – for example, if you feel your values are derided or you are just 'too old' to enjoy yourself – this may mean that there are few safe spaces in which to discuss same-sex domestic violence. The views of older lesbians and gay men as isolated, desperate and perhaps vulnerable may also render particularly invisible the potential perpetrators of domestic violence.

Elder abuse

Societal reluctance to acknowledge that older people engage in sexual activities results in the invisibility of their relationships. This means that when domestic violence happens in relationships involving older people, it tends to fall under the umbrella term 'elder abuse' (O'Keefe et al. 2007). This is especially so for LGBT elders who are more likely to keep their sexuality hidden.

Bereavement

The death of a loved one is a difficult time for anyone. Being an older LGBT person at such a time can present additional anxieties (Age UK 2010). Many of the issues discussed previously about 'coming out' apply here, as experiencing a bereavement may require constant 'coming out'. This may be especially problematic for many, especially older, LGBT individuals who are less comfortable in disclosing their sexuality to service providers. Despite recent formal recognition of same-sex partnerships, many LGBT people suffer lack of recognition of their relationships by families and, in some cases, agencies. Again, many have felt that gay-specific counselling would be desirable.

Care and the older LGBT person

For many of us, 'home' represents a sanctuary, a safe place to retreat, somewhere we can 'be ourselves'. Home can also be seen as an important site for constructing our identity, so that it becomes not just a space but also somewhere with social meaning. As we have already seen, many LGBT people experience a constrained sense of self in the public sphere, so the home may well have additional resonance. Asking for and accepting help in the home may therefore be especially hard for older LGBT people. Research has highlighted that older LGBT people receiving care in the home experience many difficulties (Pugh 2005). Many older gay men and lesbians have expressed concern that they would be subject to a disapproving or policing 'gaze', and consequently have had to de-gay or de-dyke their flat before a visit, for example by hiding 'incriminating' CDs. Other studies have begun to look into the issue of residential care homes. Heaphy et al. (2004) found that many lesbians and gay men feared getting older and having to enter care homes because they believed their sexuality would not be understood. There is evidence, for example, that many LGBT couples in care homes find their relationships are not recognised. As a result, LGBT-specific care is something desired by many older LGBT individuals. Such examples point to the fact that perhaps generic providers for older people need to make specific efforts to ensure that older lesbians, gay men and bisexuals feel included; that they feel able to access services on their own terms, without fear of discrimination; and that the information and services they receive are relevant and responsive to their circumstances and needs.

QUESTION

In what ways might older LGBT people suffer from discrimination?

CONCLUSION

Clearly, the relationship between sexual orientation and health is a complicated one – and an important one. The historical stigmatising of LGBT sexualities and the promotion of heterosexuality have served to regulate and police intimate lives. This has led to problematic health and social care provision for many lesbian and gay service users. LGBT service users do not demand special treatment. Rather, they have particular needs which require to be dealt with in appropriate ways. By thinking critically, challenging notions of 'normality' and 'acceptability' and engaging in reflective practice, you should have the skills to apply good practice to a variety of situations.

SUMMARY POINTS

- All sexual identities are socially constructed and ideas and ways of being sexual are very much tied into the culture and norms of a society. There is, therefore, no 'natural' sexuality.

- When discussing sexuality it is important to remember that all people possess a sexuality.

- Western society tends to be heteronormative, where there is both a direct and indirect assumption that everyone is heterosexual and that a particular social construct of sexuality is correct and superior to other forms of sexuality.

- LGBT people can encounter problems with health and social services that are geared for the needs of heterosexual people.

- Older LGBT people may find that they lack informal sources of social support.

- There are higher rates of mental distress and alcohol and substance use in the LGBT community and these higher rates can be attributed to the psycho-social stresses of discrimination and prejudice.

CASE STUDY

Breaking up is never easy, and for Francesca the end of her two-year relationship with Claire was hitting her hard. She had thought all was going well. Last summer had been wonderful, touring round various English music festivals before a week's holiday clubbing in Spain. They had even talked about making that next big step and perhaps moving in together. In fact, they had gone as far as looking at flats to rent. That had been mostly fun, but also annoying, especially when landlords thought she and Claire had misread the advert for the flat and not picked up it was only a single-bedroom property, and therefore not suitable for two girls to share. In fact, one landlord had been distinctly uneasy all the way through their visit and texted them shortly afterwards to say that someone else had just signed the lease for the flat, and was very emphatic that they should now look elsewhere.

Then, last August, it all went wrong. Claire had been acting a little more distant than normal for a few weeks and then suddenly in a fit of tears announced there was someone else that she had met and she had to break the relationship off. Francesca found herself becoming increasingly depressed. All the day-to-day tasks became too difficult and she began to stay in bed for as much of the day as she could. Then, last month, there had been a terrible run-in with Claire. Francesca saw her in the local shopping mall. It was strange to see her and she felt this powerful urge to talk to Claire. She only intended to say hello, but instead found herself breaking down in tears and trying to give Claire a hug. What had hurt most was Claire pushing her away. 'Not in public!' Claire had said under her breath as she walked away.

A few weeks ago she had decided to visit the local surgery to seek help for what she had decided was the depression she was experiencing. It was not always possible to see the same doctor each time and this introduced a problem for her in that she had to come out when she summarised what had been happening to her. Francesca remembered what it was like to come out the first time. It was not the actual moment of coming out that had been painful or stressful. It was actually a complete relief, and she experienced a sense of elation on telling her parents when she was in her mid-teens. What was really problematic was the build-up, the tension of rehearsing what she was going to say and her mind running through all the possible scenarios of what could happen: acceptance, rejection or denial. So, every time she visits the local surgery for an appointment she remembers those emotions and tensions, wondering how she is going to be received by the doctor when she politely corrects their assumption that it was a woman, not a man, who had left her.

QUESTIONS

Before discussing the more health-specific questions below, discuss the extent of prejudice and discrimination encountered by LGBT people in contemporary society.

1. In what ways do you think this particular case study of Francesca exemplifies any common experiences of LGBT people?
2. Why may the situation of having to come out every time Francesca visits the local doctors be difficult for her?
3. In what ways might a specific LGBT health service be of benefit for Francesca and other LGBT people?

TAKING YOUR STUDIES FURTHER

This chapter will have helped you understand many of the key terms, concepts, theories and debates relating to sexuality and health. Listed below are books that will provide deeper and more detailed discussions of the points raised in this chapter. You will also find additional resources on the companion website, including downloads of relevant material, links to useful websites, videos and other features. Please visit the companion website at https://study.sagepub.com/barryandyuill4e

RECOMMENDED READING

Fish, J. (2006) *Heterosexism in Health and Social Care*. Basingstoke: Palgrave.

Hawkes, G. (2002) *A Sociology of Sex and Sexuality*. Buckingham: Open University Press.

Richardson, D. (2000) *Rethinking Sexuality*. London: SAGE.

SOCIOLOGY OF THE BODY: CHRONIC ILLNESS AND DISABILITY

MAIN POINTS

- The body is not simply a biological entity only understood by the natural sciences.

- Perceptions of the body, what we do with our bodies and how the body is regulated are all influenced by society.

- Morality is attached to the presentation of the body in contemporary society, with thin bodies perceived as 'good' and overweight bodies perceived as 'bad'.

- Chronic illness leads to 'biographical disruption', where the 'taken-for-granted' aspects of life and identity are thrown into question.

- The medical model of disability locates the causes of disability in the individual body.

- The social model of disability sees the causes of disability as a form of social oppression and discrimination.

INTRODUCTION

The sociology of the body addresses how we use our bodies, considers how we engage with them and, fundamentally, seeks to understand the nature of the physical body. The key point to bear in mind is that the body is both 'natural' and the product of its social environment.

This chapter concentrates on the sociology of the body and what it can contribute to our understanding of health and illness. While there will be a strong emphasis on a theoretical approach to the human body, there will be equal coverage of the significance of embodiment through an examination of the impact of living with chronic illness and disability.

KEY ISSUES IN THE STUDY OF THE BODY

Until relatively recently sociologists shied away from theorising and researching the human body. The reasons for this reluctance are twofold. First, there is an unwillingness to be caught up in biological and determinist explanations of human behaviour. Sociologists have, for example, chosen to study gender rather than sex differences. Sex is often used to defend inequalities between women and men; the concept of gender, on the other hand, removes the problem of the bodily differences and draws our attention to the social construction of 'male' and 'female' in terms of the values, beliefs and expectations placed on biological women and men.

The second explanation for the general reluctance to embrace the body stems from the historical and cultural origins of the discipline itself. As Chapter 1 illustrated, the founding fathers of sociology were primarily concerned to explain the social changes brought about by urbanisation and industrialisation. Early sociological texts indicate a preoccupation with topics such as urbanisation, religion, paid work and the role of the state. Physical differences between people mattered less than inequalities of class and status. Differences such as those between women and men and between adults and children were seen as belonging to the 'natural' world, and were unchangeable and fixed. In recent times, however, sociology has developed to include topics such as sex and gender, disability, and the physical and biological aspects of our lives. In addition to changes within the discipline of sociology, a number of social and cultural shifts have taken place which have resulted in a renewed interest in the human body. The body has ceased to be the preserve of the medical and scientific world and has become a major concern for sociologists. Table 10.1 illustrates the main trends and developments.

Bodies are central to everything that we do and yet this centrality seems to have resulted in attitudes that very much take the body for granted; the body is so obvious it is hardly worth comment.

> If one thing is certain, it is that we all have a body. Everything that we do we do with our bodies – when we think, speak, listen, eat, sleep, walk, relax, work and play we 'use' our bodies. Every aspect of our lives is therefore embodied. Sometimes we may be more aware of our bodies than others but from the moment we wake, we are to a greater or lesser extent, consciously or sub-consciously relying on our bodies. (Nettleton and Watson 1998: 1)

Table 10.1 Bringing the body to the fore

Body politics: Recognition that the physical body has a social and political status such that a different body (whether that is female as opposed to male, or a body with a disability) helps determine an individual's life chances. The feminist movement and the disability movement have played a central role in attempting to ensure that people have power over their own bodies.

Demographic changes: An increasingly ageing population draws attention to the physical changes arising from the ageing process and the consequences of living with an ageing body.

The prevalence of chronic illnesses: There has been a significant change in what Nettleton and Watson refer to as 'the disease burden'. Infectious diseases have now been replaced by chronic and degenerative conditions, many of which raise important questions about how a physically changed body impacts on our sense of identity and how people live with pain and discomfort.

Consumerism: There is an increased emphasis on the appearance and health of the body. People are concerned about maintaining their bodies in good condition and purchasing goods to help them do so. In this context, 'good' suggests youthful, slim and active.

Technological changes: Physical limitations of the body can be overcome, appearance changed, organs and limbs repaired and replaced. It becomes increasingly difficult to distinguish between the 'natural' body and the 'technological' body.

The body as an expression of our identity: The body becomes a means to express an identity. Diet, exercise and lifestyles can be portrayed as 'moral' or 'immoral' and 'irresponsible'.

Source: adapted from Nettleton and Watson (1998: 4)

We have highlighted the significance of the body as a subject for students of sociology by emphasising the central role played by our physical selves in all that we do. Sociologists also seek to 'see' the body in more than purely physical and biological terms, drawing our attention to the two key 'social' aspects of the body. The first of these is the impact of environmental, cultural, social and political influences on the body, while the second is the knowledge that the body is shaped by certain dominant discourses such as medicine. Chapter 5 examines inequalities in health and presents evidence that indicates a relationship between social class and patterns of morbidity and mortality.

Social class can be used as an indicator of the types of illness people experience, as well as their life expectancy. Historical evidence reveals that body shape and stature are influenced by environmental factors. Birke (1992: 74–5) suggests an almost circular process where (a) biology, (b) environment and (c) the outcome all interact to transform one another. In her example, genetic inheritance interacts with nutrition to produce the final height of a child. Importantly, however, the final height of the child then influences the genes he or she passes on, which then interact with the environment – and so the process goes on. The second sense in which sociologists understand the body is

Embodiment refers to the experience of living through and with the physical body. Our experiences are essentially embodied. For example, we experience pleasure and pain through the body. Feelings of happiness and sadness are as physical as they are emotional.

in terms of our knowledge of the social construction of the physical. There is an inherent danger in understanding the body as only a social construction as this may impede the study of the body as a real and physical entity. Nettleton and Watson (1998: 2) point to a tendency for the sociology of the body to suffer from theoreticism, where there is little or no reference to the empirical evidence about the lived experience of **embodiment**. This chapter will overcome this with a detailed consideration of the embodied experience of living with chronic illness.

QUESTION

Can you identify how and when you are most aware of your body?

THE CIVILISED BODY: A CONTROLLED BODY AND A 'CLEAN' BODY

This section seeks to explore concepts of privacy and of the civilised, clean body. Views on what is appropriate bodily behaviour and who has access to our bodies have a key bearing on the delivery of health care as well as on our experience of illness. The physical examination of the body is central to the practice of medicine: it is this that allows practitioners to investigate whether or not the body is functioning normally. Doctors, nurses, physiotherapists, opticians and dentists are all required to touch the body, sometimes in intimate ways. Illness often entails losing some control over bodily functions. Migraine, for example, can cause uncontrollable vomiting, and food poisoning can lead to uncontrollable diarrhoea. Physical incapacity can necessitate the use of a commode, thus requiring someone to share what is not only an intimate act but also one that has overtones of being unclean. How we negotiate access to other bodies and how we think of our own are, therefore, key issues for the sociology of health.

As Nettleton and Watson (1998) have stated, we all have bodies and everything that we do, we do through them. All bodies have the same basic needs in terms of food, water and sleep. We must all remove waste from our bodies in the form of urine and faeces. Whether through illness or over-indulgence, our bodies vomit and we have little control over this. All bodies have the same basic components but differ in size, shape and colour. These are all fundamental human experiences and activities and yet, particularly in contemporary western societies, the body and its functions are regarded with a degree of shame and embarrassment.

To explore these concepts in more depth we will examine the work of Norbert Elias, first published in 1939, in relation to manners and the development of 'civilised' society. Elias's (1982) historical account of the civilised body examines the development of preferred ways of behaving and of control over the physical functions of the body. Regulation of the body came to be associated with higher social status and refinement. Nettleton (1995: 116–17) argues that the civilising of the body involves three progressive elements:

> The concept of the **civilised body** was developed by Norbert Elias. The term is used to denote a historical and cultural shift whereby the body is subject to increasing restraints that appear to limit the 'natural' body. The development of rules around eating manners is an example of how the body has become 'civilised'.

- *Socialisation*. People learn to conceal the natural functions of the body. We come to 'know' that certain functions, such as defecating or vomiting, are essentially private and potentially distasteful to others.
- *Rationalisation*. We prize our ability to control our emotions. Anger may be felt but only expressed in an acceptable way.
- *Individualisation*. Individual bodies are seen as separate from others. We demand a degree of personal 'social space' and privacy.

The development of ideas about the civilised body also demonstrates a concern to distinguish between human and bestial behaviour (Hawkes 1996: 20), and accords with Enlightenment notions about the higher self being associated with the mind and the base self with the body.

The work of Elias helps us to understand why people find intimate medical examination potentially embarrassing and why an inability to control the basic functions of the body can lead to stigmatisation. Control over our most basic bodily functions is something we require even in young children. As Nettleton suggests above, socialisation into the norms of any society entails learning that certain types of behaviour are private and potentially shameful when performed inappropriately. Mayall (1996) notes that much of the socialisation process is about teaching children to control their bodies and to be civilised. Young children are taught appropriate table manners, are toilet trained, and are taught the necessity of sitting still in preparation for schooling. Even at an early age, then, the importance of bodily control is underlined. Equally, the essentially private nature of the naked body and of sex is an implicit part of the concept of the civilised body. In her study of sex and sexuality, Hawkes (1996) argues that in medieval times nudity was not a source of shame and that sexual matters were discussed without any sense of embarrassment. She notes, too, that accompanying 'couples to the marital bed and celebration of the consummation were customs that persisted well into the seventeenth century' (1996: 22). After that period both nudity and sexual matters were moved 'behind the scenes', appropriate only in private (1996: 23).

167

QUESTION

Can you identify examples of when the body is subject to regulation and control, in both medical and non-medical settings?

How then do health practitioners deal with the potential discomfort that arises from physically intimate examinations? According to Lawler (1991), nursing staff have adopted a number of strategies to cope with potential embarrassment and shame, both on their part and on the part of the patient. A number of rules appear to govern such encounters. The first is that patients should comply with requests for examinations because they are dependent on nursing staff. Here it is helpful to refer to Parsons' model of the sick role (see Chapter 1) because it too justifies access to the patient's body on the grounds of expertise on the part of the practitioner. In addition, the practitioner's own professional code of conduct is, arguably, meant to protect the patient from potential abuse and exploitation. By maintaining a degree of professional distance, the situation may be depersonalised. Lawler (1991) also argues that patients themselves are expected to maintain a degree of modesty, while the nurse attempts to protect the patient's privacy.

Maintaining personal hygiene when ill often requires assistance with bathing, but it is common for nursing staff to allow patients the option of cleaning their own private parts. It is ironic that while much of modern health care is premised on practices such as holistic care, being attended to by a named carer, and attempts generally to break down the barriers between patients and staff, it seems that there are some circumstances when a professional and distanced stance is appreciated by both parties.

QUESTION

What are your experiences either as a patient being examined or as a practitioner undertaking an examination of a patient?

We also have to consider the public health movement, which emphasises the extent to which governments are concerned with controlling individual bodies as well as the social body. Disease and contamination of the body have been central concerns of the public health movement. Lupton (2012a), for example, writes of the economic and political implications of disease in terms of absence from work.

Our discussion of medicalisation illustrated the way in which it is not just unhealthy bodies that come under the scrutiny of the medical profession; there is an important sense in which we are all judged to be 'at risk'. The issues of cleanliness and hygiene are important illustrations of this trend, because there is considerable emphasis on preserving health through cleanliness. Lupton (2012a) provides an interesting historical account of just how our concept of cleanliness has changed over time:

> Consider the following examples of how, at varying periods in time, the body was kept clean and safe from infection and make a note of your personal reactions to them:
>
> Being 'clean' meant that those areas of the body seen by others were free of dirt.
>
> Washing was 'dry' in the sense that a cloth was used to rub the face and hands.
>
> Bathing was not an option; immersing the body in water was thought to weaken it as the liquid might invade the body.
>
> Once bathing became an accepted practice, cold bathing was preferred as it was thought to toughen and invigorate the body.
>
> The use of 'cosmetics' such as perfume to scent the body was seen as frivolous. (2012a: 33–4)

These examples of hygienic practices are in marked contrast to the values prevalent in most western societies. Personal hygiene is both desirable and, it might be argued, possible with the provision of indoor plumbing. We all sweat as a means of cooling the body down, yet the smell of sweat is shunned. Instead, we attempt either to prevent our bodies sweating (through the use of an anti-perspirant) or to mask the smell if the body does sweat (through the use of deodorant). Media images reinforce the message that bodies that are clean and perfumed are desirable bodies.

The desire for cleanliness extends beyond our bodies to our homes. The nineteenth-century push to improve the health of the nation focused primarily on instructing mothers in childcare practices and, significantly, in domestic hygiene. According to Hawkes (1996: 97), 'a good mother kept a clean home. Whiter whites were a sign of superiority'. The multitude of products that claim to be anti-bacterial or effective in combating the invisible threat of germs bears testimony to our fear of dirt and the negative moral connotations that attach to a lack of hygiene. Lupton (2012a) argues that modern standards and beliefs about cleanliness are characterised by a fear of invisible germs and viruses.

Among commentators on the sociology of the body, it appears to be accepted that the population of the United Kingdom is obsessed with hygiene and cleanliness. However, there is some evidence to suggest that this view is simplistic. Professor Hugh Pennington of the Bacteriology Department of Aberdeen University has been particularly critical of poor hygiene practices around the home. Among his main concerns is the use of washing-up bowls and reusable dishcloths.

> Professor Pennington said that placing chopping boards and knives teeming with germs together with plates and glasses in a plastic bowl created the ideal environment for the spread of bugs.

> The experts said disposable paper cloths should be used instead of tea towels that could easily spread infection.

> They also recommended using 'good old fashioned bleach' in the kitchen rather than newer anti-bacterial products that were only vaguely effective. (BBC News 2000)

There have also been major health crises that have stemmed from poor hygiene practices. In Scotland in 2002 hospital-acquired infections in general and the MRSA bug in particular led to the closure of the Victoria Infirmary, Glasgow, to all new admissions. Hugh Pennington commented that infection control was being severely compromised by the lack of basic hygiene practices, such as doctors and nurses failing to wash their hands between treating patients.

The discussion above has highlighted the ways in which bodily functions and intimate access to the body can present barriers in the caring relationship. It has been suggested that shame and embarrassment about the body are not natural but are socially cultivated, and the work of Elias has provided an insight into the development of concepts of the 'civilised body'. Our discussion now takes us on to images and perceptions of the 'perfect' body.

THE SCULPTURED BODY: CREATING PERFECTION

Images of bodily perfection, most often images of women, are powerful but never static. Whether it is the voluptuous bust, tiny waist and rounded bottom of the nineteenth century, the androgynous figure of the 1920s, the curves of Marilyn Monroe, or the taut, lean and muscular body of Madonna, images of how female bodies should look are powerful reminders of the extent to which people have aspired to the perfect body. The purpose of this discussion is to examine how and why people have tried to attain that 'good' body. A later discussion of disability and chronic illness will pose equally powerful questions about what happens when bodies are not and cannot be made perfect.

Diet is perhaps the most obvious way in which we control the size and shape of the body. As Lupton (2012a: 40) comments, 'skin tone, weight, strength of bones, condition of hair and nails are all commonly said to be directly affected by diet'. An increasingly important aspect of diet is the desire to limit the intake of food. Bordo (1990: 83) argues that types of fasting have been common throughout history, and are usually characterised by control over the body's appetites or by a religious desire to purify the flesh. However, she notes a significant shift during the late Victorian era, when 'for the first time in the West, those who could afford to eat well began systematically to deny themselves food in the pursuit of an aesthetic ideal' (Bordo 1990: 83). So began what Bordo has described as the tyranny of slenderness.

In common with others, Bordo (1990) argues that body size is underpinned by a code of morality. The possession of a slender body suggests that the individual is in control of their body and their life. To achieve the 'perfect' body requires considerable time, effort and determination. Benson (1997: 123) suggests that the body is increasingly seen as an indicator of a person's moral character:

> The bad body is fat, slack, uncared for; it demonstrates a lazy and undisciplined 'self'. The good body is sleek, thin and toned. To have such a body is to project to those around you – as well as to yourself – that you are morally as well as physically 'in shape'.

In the same vein, a muscular body has become what Bordo (1990: 94–5) describes as a 'cultural icon':

> The firm, developed body has become a symbol of correct attitude; it means that one 'cares' about oneself and how one appears to others, suggesting willpower, energy, control over infantile impulses, the ability to 'make something' of oneself.

Themes of controlling the body through willpower and discipline are frequent in accounts of people with eating disorders – a term which covers a range of behaviours from systematically starving the body, to overeating, and finally to eating and purging the body through vomiting or the use of laxatives. Although there is not the space here for a detailed discussion of eating disorders, a number of points can be made about the denial of food and the desire to assert power and autonomy. Benson (1997) describes the refusal to eat as 'an inescapably political act' because it is most often associated with asserting control and/or registering a protest. The use of hunger strikes as a political protest is common (Yuill 2007) and, at the other end of the spectrum, a child's refusal to eat is a clear sign of defying parental authority. It has been suggested, therefore, that eating disorders such as anorexia may be a way of exercising power over the body, food intake being perhaps the only area of choice open to a person. Bordo (1990) examines limiting food intake in the context of a general cultural fear of 'fat' as an indicator of losing control over the body. In this sense, bodies have to be not only slender but contained, in the sense of minimising bulges and flab (1990: 88–9):

LINK

The desire (and ability) to control and discipline the body is seen as a characteristic of postmodern society, discussed in Chapter 1.

Areas that are soft, loose, or 'wiggly' are unacceptable, even on extremely thin bodies. Cellulite management, like liposuction, has nothing to do with weight loss, and everything to do with the quest for firm bodily margins. (Bordo 1990: 90)

We have, thus far, concentrated principally on diet as a way of regulating the size and shape of the body, as well as being an indicator of a personal morality: thin bodies represent controlled and cared-for bodies; fat bodies suggest some sort of moral failing. There are, however, other ways in which the body can be managed and sculptured. Surgical intervention, most commonly in the form of cosmetic surgery to alter appearance, is an obvious example. Parts of the body can be enlarged or changed in appearance, as in the practice of breast enhancement. Far more radical, however, is the case of gender realignment, or sex change. Complex surgical procedures, combined with the use of hormones and counselling, can help a person complete the transition from male to female or vice versa. The body, and in particular the genitalia, are the most obvious indicators of our sex.

Paul Hewitt writes movingly of his own experiences as a female-to-male transsexual: 'It is not that I want to be male. I am male, and, like all transsexuals, I experience an overwhelming urge to bring the gender of my body into line with the gender of my mind' (Hewitt and Warren 1997: 75). Changing his outward appearance allows Hewitt to pass as a man. Male dress, haircuts and clothes all play an important part in signalling to others that he is male, but more fundamental changes are needed: the possession of an artificial penis and the removal of both breasts. This alone should be evidence that the body is the ultimate means of displaying who we are to others.

THE 'FAILED' BODY: ILL HEALTH AND DISEASE

We now continue these themes, but move on to an examination of the ways in which disability and chronic illness transform the body and personal identity.

Increasingly, most heavyweight newspapers carry a regular column written by someone with some form of chronic illness, providing insights into their life and the challenges that chronic illness brings. Also, with the widening use of the internet, people with chronic illnesses set up and write their own blogs. These discuss various aspects of living with a variety of illnesses (Hardey 2002; Seale 2005). Many blogs or columns are written from an 'open secret' position, in that both writer and reader know that at some point the author may well die. Over the years we have seen columns and books dealing with, for example, teenage cancer (Stephen Sutton's *Stephen's Story: A 19-Year-Old's Life Lessons on Making the Most of Your Time* (2014)) and breast cancer (Ruth Picardie's (1993) *Before I Say Goodbye*). These glimpses into the life of someone with a long-term, probably fatal condition are deeply moving, and readers feel a strong sense of attachment to the writer. Such articles and serials are also indicative of how chronic illness is moving centre stage in terms of the general awareness of health and illness. Most people in the United Kingdom now will die of a chronic illness rather than from an infectious disease – many more than in previous centuries. The increase in the number of people with chronic illnesses raises several important issues:

- The dominance of medical science and its ability to cure all is challenged; its weaknesses and limits are exposed.
- The person with a chronic illness has to reconstruct aspects of their life and identity when facing a condition that will become a fundamental part of their existence.

We can see these concerns in this extract from Picardie's *Before I Say Goodbye*, when she is corresponding with a friend about forthcoming treatment and her wider anxieties about her family:

> The latest news is that I didn't have the second lot of chemo yesterday, because my white blood cell count is still crap – they went in 'all guns blazing' (direct quote from oncologist) first time round and it was obviously OTT ... Meanwhile, my hair is falling out with amazing rapidity – I estimate total baldness will be achieved by the weekend, so the whole thing will have happened in a week. It's getting awfully expensive – had my hair cut ultra short on Monday, and reckon I will have to have it shaved on Friday. I was a bit freaked out at first – it's really alarming running your hand through your hair and handfuls coming out. Makes you look sick, feel that you are dying, etc., which I am not ... Meanwhile, I am asking everyone I know to buy me a hat. I hope I don't frighten the children – I imagine I'll look pretty weird. (1993: 1)

In this extract, Picardie records her ambivalence towards the chemotherapy treatment, which was, at that time, resulting only in hair loss. She is also battling to maintain 'normality' by seeking to minimise the impact and disruption that being bald may have on her children. These themes of identity and maintaining a 'normal life' will be explored in this section. Sociologists such as Anselm Strauss, Ilene Lubkin and Michael Bury have developed useful perspectives and ideas for understanding the many complexities and subtleties that surround people with chronic illnesses in contemporary western societies. Much research has focused on how people readapt their lives, organise resources and present themselves to the outside world.

QUESTIONS

Find some examples of people discussing their lives with a chronic illness, whether in a book, newspaper or online. Identify trends and issues in what they discuss. What insights do they give you into such a life?

In particular, we will look at the work of Bury (1991). He has devised the following concepts that help us sociologically explore chronic illness:

- biographical disruption
- adjusting to the impact of treatment regimens
- adaptation and management of illness.

Before going any further, it should be emphasised that we are not looking at a formal model or stages that people go through as their lives with a chronic illness unfold. Rather, we are looking at issues that face them at various points during their lives. The various concepts listed above should be seen as *emergent* and not *sequential*. This means that there is no ordered 'timetable' as to how a condition develops over time – what symptoms a person with a chronic illness will experience and when they will experience them. For example, with multiple sclerosis people with the condition often have no idea how the illness will develop in their life. There is almost a 'randomness' in when symptoms appear or emerge and how people will have to respond to the changes that those symptoms bring to their life when they appear.

Biographical disruption

Biographical disruption is a core concept in the sociological study of chronic illness, and has helped to illuminate and explore the lived experience of people with chronic illnesses (Williams 2000). In this section, we will look at what biographical disruption means and entails, as well as the subtleties and nuances that go along with it, before moving on to some of the criticisms that have been made.

> Biographical disruption refers to a destabilisation, questioning and reorganisation of identity after the onset of chronic illness.

First, let us turn to looking at what biographical disruption means as a concept. Think of your life as narrative, as a story that has been partially written, with past events apparently well-defined and recorded, the present unfolding, and the future a set of plans, ambitions and hopes. Now imagine that personal biography being radically altered as you learn that your body is failing: cells are under attack, or your brain is sending out a series of bizarre signals that prevent your limbs functioning as they once did. Suddenly, all that narrative, that 'biography', you have constructed for yourself and hope to build for the future is thrown into doubt. The present now has to be renegotiated (worked out), the future seems doubtful and the past is a strange place. In short, you have to face a disruption in your concept of self and in your 'own biography'. This is something that Charmaz (1983) has described as the 'loss of self', where you see your former self crumble and disappear. Frank (1995), too, has used similarly dramatic language to capture an image of the wreckage of one's life following the onset of chronic illness.

QUESTION

Think of your life as a narrative. What has been written so far and what have you plotted out for the future?

For someone with a chronic illness, biographical disruption often entails a reorganisation of their life on many levels; various ideas of self and of relationships with family, friends and colleagues will be challenged and re-evaluated. Within the biographical disruption of life the individual will have to deal with the *consequences* and *significance* of the illness (Bury 1997). We can see some of this, for example, in a study on multiple sclerosis (MS) by Boeije et al. (2002). They found that for the people in their research many parts of their lives, which they held to be important as part of their self-identity, had to be reconsidered. One useful example is that of Marc, a young man in his early thirties who was dedicated to his job and was a keen windsurfer – an activity that was a key part of his social life (Boeije et al. 2002: 886). The changes in his body brought on by the MS meant that he was unable to go to work or to socialise as he had before the onset of the condition. To deal with these issues he began to relish having free time, something he thought he would be unable to do, and he developed new hobbies with friends, such as playing cards. As Marc says:

> When I was working I was almost a workaholic. So I thought that I would go crazy sitting at home all day. But I still know how to enjoy things, it's wonderful having all these days off. Beforehand, you don't expect that to happen, but I've got such nice people around me and I often have visitors. That never seems to stop. I can open the doors with my remote control from my bedroom, which is ideal. I have contact with all kinds of people, including fellow sufferers. (Boeije et al. 2002: 886)

The actual symptoms of a condition will affect everyday life. Someone, for example, with temporal lobe epilepsy (or petit mal epilepsy, as it was formerly called) may have to live with the uncertainty of not knowing when or in what context they may have an absence (Iphofen 1996). This can make certain social situations fraught with risk in terms of safety or, more importantly, of breaking social norms. For other conditions, there are issues of self-care and managing symptoms on a daily basis. As mentioned in Chapter 1, illness also has cultural and metaphorical significance. People with chronic illness may have to respond to the way in which their culture and society perceive their condition. Certain conditions carry a social stigma when the illness is connected with undesirable states or social deviance. Younger people with arthritis feel that they are ageing prematurely (Singer 1974), while people with HIV/AIDS could be stigmatised as 'junkies', given the association of HIV/AIDS with substance use, for example. It is important to note here that it is not the person with chronic illness who is 'the problem', but rather societal attitudes and the way in which the physical environment is shaped. We will explore this highly important and fundamental issue later in this chapter, when we look at disability.

There has been some debate surrounding the assumption that biography is always disrupted after the onset of a chronic illness. Pound et al. (1998) have argued that for older people the development of a chronic illness (stroke, in their research) was in some ways expected and regarded as a 'normal crisis'. The impact of the stroke, and the consequent disruption of biography, was lessened by the fact that it was just one of many 'disruptive' issues (such as poverty and poor housing) that faced this group of people. Faircloth et al. (2004) also explored this idea of age and other factors in studying how people could minimise biographical disruption. In their study, also on stroke, they too found that age reduced the disruptive effects of stroke on older people's understandings and perceptions of who they were and their wider identity. They also found that the presence, and a history, of other illnesses (such as diabetes) and knowledge of stroke (typically seeing it happen to other people) also helped people who had experienced a stroke view it as a normal part of life. Thus, they were better set to handle the changes in their lives that having a stroke entailed. To some extent, having a stroke was part of the 'biographical flow', where chronic illness was just part of the rhythms and expectations of everyday life, especially, in this case, for older people.

Schnittker (2005) noted that age could act as a factor in lessening disruption for someone with a chronic illness generally. He found that depression as a consequence of chronic illness seemed more likely to affect people who had become chronically ill when younger rather than those who had become chronically ill when they were older. This was possibly due to older people having developed more complex emotional skills over their life course, which could help them cope with illness.

Reviewing the literature on biographical disruption, Williams (2000) has offered further refinements to this core concept. Following Pound et al. (1998), he suggested that chronic illness cannot be seen exclusively as disruption but can be viewed as continuity, where chronic illness is expected and regarded as normal due to age and class. In the case of gay men with HIV/AIDS, for instance, the onset of infection or the development of non-symptomatic HIV can also lead to an affirmation of political identity, something that Carricaburu and Pierret (1995) describe as 'biographical reinforcement'. Williams cites other examples, too numerous to mention here, but all with the same theme: that the context of someone's life has a strong bearing on how disruptive a chronic illness will be.

The work of Wouters and De Wet (2015) provides further developments in the concept of biographical disruption. Their research focused on the experiences of women in South Africa who had contracted HIV and who were receiving anti-retroviral therapy (ART), which helps to support the immune system and thereby considerably lengthen the lives of people who are HIV positive. The use of ART is one of the reasons why HIV has shifted away from being an acute illness to a long-term chronic illness.

176

They also sought to see whether Bury's concept could be applied in settings outside Europe where most of the work on it had been generated. What they found was a nuanced interplay between social context, identity and illness. HIV for the women in this study was surprisingly not as disruptive as one may have thought. The ART played a significant role in reducing the disruption as the HIV could be managed if the medication was followed. The context of their lives also contributed to their HIV status not being as disruptive as might be expected.

As with the work of Pound et al. (1998), the context of hard-lived life was crucial in shaping their biographies prior to the onset of their illness. Remember, in Pound et al.'s study, the biographies of the people in that study were dense with disruption that had nothing to do with illness, as poverty and economic hardship were the main disruptions in their lives before they experienced a stroke. The South African women's lives were also shaped by hardship, growing up during the brutal and racist apartheid era of South Africa, and by how that period in South Africa's history had left a legacy of inequality, poverty and different forms of violence. Issues of finance, as opposed to concerns with illness, emerged during the interviews that Wouters and De Wet held with the women. Feeding their families and looking after the emotional needs of others was more of a priority than dealing with the effects of being HIV positive (Wouters and De Wet 2015).

Context was present again when the researchers pursued why being diagnosed as HIV positive did not have as much of an impact as might be suspected. The context this time was the prevalence of HIV in South Africa. With such high rates of infection the women accepted that they might contract the virus, so disruption was to some extent reduced. Also, receiving a course of ART assisted in minimising the disruption by helping to manage symptoms. When questioned further, it did become apparent, however, that being HIV positive did exert an impact on their identity. The biggest change for the women was negotiating the tricky issue of disclosing their HIV status. Care had to be taken in revealing their status in case it should lead to stigma in the workplace or rejection when trying to form new relationships. Indeed, as a raft of other research has established, one of the main concerns for people with HIV is managing information about their status. Fear of being stigmatised is a constant worry, requiring care and courage with whoever that information is shared.

LINK

We discuss other health effects of apartheid in Chapter 7 on ethnicity and health.

QUESTION

Discuss the concept of biographical disruption. How accurate do you think it is in exploring the experiences of people with chronic conditions?

Impact of treatment regimens

One major adjustment that inevitably comes with a chronic illness is incorporating medical and clinical treatments into daily life. We will look here at how treatment regimens can impact on a person with a chronic illness and also why people with a chronic illness do not always go along with what they are told to do by medical experts and therapists. A key point here is that what a health professional thinks is the best form of treatment or therapy may not be accepted by someone with a chronic illness for a host of complex, but legitimate, reasons as the best way forward. For example, someone with MS may be encouraged by a therapist to use a wheelchair. This may be a sensible course of action from the therapist's perspective, as it allows the person with MS a degree of mobility that they may not currently have. For the person with MS, however, a wheelchair may signify a massive change in their life, on both a symbolic and a personal level, because using a wheelchair is a very strong indicator that they are becoming a disabled person and are no longer the person they once perceived themselves as being.

There are two main ways in which treatment regimens impact on people with a chronic illness. Treatment regimens that are part and parcel of living with chronic illness vary widely both in the form they take (for example, having to use a stoma, having regular dialysis or taking a variety of medications) and in the impact they may have (more of which later). Such impacts can be either affective (to do with people's emotions and how they see themselves) or instrumental (reorganising time and learning to manage technology and medication), though these attributes overlap to a great extent.

If we look at *affective* changes first, what we see is that treatment can alter how you think about yourself both in relation to your past biography and in relation to other people – particularly if the treatment has potentially stigmatising consequences. MacDonald (1988), for example, observed that for people with a colostomy, following treatment for rectal cancer, there was a strong tendency to conceal information about their stoma. The patients felt that the odours, noise and dealing with the bag in public places were potentially disruptive to normal social intercourse. These patients with rectal cancer were further stigmatised in a variety of ways. In addition to having to negotiate the stigma of cancer, they also broke cultural taboos concerning faeces and its disposal. As a result, social situations became fraught with risk, with patients seeking to minimise the impact of the stigma, fearing embarrassment or disgust. Overall, for these patients, there was some impairment of quality of life, even if they had managed to deal with the socially perceived 'problems' of their stomas in some way.

When someone is involved in long-term treatment or therapy there exists the problem of what Robinson (1988) terms the 'medical merry-go-round'. Here the person with a chronic illness experiences emotional highs and lows as their expectations of what treatment will deliver go up and down while they circle through various forms and stages of treatment or medication, in a way that is similar to an old-fashioned carousel ride where the horses go up and down and continually move in a circle. This can be very emotionally and physically

178

draining and exhausting. Research by Wiles et al. (2004) provides a useful example of this. Looking at people who were undergoing physiotherapy after a stroke, Wiles et al. found that clients had to manage feelings of potential disappointment when their time with the physiotherapist was at an end. Although the patients usually felt disappointment at no longer receiving 'physio', they often left with high expectations that their future recovery was going to continue and their overall function improve – something that, given the uncertainties of stroke recovery, may be unlikely to happen. Wiles et al. draw attention to the need for therapists to be wary of the emotional aspects of a client's therapy as part of the therapy process, as well as how to manage feelings of optimism and disappointment.

If we turn now to the instrumental effects of treatment regimens we can see that compliance/adherence to medication, meeting the demands of clinical appointments and using medical technology can also be very complex. Compliance/adherence to medication used to be regarded as almost a straightforward example of medicalisation within medical sociology, where the medical world took over another part of someone's private life-world. There has been a shift lately, however, in thinking about how people with chronic conditions relate to medication. Instead of being seen in 'black-and-white' terms, as meekly following what they are told to do, people are now seen as thoughtfully engaging with the medication as part of their wider adjustments to changes in the self brought about by chronic illness.

This means that it is not a simple case of the medical expert giving out advice or instructing someone in what to do and that person going meekly along with what they have been told. Such an idea is evident in Parsons' concept of the sick role, which is discussed in Chapter 1. Increasingly, as Pound et al. (2005) note, people adopt a strategic position on medication and treatment, whereby they will often see how well treatment regimens work in the context of their lives before deciding whether or not to comply. As a result, health professionals have to develop more flexible and fluid ways of interacting, adopting a variety of roles and approaches to encourage people with chronic illnesses to engage with and adopt certain treatment regimens. This may entail health professionals acting as 'educators, detectives, negotiators, salesmen, cheerleaders and policemen' (Lutfey 2005: 421) when working with clients.

Adaptation and management of illness

From the discussion so far, we see that chronic illness can have a considerable impact on a person's life. Aspects of a person's life may be thrown into question and have to be re-evaluated, while the treatment for the condition can produce a host of potentially stigmatising situations. Within this context people with chronic illnesses nevertheless seek to maintain some sense of self and identity. In the earlier extract from Picardie's *Before I Say Goodbye* (1993), there was evidence of how she dealt with hair loss by having her hair cut short in an attempt to appear 'normal'. Bury (1991) describes these responses as coping, strategy and style:

- *Coping*: is a term used in a variety of contexts, commonly when someone is coping with the illness, whether successfully or not. It can also take on emotional dimensions and relate to how someone is holding on to certain aspects of identity.
- *Strategy*: is the particular action or resources someone utilises to deal with problems created by the illness and by social responses. Strategies can range from breaking the day down into manageable chunks to avoiding the general public in order to minimise the risk of stigma.
- *Style*: is how one presents oneself to the social world in an attempt to maintain aspects of self.

DISABLED PEOPLE AND DISABILITY

As always in sociology, it is useful to explore how a particular phenomenon is defined and to critically appraise the words that are used to describe that phenomenon. The reason for this is that language is never neutral; words do not simply hang in the air and have no effect on the real world. Language, rather, is very powerful. The words used and how something is conceptualised can have very serious consequences for people, and language is much more than an exercise in 'political correctness'. The main reason is that how a social phenomenon is defined and conceptualised influences and conditions what follows in regard to how certain people are perceived by others, their standing in society, or what form of care or therapy is made available. This relationship between language or concepts and the lives of people is highly relevant for people with disabilities. Consider the following terms and expressions that are commonly used in connection with disabled people:

- cripple, crippled
- handicapped
- deformed
- invalid
- 'something wrong'
- the disabled.

Some of these words immediately appear to be offensive, at the very least. 'Cripple' and 'deformed' are probably the worst in that respect, filled with connotations of someone being less than a 'whole' person, possibly therefore worthy of pity or charity, and definitely not worthy of full social acceptance. Even though initially 'the disabled' as a term may seem to be more acceptable, it too is problematic. The definite article 'the' is at fault, as it implies that there is no person there, simply a medical condition with no personal narrative, identity or desires. Moreover, such expressions imply that everyone who is disabled has a uniform experience regardless of gender, class, ethnicity, age, sexuality or impairment. People with disabilities are seen as an undifferentiated homogeneous block. That is why terms such as 'disabled people' or 'person with disabilities' are used. These terms reintroduce the humanity and therefore rights of citizenship and broader human rights.

The above discussion is steering us towards different approaches in thinking about disability. What is being opened up here is a very fundamental question: what is disability? As we shall encounter shortly, there are two broad answers to this question. One suggests that disability is the limitations of a person because of some form of physical difference or impairment located in their body. Another, instead, refers to disability arising out of the barriers and attitudes located in society with which people with impairments are presented on a daily basis. We have here two very different accounts of what constitutes disability, one focusing on the person and the other on society. The acceptance or privileging of one answer over the other entails different understandings of disability and different relationships with disabled people.

The first answer identifies disability as occurring in the body and therefore it can be regarded as a medical condition. Interpreting disability as a medical condition implies that the individual with an impairment is almost at fault – that there is something wrong with them, and they are in some way deficient. The way to improve the lives of people with disabilities is therefore to focus on changes that can be made to their bodies. Since medical technology cannot offer complete 'cures' for many disabilities, people with disabilities have to accept the limitations on their lives, tragic as that may be. This position also infers that people with disabilities are reliant upon other people to help them, as they are limited in what they can achieve in everyday life because of their disability.

The second answer, which looks towards a social explanation, implies quite a different orientation towards disability. The fundamental premise of this approach is that the lives of people with disabilities are made difficult by the way that society, in terms of both built spaces and social attitudes, is constructed. Remove those attitudes and reorganise physical space, and the problems disabled people encounter are greatly reduced, if not no longer present. In certain respects this position shares many similarities with other groups in society who encounter or have encountered discrimination because of some socially defined difference. In the 1960s in the United States, African-Americans in some southern states, for example, encountered segregation on a daily basis, where they were not permitted by law to eat in the same restaurants as white people or sit in the same seats on a bus as white people. The only reason black people could not do these things was because of racist attitudes. So what is the difference, it could be argued, between this experience and that of disabled people not being able to access restaurants or public transport? All that is required is a different approach to design and a different mindset and there would be no problems. This does not happen because of a form of prejudice which parallels racism, in this case disablism, which perceives disabled people as being inferior and therefore excluded from the rights that everyone else enjoys. Disability here becomes an issue of civil rights that requires changes to society – changes that can be led by disabled people.

The two outlooks on disability sketched out above form the basis of the different models of disability advanced by disability activists and academics such as Oliver (1990, 1993) and Barnes (Barnes et al. 1999). The first viewpoint is referred to as the medical model and the second as the social model. Importantly, the two models are not intended by their authors to be value-free, neutral observations of the world; they are instead deliberately judgemental. The medical model is a negative and discriminatory perspective that holds a static and fatalistic understanding of disability: that's how life is, how unfair! By contrast, the social model is a positive and emancipatory perspective that seeks to offer a way for disabled people to bring about meaningful changes in their lives: life's unfair, let's go and change it and make it fair!

The medical model refers to a negative perception of disabled people that identifies disability as being located in the body of the person, related to a physical deficit, therefore requiring the disabled person to rely on the help of others. The social model focuses on disability being located in barriers created by oppressive and prejudicial social attitudes and in the design of the built environment.

Over time the **medical model of disability** has lost out to the social model in many respects. Allied health professionals, such as occupational therapists, physiotherapists and nurses, advocate the social model when working with disabled people. We can see the influence of the social model in legislation such as the Disability Discrimination Act 1995 and the Equality Act 2010, which place the onus on organisations not to discriminate against disabled people and to make buildings accessible (though in practice they are not always as accessible as they could be). There are many reasons for the success of the social model. One of the main reasons is that by refocusing the cause of disability away from the individual and towards society, the model allows for a wider understanding of the relationships between society and disabled people, exploring dynamics of power, identity, culture and oppression (Shakespeare 2006). The social model also played a fundamental role in providing a political analysis of disability, which helped in building and framing the disabled civil rights movement where disabled people organised on their own terms to challenge the prejudice and discrimination prevalent in society.

There has been growing criticism of the social model in recent years, however. The main point of departure is that the social model overemphasises the social, and holds that all of the issues that negatively impact upon the lives of disabled people are to be found in society; the upshot is that changing society would eliminate disability. What sociologists such as Tom Shakespeare (2006, 2013) and Williams (1999) have countered is that such a strong perspective on the social aspects of disability ignores the very real problems of suffering and pain caused by physical impairments and the whole subjective, personal experiences of disability. The body of disabled people, in effect, 'vanishes' in the social model. Making this observation – that the body and therefore the biological have to be taken into account – is not to reject the contribution that the social model has made in understanding the situation of disabled people in society, or to suggest that improvements in civil rights and changes in social attitudes concerning disabled people are unnecessary.

Far from it: there is still much in society that remains oppressive. It is rather to acknowledge that a more effective and holistic model of disability would include an understanding of the physical and biological aspects of disability, but importantly also an appreciation of how those biological aspects of disability interact with the social aspects. This is actually quite an important statement. Disability is not a bit of both, 50% biological and 50% social; rather, disability, and what it is to be disabled, are a state of being that emerges out of various interweaving and interacting social and biological processes. Shakespeare (2006: 55–6) captures the aforesaid very elegantly:

> The approach to disability which I propose to adopt suggests that disability is always an interaction between individual and structural factors. Rather than getting fixated on defining disability either as a deficit or a structural disadvantage, a holistic understanding is required. The experience of a disabled person results from the relationship between factors intrinsic to the individual, and extrinsic factors arising from the wider context in which he or she finds herself. Among the intrinsic factors are issues such as: the nature and severity of her impairment, her own attitudes, her personal qualities and abilities and her personality. Among the contextual factors are: the attitudes and reactions of others, the extent to which the environment is enabling or disabling, and wider cultural, social and economic issues relevant to disability in that society.

Learning or intellectual disabilities

Learning or intellectual disability provides a useful example of many of the themes discussed above, illustrating the relationships between prevailing social attitudes, disability and impairment. Estimates indicate that there are somewhere in the region of 145,000 adults and 65,000 children with severe or profound learning disabilities in England, and a further 1.2 million people with mild or moderate learning difficulties (Department of Health 2001). It is in the history of people with learning disabilities that the interactions of impairment and society are most noticeable. This illustrates the importance of Shakespeare's (2006, 2013) point, outlined in the previous section, that the wider cultural issues relevant to disability shape the lived experiences of disabled people. For people with learning disabilities, as Race (2002) outlines, there is a history of moving from reasonable tolerance in the pre-industrial age, to being regarded as problematic during the early stages of the Industrial Revolution, to being seen as a threat to the integrity of the white English race in the Victorian period and needing to be isolated from the rest of society, and finally to increasing but still incomplete acceptance today. These changes in how people with learning disabilities were understood and perceived by society were driven by developments and trends in society's attitudes to disability in one measure, but also by the wider cultural dynamics that informed the times. In the pre-industrial age, before science became the main way of understanding the world and supernatural explanations dominated, those who were considered to be fools because of impairment were regarded as possessing special and mystical insights into the nature of things and into the complexities of the human spirit. We can glimpse the position of people with learning disabilities in a different age in the plays of William Shakespeare, where often the court fool imparts wise advice gained from his 'different' perspective on the world to the King or lead characters. In the industrial and scientific times of the Industrial Revolution and the Enlightenment, people with intellectual disabilities were not so accepted. They were seen to be out of sync with the new mechanised rhythms of the workplace; they were alienated from the new techniques of mass production, and their apparent lack of reason offended rationalism. Later in the Victorian period, the Eugenics movement, a pseudo-scientific and racist approach to matters of ethnicity and what would become genetics, centred on the need for racial purity and held that the fine English stock could be contaminated by the external threat of inferior races (typically people from outside Western Europe) or the internal threat of the 'feeble minded'. At this point in history it became common to see that the 'solution' for people with learning disabilities was isolation and segregation from society in order to prevent their genes infecting the wider population.

We can witness something of this time in the genesis of the term 'Down's syndrome', which is now used to denote the condition emerging out of genetic 'damage' to chromo-some 21. When physician John Langdon Down first described the condition in the 1860s he did not apply his own name to it. He instead drew on the prevailing view of the times that there were lesser races and decided that people with Down's syndrome bore some resemblance to people from Mongolia; hence the older term 'Mongolism'. In the mind of the nine-teenth century there was a connection between people with 'lower' minds and the 'lower', in this case Far Eastern, races (Gould 1980).

LINKS

For more on history and health, see Chapter 3, where some of the general historical issues mentioned above are discussed in greater depth.

Throughout all the twists and turns mentioned in the above historical sketch, the objective reality concerning the nature of learning disability as an impairment remains in many respects 'stable'. Thus the movement of people with intellectual disabilities – from being part of the community, to being rejected, and back to being seen once more as part of the community – is dependent on changing social attitudes and not on impairment (Goodley 2001).

The above discussion has made claims that there is a move in contemporary society for people with learning disabilities to be included in the wider community. Achieving this ambition is not necessarily straightforwardly unproblematic, and many of the negative images attached to people with learning disabilities still remain. Rooney (2002), for instance, points to issues of being meaningfully part of a community. Just because someone is deemed to be in a community setting, often by virtue of not being in an institution, does not mean they are necessarily part of a community in terms of relationships with other people and local social systems. As with wider disability issues, stigma remains a defining experience for many people with learning disabilities. Full inclusion cannot be considered to have been achieved until that negative relationship has been overcome.

CONCLUSION

This chapter has shown that the human body is not just a biological entity, but is inextricably bound up with society, culture and history. Much of how we project our identity and develop a sense of self that is important and vital in our everyday interactions is performed through and with our bodies. This use of the body is becoming more central in the consumerist society in which we live, where a thin, toned body adorned in the most current of fashion styles is presented as being highly desirable. Television shows, magazines and commercials extol the supposed virtues of such an appearance. Obviously, only a very few people (usually celebrities with financial and other resources) can obtain that look, and the pressure to conform to such appearances can result in misery and suffering for many people.

The importance of the body in identity is brought into sharp relief in relation to chronic illness. Here, the emergence of symptoms and changes in the body disrupts the sense of self and can challenge how we see our lives. This can lead to all sorts of re-evaluations of identity and how to lead a life, with the destabilisation that chronic illness can bring. This 'pessimistic' take on chronic illness should, however, be tempered by research that indicates that sometimes chronic illness is 'not that bad'. Age and class, for example, can provide an emotional resilience and acceptance of chronic illness.

The body and identity are also visible in disability issues. Sociological perspectives focus on disability as the outcome of prejudicial and discriminatory social attitudes and perceptions. Bodies that do not match or that are 'different' from an able-bodied norm are devalued, and disabled people's identities are given a lesser social status. Disabled people have advanced a civil rights agenda to counteract many of the negative and oppressive structures that act against them being fairly treated in society.

SUMMARY POINTS

- The taken-for-granted status of the body has detracted from the significance of the body for students of the sociology of health.

- Human experiences are essentially embodied and this is most true of health and illness.

- The body is a bearer of values and a means of representing our identity to others.

- The civilised body is one that is controlled in terms of both bodily functions and displays of emotion.

- The limits of the physical body are constantly being extended as scientific advances allow us to alter the appearance of our bodies and to replace diseased organs.

- Ideas about the body are underpinned by normative concepts of the 'good' and 'bad' body, the former being associated with bodily perfection.

- Any form of disease, but particularly chronic and terminal conditions, brings into stark reality the limits and fallibility of the human body.

- A 'failed' body forces individuals to reassess their lives and sense of identity – though this is not necessarily a negative experience.

- Disability is a combination of environmental, social, cultural, material and physical factors. Acknowledging disability in this way asks fundamental questions of health professionals when interacting with disabled people.

CASE STUDY

James was diagnosed with rheumatoid arthritis around the time of his eighth birthday. The condition has meant that at times his mobility has been severely affected. Games and sports at school were something that he had to miss out on. Writing for long periods in exams became impossible in his final year and so he produced his work on a laptop in a room separate from the rest of his classmates. After finishing school, James wanted to enter a career in hotel management, but this proved impossible as the work involved a considerable amount of time spent on one's feet, something James could not do without being in severe pain. Instead, he chose a clerical post in the Civil Service which would allow him to be seated for much of the day and to use a PC instead of physically writing.

QUESTIONS

1. Mobility was a problem for James from an early age. What kinds of activities and experiences do you think he might have missed out on compared to other children his age?
2. How might you apply the concept of 'biographical disruption' to James' experiences as a young adult?

> 3. What kind of knowledge would you have expected James to accumulate about this condition? How would this differ from the knowledge of the clinician, and what, if any, would be its relevance to anyone treating James?

TAKING YOUR STUDIES FURTHER

This chapter will have helped you understand many of the key terms, concepts, theories and debates relating to the body. Listed below are journal articles and books that will provide deeper and more detailed discussions of the points raised in this chapter. You will also find additional resources on the companion website, including downloads of relevant material, links to useful websites, videos and other features. Please visit the companion website at https://study.sagepub.com/barryandyuill4e

RECOMMENDED READING

Bordo, S. (1990) 'Reading the slender body', in M. Jacobs, E.F. Keller and S. Shuttleworth (eds), *Body/Politics: Women and the Discourse of Science*. New York: Routledge.

Bury, M. (2001) 'Illness narratives: fact or fiction?', *Sociology of Health & Illness*, 23(3): 263–85.

Pound, P., Gompertz, P. and Ebrahim, S. (1998) 'Illness in the context of older age: the case of stroke', *Sociology of Health & Illness*, 20(4): 489–506.

Shakespeare, T. (2013) *Disability Rights and Wrongs Revisited*. London: Routledge.

Shilling, C. (2013) *The Body and Social Theory*, 3rd edn. London: SAGE.

Shilling, C. (2007) *Embodying Sociology: Retrospect, Progress and Prospects*. Oxford: Blackwell.

Williams, S.J., Bendelow, G. and Birke, L. (2003) *Debating Biology: Sociological Reflections on Health, Medicine and Society*. London: Routledge.

Wouters, E. and De Wet, K. (2015) 'Women's experience of HIV as a chronic illness in South Africa: hard-earned lives, biographical disruption and moral career', *Sociology of Health & Illness*.

HEALTH, AGEING AND THE LIFE COURSE

MAIN POINTS

- Old age and ill health are not necessarily synchronous, with the majority of older people living fit, healthy and active lives.

- Older people can be subject to ageist stereotyping and this can impact on identity and sense of self.

- It is important to understand ageing as taking place in biographical and historical time. Experiences across the life course strongly influence the health of older people.

INTRODUCTION

Globally, populations are becoming older, with more and more people living longer, a transition that is evident in just about all nations (see Figure 11.1). That trend is particularly noticeable in Asian countries and China, where the older population has expanded considerably. There are many reasons for the increase in life expectancy, but mainly it is due to the decline in acute and communicable diseases. However, some regional exceptions do exist. If you examine Figure 11.1, the life expectancy in South Africa dips in the early 2000s due to deaths in the wake of HIV/AIDS. The presence of anti-retroviral therapies (ART) will play a role in allowing people with HIV/AIDS to live longer (as we discussed in Chapter 10 on chronic illness).

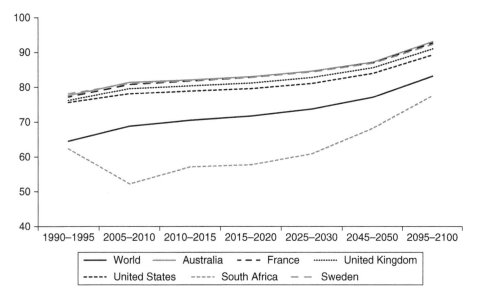

Figure 11.1   Actual and projected life expectancy in selected countries

Source: United Nations (2015)

This demographic shift raises many interesting issues and challenges both for society and for the sociological study of what it means to be an older person. As is explored in this chapter, being older is not a simple case of having grey hair, experiencing worsening health or living alone, as popular stereotypes sometimes hold. Ageing is a complex mix of personal biography, social structure and cultural perceptions of age.

AGEING IN SOCIETY: A GENERAL OVERVIEW

The body begins to age, change and develop from the moment of birth until its eventual death. This, however, should not be read as meaning that ageing is purely a biological phenomenon driven entirely by alterations to the surface layers of skin and hair paralleled by decreasing mental acuity and all-round physiological decline. Rather, ageing, as a phase of one's life, is the product of three factors that all weave together: biology, psychology and the social. Each of these factors can exert an influence on the others. So, for example, going grey may be a physical sign of ageing in some sense, but it depends on the society of which one is a member as to whether having grey hair means someone is deemed to be 'old' and should be treated in a different way from someone who does not have grey hair. It is through the social that experiences of, perceptions about and attitudes towards what it is to be old and what is regarded as being old are mediated and created. Similarly, a society can exert such pressure and stress on someone that this hastens their biological ageing. Among the more overt social aspects of ageing in society are certain negative attitudes expressed by individuals. It is to a discussion of **ageism** that our attention turns next.

Ageism

Ageism comprises: (1) a set of beliefs originating in biological variation related to the ageing process; (2) the actions of corporate bodies and their agents, and the resulting views of ordinary people. It follows that:

1. Ageism generates and reinforces a fear and denigration of the ageing process, and stereotyping presumptions regarding competence and the need for protection;

2. In particular, ageism legitimates the use of chronological age to mark out classes of people who are systematically denied resources and opportunities that others enjoy, and who suffer the consequences of such denigration, ranging from well-meaning patronage to unambiguous vilification. (Bytheway and Johnson 1990, cited in Bytheway 1995: 14)

In other chapters we have looked at discrimination and prejudice in the form of sexism and racism. We have seen how socially created perceptions of people's characteristics (their sex or ethnicity) act as barriers that prevent women and people from ethnic minority groups having a full and equal place in society. Such barriers can have a negative and harmful effect on their health.

Ageism is yet another example of the many prejudices that exist within society. In popular culture there are many examples of this stereotype. A useful example is, arguably, Abe Simpson, the grandpa character in *The Simpsons*. In the episodes in which Abe appears, the comedy content is generated by Abe falling asleep at inopportune moments or embarking on long rambling stories about his youth. Instances such as these match popular stereotypes that all old people are 'demented' and in poor health.

Ageism is, however, more than just finding old people amusing. It can take many other forms as well. At its worst it can be structurally located and act as a barrier to older people receiving appropriate health care. Age Concern England (ACE 2002b) has noted the presence of two forms of ageism within the NHS. The first is *direct ageism*, namely instances when actual policy or guidelines prevent someone from receiving appropriate health care based directly on their age. This is a very overt and easy-to-identify form of discrimination. The other form of ageism, *indirect ageism*, is more subtle and is concerned with attitudes and assumptions that the health of older people is less important than that of younger people.

QUESTIONS

Identify positive and negative portrayals of older people in society. Which type of image is more frequently visible? Why do you think there is prejudice and discrimination against old people in current society?

BODIES AND AGEING

Despite the fact that this is the fate of us all, old age is often associated with negative images and attitudes. The earlier discussion of the sociology of the body illustrated the importance of our physical self for our sense of identity, and from this it is possible to see that the visible signs of ageing (greying hair and developing wrinkles, for example) act as a set of symbols, which can be read in often prejudicial and negative ways in society. This is especially so in a consumer society where an old body is often perceived as a less socially valued and acceptable body than a young, fit, fat-free and athletic body. Indeed, the ever-increasing range of cosmetics offering to hold back the onset of the signs of ageing is another way in which both the body is commodified (essentially one is compelled to purchase a youthful face and body) and youth is prioritised. Youth is clearly associated with notions of optimum physical performance (hence sports people are 'old' in their mid-thirties), cognitive ability and attractiveness. In contrast, old age is seen as a period of decline marked, for example, by loss of height and by wrinkled skin. This social impulse to maintain youth is especially problematic for women, who, unlike men, are likely to be judged on their physical appearance – their looks – rather on any other criteria.

The continuing importance of the body and images of ageing can also be seen in the next example. One of the most important activities that we do with our bodies is to dress and present it with clothes that accord with what we wish to say about ourselves and what we believe to be socially appropriate. This can be a difficult balancing act at any stage of one's life, given the strong pressure to meet certain consumerist and cultural expectations. There are, though, certain issues that older people have to negotiate when they choose what to wear. Twigg (2007, 2013) draws our attention to how clothing is 'age ordered', with certain styles of clothes deemed both age appropriate and a signifier of age. In some respects, this can be seen as an informal policing of how older people (women in particular) present themselves as they grow older. Often this means a toning down of style and opting for less 'flamboyant' styles. Twigg (2007: 296) uses an example from research by Holland (2004) to illustrate this point. Here, women who have an alternative style of dress (for example, grunge and Goth styles involving dreadlocks, piercings and tattoos) indicated a sense of apprehension about having to alter their appearance as they grew older. The women in this study were worried that their alternative stylistic difference, which was an important part of their youthful identity, would be seen as being 'grotesque' if they maintained it into their middle years and beyond. The two phrases that sum up the association between youth, attractiveness and age are 'growing old gracefully' and 'mutton dressed as lamb' (Fairhurst 1998: 261). Both phrases make assumptions about age-appropriate actions and appearance. Mutton is older, tougher meat than youthful and tender lamb. Fairhurst's respondents all interpreted 'mutton dressed as lamb' as the wearing of 'inappropriate clothes, hair, make-up or jewellery' (1998: 262).

Featherstone and Hepworth (1993) also draw our attention to the largely negative terms used to describe older people. Such words include 'wrinkly', 'gaga', 'biddy', 'fogey' and 'geriatric' (1993: 308). The biological process of ageing is 'shaped or constructed in terms of symbolic imagery, both verbal and non verbal' (1993: 308). Words and images are used as stereotypes to make sense of and describe the experiences of older people. The danger of such stereotypes is that they fail to reflect the complexity and diversity of people's experiences of ageing.

These negative images of old age can permeate all aspects of ageing in society. One of the most common stereotypes is that old age is synonymous with decline and dependency, and that ageing is *itself* a disease or illness. These assumptions provide a useful starting point for a discussion of the assumed association between old age and ill health. As we will go on to discuss, many older people, on the contrary, enjoy a life relatively free from sickness and dependency. The same negative stereotyping of individuals on the basis of sickness and dependency can, arguably, be seen in relation to people with disabilities. Such an association may, therefore, lead us to conclude that it is the assumption of dependency and of an inability to perform socially that is the source of the discrimination, rather than the actual age of the person.

Thus far we have given consideration to images of old age. The following section is concerned with placing those images within a theoretical context. The aim of this discussion is to illustrate through a sociological analysis that, much more than simply a physiological experience, age is fundamentally a social experience.

SOCIOLOGICAL THEORIES OF AGEING

Sociology offers a number of perspectives, all of which seek to explain the social situation, status and role of older people. **Disengagement theory** offers what might appear in the twenty-first century a rather dated perspective on ageing and the role of older people. Cumming and Henry (1961) suggested that as people reach old age they gradually disengage from society, in terms of their social contacts, roles and responsibilities. The process of disengagement prepares the older person and society in general for the ultimate disengagement in the form of death or incapacity (Bond et al. 2007). Disengagement theory is based on a broader functionalist perspective of society with its emphasis on the roles, responsibilities and values that ensure the smooth running of the social structure. By disengaging, for example through retirement from the paid workforce, individuals cease to be essential to the functioning of the social structure. On this basis, their death does not result in any significant disruption since older people have ceased to be part of the workforce.

Disengagement theory states that older people relinquish their roles in society so as to minimise social disruption as they approach their final years.

Bond et al. (2007) highlight a number of problems with this perspective on ageing. They argue, first, that disengagement theory condones the social isolation and marginalisation of older people, which for many results in poverty and loneliness. Second, they suggest that this theory is based on an assumption that disengagement is a natural and inevitable occurrence. It is possible to argue that the theory is essentially ageist in the sense that it assumes identical experiences for all older people. However, as Bond et al. (2007) point out, many older people may still be actively engaged in society, while for others old age is part of a life-long experience of non-engagement and social isolation. The final criticism that can be made of disengagement theory is its failure to appreciate that certain social practices (such as enforced retirement from the paid workforce) and cultural values (ageism) combine to ensure that disengagement does become the experience of many older people. In this sense, we can perhaps appreciate that disengagement is the consequence of a specific set of social arrangements rather than a natural and inevitable part of the experience of ageing.

> **LINK**
>
> Disengagement theory is closely related to the functionalist perspective outlined in Chapter 1.

In contrast to disengagement theory, an alternative explanation of the experience of older people centres on the social creation of dependency. The essence of **dependency theory** is that older people are constructed as dependent on the state, primarily through exclusion from the paid workforce. Such exclusion also means that older people are further isolated from a wide variety of social settings, relationships and networks. Data indicate that older people constitute one of the groups most at risk of poverty because of their dependence largely on welfare benefits. The potential effects of retirement are, according to Bond et al., poverty and restricted 'access to social resources in the form of a reduction in social relationships' (1993: 34).

> Dependency theory claims that older people's lives are restricted by poverty and not being able to access social and cultural resources.

So far, the discussion has focused on what may be seen as pessimistic perspectives on ageing. We shall now turn to what might be regarded as more optimistic perspectives – where growing older opens up the possibilities of a phase in one's life that is filled with rich and rewarding experiences, free of the binds of work and other commitments. Such perspectives also draw our attention to some of the complexities of growing older in contemporary society, brought about by changes in welfare provision and the all-pervasive influence of consumer culture offering a range of possibilities on *how* to be an older person. Here, older people are seen to have more freedom to choose and decide their own identities and lifestyles.

Key to this more optimistic perspective is the work of Laslett (1987, 1989) and, more recently, Higgs and Gilleard (2015) and the concept of the **Third Age**. The concept of the Third Age calls for a reworking of how society views the different stages of moving through life. Essentially, the Third Age involves a transition from various states of dependence to independence and from responsibility to increasing freedom and flexibility. So, the First Age is childhood, when we

> Third Age theory points to old age as being a 'golden age' where enriching and rewarding experiences are available due to freedom from family and work commitments mediated by a consumerist society.

are dependent on our parents. The Second Age is the independence of being a mature person and being able to provide for ourselves, but perhaps being hemmed in by the responsibilities of raising a family and holding down a job. The Third Age is a period of life between later middle age and early older age. It is marked by increasing freedom from the constraints of work and family concerns, and can also be a 'golden age' occupied with activities that lead to a sense of fulfilment, self-realisation and personal growth. More recently, Laslett (1996) has added a Fourth Age, where physical decline and health problems begin to dominate the experiences of people in deeper old age, that is those over the age of 75.

The Third Age has been made possible by the increasing numbers, affluence and health of older people. This, combined with a consumer culture which blurs many of the distinctions between the age groups, has allowed older people to escape the social expectations of how they should lead their lives and to strike out and create identities of their own.

There are, however, criticisms of this approach. For example, Bury (2000) has raised objections that the research is 'data light', meaning that more research has to be carried out to see whether this Third Age is actually happening, or whether it is more of an idea of what could happen given the changes indicated above. Another criticism is that this phase of self-realisation after one has retired is only open to those with the financial means to accomplish it. One could argue that poverty still affects the lives of many older people, thus effectively preventing them from engaging in the consumerist activities that are so much part of the Third Age. Just over 20% of pensioners are living in poverty (ONS 2005a), though this is worse for older people from ethnic minority backgrounds and people in deeper old age.

QUESTION

Which sociological theory of ageing do you find the most persuasive, and why?

HEALTH AND THE LIFE COURSE

As was outlined above, there is often an almost taken-for-granted association between ageing, disability and ill health. The reality is far different, with many older people living healthy, active lives, especially the 'younger' old. A closer examination of these figures does, however, reveal some subtle but important differences. In terms of gender, older women experience more health problems than men of the same age. It is also clear that some distinction should be made between age groups within the catch-all category of old age. Field (1992) draws a distinction between the 'young old' and the 'old old', the former below age 75 and the latter over 85. Although the cut-off points might seem a little arbitrary, they are nevertheless helpful in identifying a trend towards increased levels of disability and ill health among older people over the age of 75 (1992: 276).

Being old is simply – and obviously – not just always having been a certain age for all one's life. Older age is just another of the many elements and phases that go to make up one's life. How that life is lived, however, greatly influences health in the older years, in terms of both developing long-term illness or disability, for example, and shaping how illness and health are experienced and perceived. A useful concept in trying to understand this relationship between health and old age is that of the **life course** (Hockey and James 2003). In the past, moving through life was conceptualised as being similar to a cycle and commonly expressed using the term **life cycle**. Aspects of moving through life in this context were seen as inescapable certainties in life encountered by every generation. This included such events as school, work, marriage and starting a family. Overall, life-cycle approaches conceive life as being a set of rigid stages that one goes through without any variance or personal choice. In contrast, life in this current phase of modernity has become increasingly complex, fluid and fragmented. The certainties that are implied in a life-cycle approach are no longer with us and there are now great variations in how people experience and choose to live their lives. So, for example, people increasingly do not always enter into marriage or may delay having children, if they make that decision at all. By seeing life as a *course* that one takes through life where one has a certain latitude in making choices, rather than a *cycle* over which one has little control, such variety can be easier to understand.

> Life course is a way of conceptualising the passage of life that better recognises the increasing fluidity and fragmentation of contemporary society, and the interaction of individual agency and social structure.
>
> Life cycle is a concept borrowed from natural science, implying a series of set rigid stages that humans move through in their lives.

Regarding ageing in the context of both 'biographical' and 'historical' time is important to the life-course approach (Bury 2000). Biographical time refers to the personal events in your life: for example, developing relationships, or choosing to go travelling, or what you did at university. Historical time refers to the events and social attitudes that mark particular phases in history: for example, the Second World War, or the changes in attitudes towards sexuality that took place in the 1960s. Though biographical time and historical time may seem quite different, they do relate to each other. Historical time can set the scene for what happens and unfolds in biographical time, giving a particular generation a shared set of beliefs and common experiences.

QUESTION

Sketch out your life course so far. Identify both your biographical time and the historical time in which you live. What aspects of historical time help shape the identity of your generation?

Thinking of ageing in this way helps us to understand older people's health in two main respects. First, acknowledging a biographical element allows us to see that not all older people are a homogeneous social group and alike in all manner of ways. Rather, it draws attention to the importance of difference and how people can age in the same historical time but do so in their own individual ways, and how events in their past affect their health in the present. Second, the historical element can help us understand that people are part of a particular generation and that the experience of being part of that generation (this is called a *cohort effect*) shapes their health beliefs and attitudes towards illness. Ultimately, though, it is the human body on which the experiences of both biographical and historical time will be 'recorded', in terms of good or bad health in older age. Blane et al. (2004: 2171) usefully summarise this point:

> The body can be seen as a mechanism which stores the past benefits and dis-benefits to which it has been exposed, either because damage at a critical period of development causes irreparable loss or because the effects of various types of damage accumulate over time.

So, for example, coming from a deprived background in childhood and working in an occupation that was tightly supervised and low in control could lead to poor health for an older person. Conversely, the opposite – material stability and an enjoyable career – is much more likely to mean good health for an older person. These are themes that we have explored in other chapters and that indicate, once more, how social influences, such as class, strongly influence health. Berney et al. (2000), for instance, found that both negative material and psycho-social factors from childhood onwards can greatly impact on our health as we become older. From the residential and occupational histories of 294 people aged between 63 and 78 they found differences in social class and gender for health that were related to the lived and working experiences of the people in the study.

LINK

See Chapter 10 on the body for more discussion of the sociological perspectives on the body and chronic illness.

A useful illustration of how life-course experiences and events impact on health can be found in the following extract from research by Sanders et al. (2002) into the experiences of older people with painful joints brought about by osteoarthritis. What is evident here is how this interviewee clearly saw her current poor health as the outcome of the hardship that had been a defining feature of her life:

> I've always done a job that involves a lot of steps and kneeling, and I've always worked because we had this old house that was condemned and you couldn't get new houses during the war, and when my husband came out of the army, we didn't have much money, he was on the buildings so ... I used to do part-time work. And I done over there 15 years picking mushrooms across the road part

time while the children were at school. And after that finished I went in different shops just working odd hours so that I was here when the children were here. Whether it was the wear and tear on the knees. But anyway, after about 20 years, I was walking on two sticks, you know during the time I was working. (int. 8, 82 years, occupational class IV) (Sanders et al. 2002: 235)

The life course also shapes how older people come to view and experience illness. In Chapter 10, when we looked at chronic illness, we noted the research of Pound et al. (1998). They found that for the older people in their study who had survived a stroke, possible disruption to their lives was lessened by their attitudes. As a generation, their experiences of historical time had been of self-denial and coping with the problems life presented to them due to living through the privations of the Second World War. It was these events that forged a common stoical approach to life. For this generation, a health problem was no different from the many other problems they expected to encounter.

DEMENTIA

As has been stressed throughout this chapter, being an older person does not automatically entail being ill. This is a popular misconception, for the majority of older people enjoy fulfilling and healthy lives. There are, however, certain conditions that do affect older people more than other sections of the population. One of these is dementia. The World Health Organisation (WHO 2015) indicates that 47.5 million people have dementia and predict that there will be 7.7 million new cases every year, and that this is a major cause of disability in older age. Dementia refers to a variety of degenerative conditions affecting the higher functions of the brain, with memory loss being one of the most unsettling symptoms both for people with dementia and for their families. Out of the 100 different forms of dementia the most common are Alzheimer's disease, vascular dementia, and dementia with Lewy bodies. In this section we shall mainly focus on Alzheimer's disease.

Dementia demonstrates a point that was made earlier: that ageing is the result of social, biological and psychological influences. Undoubtedly dementia has a biological basis, with a variety of causes including, for example, changes in the brain chemistry, restriction of oxygen to the brain, and degeneration of nerve cells and brain tissue. It also has psychological aspects, the most notable being memory impairment. Some aspects of dementia are, however, very social in their effects and create issues for maintaining a sense of who we are and how we relate to other people. It is to these issues that we now turn.

As a degenerative condition the effects of dementia unfold over time, beginning with disturbances in memory and progressing to substantial or complete memory loss in addition to physical frailty, speech impairment and emotional disturbance. This corrosion of memory and intellectual function can cause a potential destabilising of self and identity. In effect, someone can lose the memories of their life and the facets of their personality that make them who they are, and this has implications for their ability to function as a social being. Much of how we communicate with others is based on how we present ourselves in conversations, for example. During such interactions, what we say, and how we respond to the prompts and questions of others, communicate how we wish to be seen. Dementia can make this whole situation problematic. Either the person with dementia finds it difficult to engage in the expected way or the person they are interacting with is unable to adapt to the person with dementia.

People in the early stages of dementia have an awareness of the changes and transformations that are taking place in their lives as the condition begins to alter their memory and other cognitive functions. This is a difficult and worrying phase, not just because of the changes they detect in themselves, but also because of the changes in how other people react to them. Langdon et al. (2007) found that a variety of issues could cause concern for people in the early stages of dementia. For example, the actual name of the condition could cause upset. 'Dementia' sounds very similar to the word 'demented', with its implications of being 'without mind'. This could, according to the people in the study, lead to them being viewed by others as 'short on top', 'a bit funny' or 'crackers'. Being seen negatively, or being stigmatised, by others could cause unease in other ways too. Revealing their diagnosis was fraught with risk as it was feared that other people would not really understand the condition, as this extract from a woman with dementia illustrates:

> I haven't told anyone. I think they will treat me differently. I wouldn't be upset though, it depends what they know. If they have heard about it and don't understand they would treat me differently. They think it's something bad – they would scorn you and not want to come near you and fully believe you are like that. (Langdon et al. 2007: 995)

How dementia is perceived is also critical in how we care for people with dementia. In Chapter 16, where we discuss how medical technologies are changing approaches to the care of people with long-term conditions, we discuss the contradictions surrounding people with dementia and technology. New technologies can either be liberating or restrictive for older people. For Wigg (2012), it was how care institutions understood dementia that was vital. In her research focusing on two different institutional settings, she found the institution that medicalised wandering often used technology to constrain residents with dementia, while the other institution, which offered a different understanding of people with dementia – namely that they needed freedom – used technology to enable that freedom to be as safe as possible.

LINK

See Chapter 8 on stigma and how social attitudes can have an adverse effect on people's sense of identity.

Ultimately, the almost complete loss of memory leads to a 'social death', where the physical body is still alive but the self is, in many ways, no longer there. One has to take care not to see 'social death' as an absolute state. Often it can depend on the views of other people, particularly relatives and carers, who, for a variety of legitimate and personal reasons, may not share an 'objective' assessment that a loved one has undergone a 'social death'. Also, as Sabat (2001) points out, for people with Alzheimer's disease, personhood and the self are not completely 'wiped out'. He stresses that many aspects of some form of self continue to be present; that ignoring them is to deny the person's humanity; and that as much as possible should be done to support and nurture the sense of self of someone with dementia.

Sweeting and Gilhooly (1997) found many complexities and subtleties in how carers managed their encounters and relationships with a spouse or family member with dementia. Their research uncovered various strategies that carers had developed, focusing on a combination of believing and behaving as if a loved one was socially dead. This could mean stating openly that the person with dementia might be better off if they passed away, for instance, while perhaps caring for that person on a physical rather than a social or emotional level. Other carers in the survey adopted a different strategy: while accepting that the person they were caring for was socially dead, their behaviour towards that person was otherwise. This entailed carrying on as much as possible with life as it had been prior to the onset of dementia. For example, they would make sure that the person with dementia was always included in social interaction and that familiar activities, such as playing bingo, still went ahead. A third group believed and behaved as if the person with dementia was not socially dead.

The above discussion has sought to highlight the range, extent and consequences of disease and disability among older people. It is clear that while there are specific conditions associated with the onset of old age, many people experience an old age relatively free of such complaints. Significantly, the consequences of disease and acute conditions may be considerably different for older people than for the younger population. Older people have a greater tendency to experience multiple pathologies, with each condition compounding the one before. Their health experiences have also to be considered within a social context where ageing is seen in negative terms and assumptions are made about the inevitability of disease and decline as part of the ageing process.

CONCLUSION

The main message both from this discussion and from current research is that old age does not automatically equate with infirmity, disability or poor health. Indeed, the majority of older people lead active and healthy lives. What do create issues and challenges for older people are the negative stereotypes and images attached to being old in contemporary society. Ageist attitudes still persist, whether these are expressed in the actions of private individuals or institutions.

What it means to be older in the early part of the twenty-first century is quite different from other times. Being older now can be (for those with the requisite resources) a phase in life where ambitions and life goals can be realised. Old age does not automatically mean poverty or deprivation. The increasing numbers of older people allied with the rise of a consumerist society, through which they can express their identity and sense of self, will hopefully lead to a re-evaluation of how older people are perceived and understood.

SUMMARY POINTS

- Old age is an inevitable phase of human lives, yet can be subject to negative ageist attitudes.

- The vast majority of older people enjoy healthy active lives and it is incorrect to assume that old age automatically means poor health.

- What it is to be old in contemporary society is changing, with many older people enjoying a 'golden age' in their lives made possible by access to consumer culture.

- The life course is a combination of historical and biographical time.

- Older people's lives are influenced by their experiences over their life course. Those with employment histories that are low in control and status tend to have poorer health as they age.

CASE STUDY

Joan's first memories as a very young child aged 5 are of an air raid during the Second World War when she was growing up in Glasgow. She remembers the sound of the sirens and the deafening explosion of a bomb falling on her street. She also remembers her mother constantly telling her off for wasting things, whether it was food, clothing or just about anything. But that was all part of the scarcity of the war years and in the rest of the 1940s when she was growing up. This culture of thrift and saving up for a rainy day made a big impression on her. These were to be values she would hold throughout her life.

In early 1961 she met Dave, who asked her to marry him a year later. Life in the 1960s was a great deal more pleasurable than it had been previously. Dave and Joan managed to find themselves well-paid jobs and, even though Joan still saved and was always reluctant to buy anything she considered unnecessary, they both enjoyed themselves. Music was a particular past-time. First it was the Beatles, and then some of the more obscure and alternative American bands as the 1960s progressed. Despite her thrift, Joan had one passion: clothes. She remembered her own mum as only having one or two outfits, but now there was so much choice and each season had new styles, and there was so much more to buy than ever before.

Life carried on in this vein into the 1970s. Now in their early 30s Dave and Joan began a family of their own. All went well, Dave had promotion at work and they gained a modest level of affluence. Not enough, perhaps, to regard themselves as well-off, but definitely as comfortable. Life progressed reasonably well during the 1980s, but Joan and Dave noticed that the Conservative government of the day was making changes to the welfare state, and many of the sureties of state provision that they assumed would be there as they grew older were beginning to be rolled back. However, the ability to save and be good with money, which they learned in her early life, served Joan well. She made sure that enough money was put away each month in a private pension plan and other investments.

In the early 2000s both Joan and Dave retired. With their children now mature adults leading their own lives and away from home, Joan and Dave found that they had both the free time and the financial resources to do something with that time. Joan found that she could rekindle her youthful penchant for clothes and dressed very stylishly, although she always felt tentative about trying on anything that was too 'young' for her. She and Dave also began to travel. They had a holiday in San Francisco. This allowed them to realise a lifetime ambition: visiting the city where so many of their favourite bands came from during the 1960s.

Lately, as Joan is now in her early seventies, she's noticed that she is beginning to feel a little tired more often, and finding it much harder both to move around her house and go about in town. This is unsettling for her as she always liked to be active. She also dislikes the idea of how other people act towards her. The other day someone called her an OAP – that made her feel old. But, as she herself always points out, life is what you make it.

QUESTIONS

1. Which of the three sociological theories concerning ageing best fits this case study?
2. Identify how Joan's experiences in both biographical and historical time have influenced her life.
3. In what ways has consumerism been a part of Joan's life?
4. Why is the presentation of the body so important in contemporary society?

TAKING YOUR STUDIES FURTHER

This chapter will have helped you understand many of the key terms, concepts, theories and debates relating to health, ageing and the life course. Listed below are books that will provide deeper and more detailed discussions of the points raised in this chapter. You will also find additional resources on the companion website, including downloads of relevant material, links to useful websites, videos and other features. Please visit the companion website at https://study.sagepub.com/barryandyuill4e

RECOMMENDED READING

Higgs, P. and Gilleard, C. (2015) *Rethinking Old Age: Theorising the Fourth Age*. London: Palgrave Macmillan.

Twigg, J. (2013) *Fashion and Age: Dress, the Body and Later Life*. London: Bloomsbury.

SECTION 3

CONTEXTS

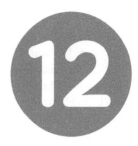

PLACES OF CARE

MAIN POINTS

- Health and social care occurs in distinct places, and these places can exert influences over that care and the quality of life for the people receiving that care.

- Many sociological theories draw attention to the problems of institutional care, which at worst can result in a loss of identity and residents becoming institutionalised.

- Recent shifts towards community care bring fresh challenges. There exist problems in defining community, and evidence suggests that community involvement is giving way to increasing individualism.

- Informal care given by friends and family is an important feature of supporting and looking after people in the community.

- The act of caring can bring about changes in the home and in relationships between those who receive and those who give care.

INTRODUCTION

All health care takes place in some spatial context or location, whether it is a hospital, an institution or the community. Each of these contexts brings with it a range of issues and challenges, all of which are open to sociological interpretation. This chapter will begin by looking at organisations generally and evaluate some of the major theories that attempt to understand institutions. Max Weber's classic theory of rationality and bureaucracy will be outlined, followed by Michel Foucault's views on the organisation of physical space and surveillance. How people subvert and manage to bend the rules will be examined next.

Where health care takes place is often decided by **social policy**, as we discuss in Chapter 13, and in some countries there has been a shift towards caring for people in the community as opposed to institutional settings. Critiques of institutional or asylum care will be discussed, focusing on the work of Foucault and Andrew Scull. More attention will be given to Erving Goffman's seminal work on institutionalisation and the negative effects of institutional care. Care in the community was proposed as an alternative and better form of care. However, it too is problematic. One difficulty is in trying to define what a community really is, with multiple and different uses of the concept in existence. Even if a definition can be agreed upon, there still exists a debate about whether **community care** actually changes anything, and some comments will be made on how the community may just be an extension of the institution. Finally, there will be some discussion of the many issues facing carers in the community, highlighting what care involves and some of the problems facing carers.

ORGANISATIONS

For many people the hospital is still the expected place or context for the provision of health care. Like many other examples of large organisations, hospitals have complex bureaucracies, operate surveillance, and often involve the management of thousands of bodies. Unlike other examples of large organisations, however, they are expected to effect a positive physical or mental change in some of the people who enter through the front doors. This means that although we can use an array of sociological perspectives to understand large institutions, we must also pay attention to the differences that arise from them making life-or-death decisions about people. Attention will be given to the classic work of Weber on bureaucracy and organisations. How the physical layout of a hospital and use of surveillance affect patients and staff will be examined with reference to the work of Foucault. How people 'subvert' organisations will also be discussed.

Weber, organisations and bureaucracy

The ideas of Weber (1997, 2001) about rationality are a useful starting point. Weber, writing at the turn of the twentieth century, saw all human activity as purposeful, and in investigating society it is important to try to identify what meanings people attach to what they do; he termed this *Verstehen*, or understanding. To this end he identified the following three forms of action:

- *Affective or emotional action.* This is action that results from an individual emotional state at a given time. If we feel happy and caring we may wish to spend longer with a patient or be more caring than we might if our mood was bad.
- *Traditional action.* We engage in certain forms of activity because we always have, to the extent that we may be unaware that we are doing it. An example of this could be the British habit of saying 'sorry' or 'cheers' in a variety of situations even though we might not actually want to apologise or wish someone good health.
- *Rational action.* This is purposeful activity where there is an intended outcome to our actions. To achieve particular ends we must also take into account what we need

and what is the best way of reaching our intended outcome. An occupational therapist devising a treatment plan, working out what goals a client can reach and what is required to reach those goals, is an example of this.

For Weber the key to understanding the modern capitalist period was the increase of rationalisation in every aspect of life. He saw a move away from spontaneity and the outward expression of emotion towards a society in which every aspect is governed by rules, procedures or non-spontaneous practices, all grounded in logical, rational science. To this end, he characterised mankind's condition in modernity as living in an 'iron cage'.

Weber's analysis of bureaucracy and organisations is distilled into what he termed an *ideal type*. By ideal type he does not mean what an organisation should be, but rather a pure form by which to measure a particular organisation. The closer to this ideal, the more effective the organisation will be:

- *Everybody knows what they are meant to do.* Everyone in an organisation should have a clear knowledge of what they are meant to do and what their responsibilities are.
- *It's clear who is in charge and who you are accountable to.* Effective organisation requires effective leadership, which operates in a clear-cut, hierarchical manner.
- *Everybody follows the rules.* There are clear procedures and guidelines for whatever is undertaken within the institution.
- *Those in an organisation act with as little emotion as possible.* Decisions are based on the rules and not on personal whims or desires.
- *Your position is a result of how well you can do the job.* This reflects your knowledge and expertise.
- *Work and home are entirely separate spheres.* No aspect of the organisation is owned by an individual and what happens in work cannot be used for private gain.

QUESTIONS

Do you recognise any of Weber's ideas in places where you have worked or had placements? If you do, did these make for efficient organisation?

Physical layout, surveillance and Foucault

Every hospital is a specifically designed building, with certain features that aid its particular function. In hospitals we find rooms that are designed or designated as treatment rooms, operating theatres or consultation rooms. This may seem a

LINK

Chapter 1 discusses the ideas of Foucault further.

useful and logical way of organising space so as to manage the complexities and functions of hospital work. Foucault (1970, 1979a), however, argues that the design of architectural space is not always for some neutral utilitarian function, but often reflects power balances, authority and ways of controlling people. Prior (1993) discusses a mental health hospital built in the 1950s where there existed separate wards for black and white people, with fewer separate facilities for black people. This is a clear example of how prevailing racist attitudes at the time were made 'concrete' in the construction of a building, with the intention to enforce a particular racist discourse on the people who were sent there for 'care'. Modern-day hospitals may not possess such obvious examples of control, but space is managed for specific reasons. In NHS hospitals, in particular, most space is highly impersonal, with people on large open wards. Senior figures often have their own spaces that are at a distance from the rest of the staff to indicate their higher power and status.

QUESTIONS

Next time you are in a hospital or a surgery, look at the layout of physical space. Are there any power relationships that you can detect? Is the space organised so as to facilitate control over those who use it?

The most useful aspect of Foucault's work is on **surveillance**. Part of every modern organisation depends on, and subjects bodies to, surveillance. Surveillance can be seen to exist in two different forms:

Direct observation

This is where people are directly monitored or observed either by a superior or by someone in a position of authority or responsibility. Again, think of a hospital ward and how the actual space (see previous comments) is set out so that someone can monitor what is going on. In addition to making sure that the patients are receiving care and their health is not at risk, surveillance also checks that they are behaving themselves and acting in a manner that complies with the rules of the institution. There is also surveillance of staff, to make sure that they are working and performing their tasks. This may sound innocuous, but Foucault maintains that it creates a form of control whereby people become compliant to forms of authority or power.

Written records

An increasing and ever-growing aspect of contemporary life is the vast amount of data, whether electronic or written, that is kept about us. Each of us accrues numerous records concerning tax, educational attainment, criminal records, career progress, health, and so on. These records are a more insidious method of control, as what is written down can have a dramatic effect on areas such as career and employment. In a healthcare context, vast amounts of information can be kept about an individual. This information could have a bearing on how well someone is cared for and treated when they have, for example, potentially stigmatising conditions such as HIV or some form of mental illness.

Blau and informal routines

This outline of the various theories about organisations so far may give the impression that either we are like *Star Trek*'s 'The Borg', living as completely perfect rational, emotionless drones working for the greater good of the collective or organisation, or we are being constantly monitored. However, other studies, and Foucault himself, noted that people develop ways of subverting the routines and overall controls of organisations. The more sociologists studied organisations, the more they found layers of subtlety and nuance that were missing from Weber's account.

Peter Blau (1963), for example, found that instead of workers rigidly sticking to the rules and complying with the bureaucracy, a whole host of informal working practices can develop. These informal practices, *contra* Weber, can actually improve the overall working of an institution. Often the complexities of what an organisation has to deal with cannot be covered by contingencies in the bureaucracy and a certain flexibility is required, though never officially sanctioned. Workers may prefer these informal working practices as they can act as a relief or as a way of overcoming the effects of working for a potentially suffocating, alienating bureaucracy.

Technological changes can also have an effect on organisations and bureaucracies. The recent and massive expansion of the internet and computer-based technologies promises to change our working and private lives.

QUESTIONS

Have you encountered examples of working where informal routines were used that went against the formal rules? Do you think the informal routines produced a better, more efficient outcome than the formal rules?

INSTITUTIONS

Research has indicated that institutional care can be damaging to the health and identity of those being looked after. Writers such as Goffman, and more recently Prior (1993), have noted that individuals can become institutionalised by their extended stay inside long-term places of care.

Institutions, or asylums as they were formerly known, have long been a feature of care within western countries and their contribution to providing effective care has been much debated. Some authors assert that by a rational progress various innovators develop new and more humane and effective techniques, while other authors note that institutions fit into the existing patterns of social control and act as agents for dominant social groups or the needs of capitalism. The writers Foucault and Scull were proponents of this view.

Foucault's critique of institutions

For Foucault, the history and development of the asylum or institutional care are linked with the growth of surveillance, discipline and notions of scientific rationality from the period of the Enlightenment onwards. He concentrates on how the focus of the 'other' shifted away from the lepers of the Middle Ages, who had been excluded from society, to the mad in the modern period. In the medieval period, leprosy and lepers were a pariah group, the 'other' of society, routinely excluded from social acceptance and admittance to everyday life. People who were mentally ill were regarded as possessed by demons or witchcraft. Later, the emphasis on scientific rationality and scientific investigation during the Enlightenment led to increasing classification, and consequently increasing control of the population. The mad, those designated as irrational and lacking in reason, now came under particular scrutiny. Such a group posed a challenge to the new orthodoxy of rationality, and so it was they who were separated from society, this time not to leper colonies but to asylums and other places of containment (Pilgrim and Rogers 2014; Turner and Samson 1995).

Foucault highlights the use in the nineteenth century of English philosopher Jeremy Bentham's (1748–1832) Panopticon design for asylums. The Panopticon (the all-seeing eye) allows for the continual regulation and surveillance of inmates. A central tower allows observation of every cell whenever a guard or warden wishes. This gives the authorities great power to classify and control those in their charge.

Foucault is critical of what on the surface are seen as liberal and progressive forms of treatment. Figures such as William Tuke and Philippe Pinel are often credited with bringing the treatment of mentally ill people out of the Dark Ages and into the Enlightenment. Tuke founded his famous Retreat near York in 1796, where kindness and benevolence were to be the moral basis of treatment in place of the degrading, inhuman treatment that had existed before. Tuke wanted a 'desire for esteem' to replace 'the principle of fear' (Morgan et al. 1985: 152). A few years earlier, in 1792, Pinel had unchained the inmates of the Bicêtre asylum south of Paris and founded his *traitement moral*. For Foucault, though, these were not the humanitarian breakthroughs that they are sometimes represented as being. For him, it was the replacement of one form of control (physical) by another (moral). The mad were no longer bound with chains but with strict regimes and routines backed up by moral and religious teachings, a more subtle and insidious, but just as effective, form of control (Samson 1995). The purpose of these moral controls was to turn those in the asylum into 'docile bodies': manageable, controlled entities who posed no threat to the authorities.

Scull's critique of institutions

The Marxist writer Andrew Scull (1979) takes a different position from that of Foucault in that he concentrates on the needs of capitalism, on the medical profession and on the effects of urbanisation on the development of the asylum. For him, the asylum was a 'dumping ground' for those superfluous to the needs of capitalism who did not fit into the new market-led economies that developed during the nineteenth century. The poor and unemployed who were capable of working were sent to the workhouses, while those who were incapable were sent to the new asylums. Thus the removal of potentially awkward members of society allowed for the smooth accumulation of capital.

LINK

Chapter 1 discusses Marxist ideas further.

Scull also draws attention to the opportunistic nature of the emerging medical profession. By absorbing Tuke's ideas on moral treatment into its body of scientific knowledge, the profession was able to persuade Parliament to pass the County Asylums Act and the Lunacy Act of 1845. This gave the medical profession a monopoly in the field of madness, and since they now had the power to define madness, as well as control it, they could ensure a steady clientele for their services (Pilgrim and Rogers 2014; Turner and Samson 1995). Throughout the nineteenth century there were substantial increases in the number of people inside asylums or classed as insane:

- In 1849 there were 27,000 inmates in 23 asylums.
- In 1909 there were 105,000 inmates in 97 asylums.

Both Foucault and Scull offer a view of the rise of the asylum that counters notions of a steady, value-free evolution of care for mentally ill people. For these writers, wider social and cultural forces influence and shape the development of institutions and asylums.

Goffman's critique of institutions

Whatever the origins of asylum care historically, there was a reappraisal of the effectiveness of institutions in the twentieth century, especially in the post-war period. During the 1960s the 'anti-psychiatry movement', which included writers such as R.D. Laing and Thomas Szasz, started to challenge assumptions about the nature of mental illness and its treatment, favouring a more open, patient-centred approach. Alongside this challenge to psychiatry, Goffman questioned the role of the asylum. In his seminal text *Asylums* (1961) he sought to delve beneath the surface of psychiatric institutions and expose the problems that asylum and institutional care could create. His basic premise was that the needs of the institution came before the needs of the patient, and this resulted in a change of identity for the patient. In becoming institutionalised, the patient's whole personality is transformed into a shadow of its former self, and motivation, independence and individuality are lost.

Goffman begins his analysis by observing that we live in a world of institutions, whether workplaces or religious, educational or military establishments. However, there are some institutions in society that are different. These he terms 'total institutions'. In these all the normally separate parts of daily life (such as eating, sleeping or leisure activities) take place in one setting: 'He suggested that the key process – the totality – was established by collapsing the normally separate social spheres of work, home and leisure, into one monolithic social experience' (Morgan et al. 1985: 157). As a result patients inside a mental hospital can lead lives as a 'batch' – a term Goffman borrows from animal husbandry. Individuality is attacked and degraded as they become part of a homogeneous group that carries out daily tasks and functions as part of a timetabled mass.

The loss of personality and sense of self begins on admission to a mental hospital when the patient embarks on what Goffman terms a 'moral career' (see Figure 12.1). The first stage is the removal of the patient's sense of identity, which he terms the 'mortification of self'. This is followed by the 'reorganisation of self', which sees the institution replacing what it has taken away. This process may be carried out deliberately, for example in prisons, where the prisoner has his belongings and personal clothes removed and replaced by a standard prison uniform. Or it may be less deliberate, such as a mentally ill patient being provided with clothing from a hospital communal clothes store. This nevertheless has a similar effect to the prison uniform, for it is the removal and denial of clothing as self-expression and its replacement with clothing that suits the needs of the institution rather than the person. Goffman describes quite elegantly how the patient responds to this reorganisation of self. Goffman allows for the patient to respond in a variety of ways rather than becoming automatically institutionalised. He noted that patients can adopt various strategies for dealing with life in an institution and can develop different ways of surviving in the 'underlife' of institutions. There are five broad responses that a patient can make to life in an institution:

- *Colonisation.* The patient adapts unenthusiastically to their new situation.
- *Conversion.* The patient accepts what has happened and becomes institutionalised.
- *Withdrawal.* As far as possible all contact is minimised.
- *Intransigence.* The patient resists attempts to convert their behaviour. This resistance can be quite aggressive.
- *Playing it cool.* This adaptation maximises the chances of surviving the institution with much sense of self and identity intact. It involves minimising visibility and staying out of trouble.

The 1973 film *Papillon* (French for butterfly, with its connotations of freedom) provides an example of how people respond to life in an institution. Starring Steve McQueen and Dustin Hoffman, the film deals with the lives of two prisoners in the French penal colony of Devil's Island. Throughout the movie the harsh authoritarian regime seeks to

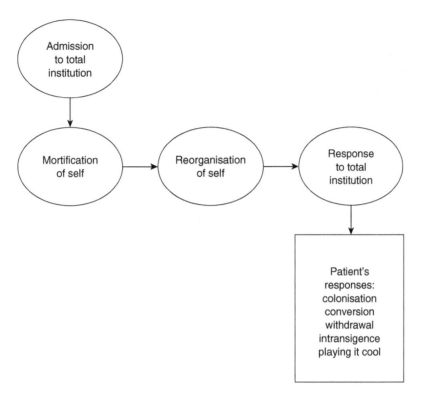

Figure 12.1 Institutionalisation

force all inmates to become compliant to its authority. In the final scene McQueen displays his opposition and *intransigence* by making a daring escape bid, while Hoffman displays his *conversion* by declining to escape, being content with life in the prison. Other cinematic representations of institutionalised life can be found in *The Shawshank Redemption* and, of course, *One Flew over the Cuckoo's Nest*.

LINK

See Chapter 13 for more information on community care and changes in health and social policy.

THE COMMUNITY

The preceding section highlighted many of the problems that can arise from institutional care: dependency of clients on the institution, iatrogenic effects of care, difficulties in returning people to life outside the institution. This may imply that life and care in the community, on the other hand, is problem-free and inherently good. Unfortunately, much research has indicated that this is not the case. As with institutional care, there exist many problems with life in the community. In the early days of community care in the United Kingdom, GP David Widgery (1991) described returning people to the community as the 'sociological equivalent of Siberia' – the idea being that people could disappear without trace and adequate support. In addition to the problems of finance and service provision, there are problems of trying to understand what the term 'community' means.

What is a community?

Many British readers of this textbook may have an idea of a community as something similar to the depiction of life in popular soaps such as *EastEnders* or *Coronation Street*, where mainly working-class people live interdependent lives in a self-contained area. Occasionally the characters in these dramas may fall out, have arguments or even shoot one another, but essentially there is some form of social cohesion underpinning all inter-actions. If this were the case in reality, then care in the community would make sense, as people could be returned to an area that was rich in mutual aid and neighbourly goodwill and support. This form of community was depicted in the classic research of Young and Willmott (1961) into an 'urban village' in the working-class East End of London. In the brick-built, back-to-back streets they found strong examples of mutual aid and a community that cared for its members. Dense social networks were maintained by a 'mother–daughter link' and, around this fulcrum, support for family members and neighbours was organised.

Such examples are, however, increasingly rare at the beginning of the twenty-first century. High unemployment, drug-related issues and social disintegration now blight many communities. The fabric of many areas has been altered by changes in social planning and post-war redevelopment. The chances of being part of a protective, supporting community are greatly reduced. Other trends, such as the trio of globalisation, individualisation and det-raditionalisation, have been identified by Crow et al. (2002) as being inimical to the continu-ation of neighbourliness and community. In the United States, the highly influential work of Putnam has identified that increasingly Americans are becoming detached from civic society and are less community-oriented. Putnam provides a useful metaphor to illustrate this decline in the title of his book *Bowling Alone* (2000). In the 1950s and 1960s in the United States many Americans belonged to bowling leagues and regularly played and socialised as part of bowling teams. Participation in such leagues and teams has dramatically declined since then and, as Putnam argues, Americans are no longer bowling together but bowling alone.

QUESTION

Do you think other countries are also becoming less community-oriented, with people concentrating on their own lives as opposed to participating in community events?

An initial problem is trying to offer a definition of **community**. There have been many attempts to provide one, but the main problem is that the term covers a heterogeneous collection of interactions, situations and forms. If we look at the following shortlist of what are referred to as communities, we can see some problems:

- student community
- gay community
- business community
- black community
- Protestant community.

QUESTIONS

What community or communities do you feel you belong to? What do you share in common with other people in those communities?

Recently, the multinational coffee chain Starbucks has been marketing its cafés as a form of community–home environment, a move that received a strong rebuke from anti-capitalist Naomi Klein: 'Starbucks pretends to sell us community, but they're selling coffee. This is a betrayal. Community is a strong and powerful idea, and I don't want it stolen from me' (BBC News 2001). What all this demonstrates is that the notion, concept and ownership of 'community' are highly complex and contested. On the above list we can find groups of people who claim to be part of a community, but their reasons for claiming membership are varied. In some cases the claim is based on characteristics such as race, in others it is lifestyle, while religion or occupation may be the underlying reasons for others. In some cases these terms will reflect a distinct geographical area (for example, the 'Protestant community' may refer to people of a Protestant background living in the Shankill Road in Belfast). In other cases it may not refer to a distinct location. The business community will draw membership from people living and working in a variety of settings. At other times a claim to belong to a community is made because of a choice (people choose to study at university, therefore their membership of the student community is voluntary). For some, membership is based on an ascribed characteristic (because of skin colour, for example, someone may find themselves 'automatically' belonging to a particular community).

We should consider global influences on community as well. Modern lives are increasingly infused with influences from beyond their immediate location and this too affects how people see those in their immediate surroundings. Savage et al.'s (2005) work on globalisation and belonging points to how the local is infused with global imaginings and meanings. Even though one may live in a particular locality, the liquidity of global flows of information and goods, the symbolic resources that globalisation provides, overlay and enrich the experiences of the spatially situated practices of that local landscape. This can, for example, mean communicating with people on the internet, or the influences on what clothes one wears or the food one eats.

QUESTIONS

What examples of globalisation do you encounter in your daily life? Discuss whether or not globalisation is reordering and changing local communities and environments.

In an attempt to overcome these definitional problems we can look at some useful older work by Bell and Newby (1976). They identified three ways in which the concept of community is used:

- as a topographical (geographical) expression
- as a local social system with interconnections between local people and social institutions
- as a human association with no logical connection with places or local social systems.

This may sound interesting in terms of trying to crack an academic problem, but when one turns to applying the conclusions to the real world, to people living in the community, then a few opposite points can be raised:

- What community do they belong to?
- Will someone care for ill or disabled members of the community?
- Will that community take care of people in need?
- Who else belongs to that community?
- Who represents that community?

After considering these issues, another question arises: does caring for people in the community necessarily improve health and avoid the potential problems inherent in institutions? Work by Prior (1993) indicated that in many ways the problems that arise inside institutions are present in communities too. The thrust of his argument, arising out of research into community care in Northern Ireland, was that even though the location of care had shifted from institutions to the community, the actual substance of patients' daily lives had altered only slightly:

For when all was said and done, they attended the same day centres as previously, they saw the same social workers, spoke to the same nurses (albeit wearing everyday clothes rather than uniforms), and usually lived with exactly the same individuals as they had done in hospital. For most people it was only the dwellings that were different. (Prior 1993: 192)

For many ex-patients, the places they were relocated to still retained many of the features of an institution, with, for example, locked doors or upper-storey windows that could only be partially opened. However, it was more than just the design features of the buildings that echoed the institutions they had come from. The daily routine and the staff they saw also mimicked their experiences in an institution. Life was still lived according to timetables and they saw the same array of mental health workers. Even social events took place in the same locations as they had when the patients were in institutional care.

QUESTIONS

How did you react to the preceding paragraph? What do you think of group homes: are they a break from the institution or just the institution in another format? What does this say about attempts to provide better care for those that require it?

One underlying point noted by Prior is that even though changes in discourse and treatment philosophies may change practices in treating mental illness, these changes do not necessarily entail any dramatic shift in the overall circumstances of the patient. It was hoped that the movement away from care in institutions to care in the community would herald a new era of tailored, dignified treatment that would break down barriers and allow people with mental health problems to become part of the community once more. As Prior notes, however, all that happened for many patients was a change of dwelling. This move might also be into an area that does not regard former mental healthcare patients as part of their particular community, or welcome them into it.

CARE AND CARERS

The previous paragraph illustrates one of the many ways in which the concept of care is used. Here it is in the context of policy, whereby a particular piece of policy lays out regulations or intentions about how care and caring for people

> Informal care is a combination of service and affection, provided on the basis of kinship or friendship. It is also mainly unpaid.

should be carried out. But for most of us the talk of care, especially in an informal context, evokes images of emotions and feelings. However, for those engaged in care work, caring is not just a state of emotionality; it involves onerous work and great physical exertion. Sometimes, caregiving informs ideas about gender roles, especially women's roles. The many facets of care and the way in which the concept of caring is used can make defining care difficult. That is not to say that it has not been attempted. Graham (1983) provides a useful definition of **informal care**. She sees care as being a combination of service and affection. *Service* relates to the 'doing' part of caring, including all the physical aspects, such as lifting and handling, washing and bathing, collecting messages and preparing meals. *Affection* relates to the 'feeling' part of caring; this includes love and compassion.

For most people informal care is provided and received on the basis of kinship or family ties (Qureshi and Walker 1989). As care can often involve intimate or physical contact, most people would like care to be provided by a family member, in this order of preference:

- spouse
- relative in lifelong joint household
- daughter
- daughter-in-law
- son
- other relative
- non-relative.

Reciprocity is another factor involved in kinship care: kin have either cared for or will care for other kin.

GENDER, CLASS AND CAREGIVING

Much of the literature on care indicates that women are the primary caregivers within the family and society as a whole (Lee 1998; Malin et al. 1999). Summarising research, Twigg and Atkin (1994) point to how women are expected to care and how gender makes a difference when it comes to receiving additional support. Men find it easier to access services and are in some ways expected to put up with less than female carers. Morris (1989, cited in Parker 1993) observed that men are less able to take on the caring role. However, one must be careful to avoid the simplistic assumption that all men and all women have uniform experiences. Drawing on the 1985 General Household Survey, and following points made by Graham (1991) that class and race need to be taken into account, Arber and Ginn (1992) indicate that care is multidimensional, with many criss-crossing structural factors. They found quantitative and qualitative differences between men and women according to their class location. The level of physical impairment was only one factor that affected the care experience of households from different class backgrounds; other factors were their ability to access and use different material, financial and cultural resources. Middle-class households had more money available to 'lighten the load' of care. This could be, for example, by building a 'granny flat', or buying aids and adaptations. There was also evidence that middle-class households utilised social services more and were better at obtaining desired outcomes than the working-class households in this study. There was also a class and gender difference. Working-class men were much more likely to be involved in care, looking after someone at home, than were their middle-class counterparts. Looking after someone at home was seen as more demanding, as it restricted employment and leisure opportunities.

LINK

Chapter 10 discusses disability in more detail.

Experiences of care

The experience of care can vary from being fulfilling and satisfying to being draining and restrictive. As mentioned earlier, affection and feelings of compassion are major reasons for people taking on care work. By demonstrating affection and compassion, the carer can realise a sense of purpose and achievement. For many carers, however, there are multiple problems, often to do with restriction of activity, time and money.

Tozer (1999) noted in her research on families with two or more disabled children that the parental carers reported that family life was restricted and they were sometimes left feeling isolated. Dearden and Becker (2000) identified similar findings for young carers. They reported that educational opportunities were restricted for young people involved in care. Feelings of restriction are commonly noted in research findings. Summarising research, Twigg and Atkin (1994) observed that the problem was not so much restriction caused by carrying out care tasks, though that was important, but generalised feelings of anxiety at leaving the person being cared for on their own. Worries were expressed about safety, or about an unforeseen circumstance arising.

One of the commonest problems facing carers and the people they care for is poverty and financial hardship.

The experience of care: the home and the body

Care brings about many changes and challenges and can unsettle assumptions about two important areas of our lives: how we relate to our home and how we relate to our body. What we shall see in the following discussion is how care leads to a reordering of what home means and how carers interact with the bodies of their loved ones when they are caring for them.

First, let us consider and think about what is meant by 'home' as a concept, because 'home' is not just simply a building (a house, in other words) or a place where someone lives, but also an important symbolic and emotional resource. In reviewing the literature from a variety of disciplines on the concept of home, Mallett (2004) draws our attention to how 'home' offers multiple meanings:

- *Memory*. Home is a place where memories reside, though not necessarily tied to a strict chronology or personal narrative. One obvious example of this is the placing of photographs around the home. Photographs in the home capture more than an image of someone; they also capture a particular historical moment or significant person in someone's life. The further one moves in time away from when the image was taken, the more it becomes a memory of that moment or person, and part of the personal narrative.
- *Family*. Traditionally, home and family went hand in hand, as the family home and the family house were the same thing. Currently, though, given changes in family structures and the increasing number of people living alone, this is not always the case. Especially following divorce and separation, we may have several homes.
- *Haven*. Home is somewhere private that is apart from public life, for example somewhere away from the pressures of work. However, this is increasingly being challenged by the rise of home working.
- *Gender*. Often home is seen as being a female place (though critically one where male authority is ultimately paramount), where women enact their required social roles of home-making and nurturing, with certain spaces in the home being gendered: for example, the kitchen as a feminine space and the garage as a masculine space.
- *Identity*. Homes act as a projection or idea of self and who we think we are. In choosing types of decoration, ornaments and furniture we are, in many ways, externalising and putting into objects our sense of self.

QUESTIONS

Discuss the importance of place to identity. What trends, if any, can you observe in society that emphasise homes and houses as an important aspect of self?

We must, therefore, be aware that 'home' is a very complex concept and that when care comes into the equation many of the above ideas of what home is can lead to challenges and potential problems. A useful example of this can be found in the research of Angus et al. (2005). They found that the various practices and activities associated with caring could transform and disrupt a household, especially the emotional and symbolic characteristics of a home. This arises (unintentionally) out of the actions of health and social care professionals who are required to make the home more functional (for instance, to make it easier

220

for the person who is being cared for to move about or to use the kitchen) so as to allow the cared-for person to remain in their own home. To do this often means moving furniture or putting in new pieces of equipment. Consequently, this can change how the home is perceived as the various symbolic aspects are disrupted and rearranged. In effect, the home can become a different place, which is no longer the physical and material representation of identity and self. These changes in the home may mirror the changes in the person, with the loss of self that is brought about by illness being visible in the loss of self as represented by the rearrangement of the home. The introduction of technology into health and social care also contributes to the reordering of the home, a point we discuss in Chapter 16 on health technologies.

Another aspect of being cared for in the home comes with the involvement of health professionals from the formal care sector. Although health professionals bring valuable skills and experiences to the person who is being cared for, their presence signals another change for the home in a very important way: the home becomes a place of work. The changes in how health and social care are organised, with ever more focus on the community, mean that for health professionals the boundaries of their place of work have become increasingly fluid. They are no longer tied to a single location, but instead move between multiple locations, such as hospitals, community support offices, GP surgeries and people's homes. Again, this is disruptive of the symbolic qualities of home. Normally, when someone calls on someone else in their home it is for socialising, or is part of being friends, but when a health or social care professional arrives at someone's house they are not there for informal social interaction but to do their job.

CASE STUDY

Mrs Robertson, aged 86, has recently returned home after an operation on a herniated disc that had been causing her some back pain for a considerable time. The operation was very successful, but it will take a few weeks for the discomfort to subside and for her to regain full mobility as she has to use a walking stick. To make life easier, her son has rearranged her living room so that she has more room to walk about and has purchased a high-backed chair to help support her back. In the kitchen, because Mrs Robertson finds it hard to bend down or stretch up to find cooking equipment or packs and cans of food, her son has placed many of these items on the kitchen work surfaces. In many respects, the actions of her son have made life considerably easier for her on a physical functional level. On an emotional level, however, these changes are causing Mrs Robertson distress and anxiety. The neat, ordered home, with the furniture arranged in particular ways, has taken her years to achieve and acts as a strong source of personal identity for her. But with everything in the living room pushed to the walls, it looks, to her, a complete mess and she finds it very embarrassing when friends and neighbours call round for a visit.

The kitchen too was often a source of pride but now it just looks messy, with many objects that should be in cupboards now out in the open. All in all, she finds the changes in her home as much a problem as the problems with her back, but, worst of all, seeing her home this way makes her feel old, something she does not like.

Much of the physical act of caring for someone involves close physical contact and interacting with someone's body, and research by Twigg (2006) notes that this can lead to many challenges. Often care is quite intimate in what it can involve: for example, it can mean helping someone to cut their toenails or assisting them in using a toilet, or washing and dressing them. These activities may seem quite functional, in that they are necessary to maintain the hygiene and the general wellbeing of someone requiring care. For the person (often a partner or a close family member) who performs the care, however, these activities come with an emotional cost. In Chapter 10 on the body we saw how the body is not just a biological entity but is also important to our sense of self and to how we relate to others. Part of this involves strong social and personal norms concerning which parts of our body we permit others to see and touch. Allowing someone to touch intimate places, such as the genitals, is a very special and symbolic act denoting that we see that individual in a particular way. Thus, the touching becomes part of how we relate to someone on an emotional level, the act of touching being a bodily manifestation of the inner emotions of affection and love, for example. This relationship between emotions and the body is disrupted when the act of touching no longer takes place to demonstrate affection but to maintain the functionality of the body. Many carers report that they begin to see and relate to the body of the person they are caring for, particularly if is their partner, in a different way. The affectionate intimacy may be replaced with a functional intimacy. This can have an impact on the relationship between the carer and the person they are caring for, as they may no longer see that person as a sexualised human being or the person they relate to in that way.

QUESTIONS

What taboos and norms surround the body in contemporary society, especially when it comes to touching and looking at the body? Is there a contradiction between the functional needs of care and the emotional needs of a relationship?

CONCLUSION

Providing a place to care for people who require assistance, support and someone to look after them has been, and no doubt always will be, a challenging issue for society. What we have reviewed here are various attempts to provide that care, and the often unintentional problems that consequently arise.

Sociological perspectives on the rise of the asylum are mainly critical, on various grounds. This can range from seeing asylums as a 'bricks-and-mortar' manifestation of the power of certain groups in society, to viewing them as a dumping ground for those who are surplus to capitalism's requirements. Sometimes it is the institutional requirements – needing to organise large groups of people to ensure that they are fed and clothed, for example – which lead to an established identity being degraded and transformed into an identity that is compliant and easy to manage for an institution.

Shifts in government policy within the United Kingdom have seen an increasing focus on care in the community. This can be viewed as an appealing alternative to some of the issues noted above. In reality, however, community care brings fresh challenges. The actual existence of community, in the sense of a definable entity which will offer care and support for those requiring assistance, is questionable. Various impulses and processes, such as greater emphasis on individualism, are causing a move away from civic involvement and being 'community minded'. This brings into relief who will be doing the care work. Often, in reality, this will mean care being provided by friends and families. Though this brings its own rewards, carers can experience financial difficulties as well as disturbances in their relationship with the person for whom they are providing care.

How all these problems are to be resolved is still open to question. What this chapter clearly draws our attention to is that looking after someone and providing appropriate care is highly complex and multidimensional, in both the physical and financial resourcing of care and the demanding emotional work that accompanies informal care.

SUMMARY POINTS

- Various theories attempt to understand organisations. Weber stresses rationality and bureaucracy; Foucault emphasises surveillance and physical space; Blau notes the existence of informal routines.

- Institutional care has been strongly criticised on the grounds that institutions act as a method of social control or a 'dumping ground' for so-called undesirables.

- Goffman critiques institutions for causing institutionalisation – an assault on self and identity.

- Defining community can be hard, with definitions including places or shared characteristics such as ethnicity or class.

- Care in the community may create further problems and may not necessarily avoid the problems of institutional care.

- Providing care in the home can alter the symbolic and emotional elements of a home.

- The close contact of physical care provided by an informal carer can impinge on their affective relationship with a loved one.

CASE STUDY

Bill was admitted to Culliere Hospital 25 years ago, having been diagnosed with a psychotic condition. Initially he was quite ill and had phases of believing that he could hear the thoughts of other people and that they were saying unpleasant things about him. After years of treatment and care the symptoms became manageable and their frequency declined, to the point that he no longer seems very ill any more. Over the years his role within the hospital has changed. He quite often assists with some of the group therapy sessions and has some responsibility for maintaining and tidying the art room. Bill was given that duty because he enjoys painting and is quite an accomplished watercolourist. Some of his work is hung in hospitals throughout the region. On Wednesdays and Sundays he even takes classes with some of the day patients, teaching them the basics of using watercolours. His skilled painting and control over the art room has sometimes led new members of staff to think that he is a part-time member of staff, perhaps a retired art teacher who wants to help in the hospital.

In many ways Bill feels happy and fulfilled in what he does and has expressed no desire to return to his family. However, recently the local health trust has been attempting to reduce the number of long-term patients in the hospital, with an eye to possibly closing the facility down altogether. To this end it has been decided by the hospital and social services that Bill is well enough to live in the community. This has made him feel highly anxious. He does not want to lose his art room or the chance to take classes. On three occasions now he has been taken to a halfway house to see if he would like it there. His initial impressions were all negative. There was no art room and the neighbours in the street did not look particularly friendly, with some actually appearing quite hostile. To settle him in he was told that he would still see the same occupational therapist as he had in the hospital, and that it would be possible for him to continue to hold his art classes in the hospital. This reassured him slightly, but ultimately Bill really wanted to stay at Culliere. After all, for him it was home.

QUESTIONS

1. How has the stay in Culliere Hospital affected Bill?
2. Do you think moving him would help his mental health?
3. Why might the local community not welcome the siting of a halfway home in their area?
4. Where do you think people are best treated or cared for?

TAKING YOUR STUDIES FURTHER

This chapter will have helped you understand many of the key terms, concepts, theories and debates relating to institutions and community care. Listed below are books and a journal article that will provide deeper and more detailed discussions of the points raised in this chapter. You will also find additional resources on the companion website, including downloads of relevant material, links to useful websites, videos and other features. Please visit the companion website at https://study.sagepub.com/barryandyuill4e

RECOMMENDED READING

Angus, J., Kontos, P., Dyck, I., McKeever, P. and Poland, B. (2005) 'The personal significance of home: habitus and the experience of receiving long-term care', *Sociology of Health & Illness*, 27(2): 161–87.

Goffman, E. (1975) *Asylums: Essays on the Social Situation of Mental Patients and Other Inmates*. Harmondsworth: Penguin.

Twigg, J. (2006) *The Body in Health and Social Care*. Basingstoke: Palgrave Macmillan.

HEALTH POLICY

MAIN POINTS

- Health policy can be difficult to define and is best thought of as a contested term.

- Health policy is not simply what a government enacts.

- It is better to think of health policy as a web of decisions and actions.

- Health policy is the outcome of a variety of processes.

- The evidence suggests that we need to address wider structural inequalities in society that may go beyond what we traditionally regarded as health policy in order to tackle the deeper causes of poor health and wellbeing.

- Neoliberalism is a globally dominant political ideology.

INTRODUCTION

One interesting part of studying health and wellbeing is exploring just how and, more importantly, *why* certain countries develop certain forms of health policy. After all, as was mentioned in Chapter 1, when people become ill they do not turn to a sociologist to help them analyse how their ill health is the result of the intersection of their social position and their biology, but it is to the medical profession that they turn in order to seek a cure. How that medical profession, and all the other aspects of health care that someone may access, are configured is the result of particular policy decisions made by governments and other groups in a society. It is what health policy is, how it comes into being and what future direction health policies may take that are the main focus of this chapter.

What we *do not* undertake in this chapter is a specific analysis of one country's health policies in any great depth. Instead, the focus falls on the deeper processes that lie beneath the formation of health policies, exploring what shapes policy in the first place. We also wish to highlight that what is traditionally thought of as health policy – an emphasis on hospitals, health professionals and treating illness – may not be the best way to tackle the health problems of the twenty-first century. The main lesson of the other chapters in this book is that contemporary health problems are increasingly *social* in origin. If you accept that premise, then it logically follows that policies that aim to improve health and wellbeing concentrate on what it is about how society is constructed that creates the conditions for poor health and wellbeing. Having that emphasis on dealing with the social causes of poor health and wellbeing means that we can prevent problems before they arise.

WHAT IS HEALTH POLICY?

Trying to define health policy is notoriously challenging. When we think of health policy what can often come to mind are, on the one hand, the institutional and structural arrangements (the building of hospitals, how health services are paid for, and so on) by which health care is delivered. The exact detail and form of those arrangements varies considerably by country. So, for example, in European countries it is the state that bears responsibility for the provision of health care, although the exact form of that state or public provision is quite variable. In the United Kingdom, the National Health Service (NHS) operates free at the point of delivery, where anyone seeking treatment or a consultation with a doctor is not required to pay for that service. In France, the state provides health care but access to the health service is not free. A fee of 23 euros is charged for each visit to the general practitioner. Other countries provide a mix of public and **private sector** health care. For example, in the USA roughly half of all health care is provided by the state and the other half by the private sector. A similar composition of health care is evident in South Africa, where the public and private sectors provide roughly half each of overall health care, although the public sector is often criticised there for being underfunded (see Table 13.1 later for some international comparisons).

On the other hand, when we think of health policy it might be the acts and pieces of legislation or written policy documents that come to mind. Some examples of legislation and policy documents are provided in the box below.

EXAMPLES OF HEALTH POLICY DOCUMENTS AND LEGISLATION

The Beveridge Report (Beveridge 1942) – The official title was 'Social Insurance and Allied Services', but this landmark document, which became known as The Beveridge Report after its author, the Liberal peer Lord Beveridge, laid the foundations of the welfare state in the United Kingdom following the Second World War. The Report outlined how the British state could support its citizens from the 'cradle to the grave' in order to reward them for their war-time sacrifices and also to build a better Britain with a healthy, well-educated, motivated workforce. This support was to be provided in the form of education, social housing, social security in times of unemployment, and universal health care was to free to everyone at the point of access. Various other acts and other pieces of legislation came into play after the war, but in 1948 the National Health Service was created.

The Patient Protection and Affordable Care Act (PPACA) (2010) – Also known as the Affordable Care Act, but more commonly referred to as Obamacare, this is an American piece of legislation that seeks to address two areas of concern in American health care: high costs and lack of health insurance coverage.

Given that there is so much diversity in what constitutes health policy in different countries and how we might conceptualise health policy, trying to establish a simple clear definition is problematic. As Baggott (2015) notes, multiple competing and contending definitions of health policy exist. To overcome this problem, Ham (2009: 131–2) recommends the use of an older definition provided by Easton (1953: 130), who perceives policy as a 'web of decisions and actions' that are concerned with the allocation of values. In this context, 'values' refer to what a government can distribute and provide for its citizens.

Ham proceeds to draw out the implications of how Easton understands policy:

Public provision or public sector is the services and resources provided by the government, which usually funds those services and resources through general or specific forms of taxation.

Private provision, or private sector, means the services and resources provided by companies, firms or corporations, which usually fund those services and resources through selling them on the open market.

1. *A study of policy also requires a study of the actions that flow from a decision concerning policy.* What is intended by the originators of policy does not necessarily mean that is how the policy actually unfolds on the ground. Policies are open to reinterpretation and adaptation by the people who have to carry them out and implement them. As a consequence, the shape a policy takes in the ward or public health department can be quite different from how it was intended.

2. *Policy is rarely contained in one piece of policy* and is better understood and seen in the context of other policies, hence the 'web of decisions' in the above definition. Health policy therefore emerges from a variety of policies, decisions and actions.

3. *Policy is never static and is subject to change.* This change can arise for a number of reasons, including the experiences of how a policy is enacted and what happens to that policy in practice. Also, as we discuss later, policy is open to political intervention, and different political parties can significantly alter the decisions made about policy.

4. *What is not decided on and not done can be just as important as what is decided and what is done.* Ham adds this to his analysis of Easton. What he means here is that it is equally as interesting to explore what is *not* done as much as what is actually done. Sometimes policy makers prefer to maintain what is in place, and the way that resources are already allocated, rather make any radical changes.

5. *Sometimes actions need to be studied when no decision has been made.* Not all policy comes from the top, decided by the politicians or the bureaucrats. Workers or health professionals lower down an organisation can engage in activities and actions that have not been decided further up and perhaps come about as a response to issues in service delivery or what they encounter in their daily practice that may not have been considered further up the organisation.

Trying to establish just how health policy is formulated and devised can also be a daunting task. Part of that problem is that health policy is not as transparent as it could be, so we do not really know what goes on behind the closed doors of government departments or think tanks or the various other actors who contribute to policy. Older models of health policy formation that stress a rational step-by-step approach, where policy evolves incrementally, while useful, tend not to capture the complexity of how policy is made in the modern world. For example, Crinson (2009) discusses how Braybrooke and Lindholm's (1963) linear and neatly organised model of policy formation is giving way to March and Olsen's (1976) model, which emphasised chaos and uncertainty.

Health policy is therefore rarely purely the outcome of a group of wise people rationally discussing peer-reviewed and thorough evidence and thereafter devising an appropriate policy. As various commentators have noted, a variety of processes and factors influences and shapes health policy. Figure 13.1 represents a synthesis of the various processes at play, although this list is not exhaustive and other processes can emerge in specific contexts. How they all meld together depends very much on where you are and when. Some processes and factors can exert a strong pull at certain times and less so at others, and one (or more) process and factor may prevent another process from unfolding how it might have done otherwise. For example, a political party may come to power whose political **ideology** holds that health care should be free for everyone, but the economic constraints in which they have to operate prevent them from enacting their ideological position. As a result, they may be required on pragmatic grounds to introduce charging for certain aspects of health care.

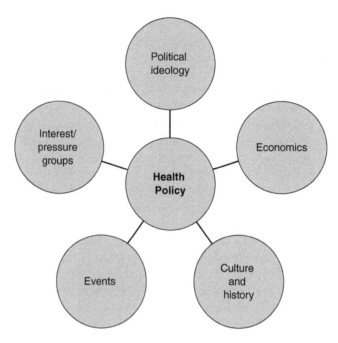

Figure 13.1   Processes and factors that influence the formation of health policy

Economics: This is possibly one of the enduring and (generally speaking) more powerful influences on policy. What can be achieved and what is possible is often enabled or limited by what finances are available. In any nation state, issues of cost and affordability of health care are often the focus of debate and discussion: where the money to pay for health comes from, what the priorities for spending are, or how best costs can be contained or reduced.

One point to note about healthcare expenditure is that no simple correlation between high expenditure on health care and improvement in health, mainly in terms of extending life expectancy, exists. In Table 13.1 expenditure data relating to the countries mentioned in this chapter are laid out. What is evident is that spending a great deal of money, as the Americans do ($9,146 per capita), does not seem to give them a life expectancy advantage over their South American neighbour Chile, which spends considerably less ($1,678 per capita), with life expectancies of 79 and 81 years respectively. This echoes a point that Wilkinson and Pickett (2010) make: after national income per capita has exceeded somewhere around $10,000, it is not how wealthy a nation is, but the extent of income inequality that influences life expectancy. The data in Table 13.1 also indicate another interesting point: in high-income countries such as the United States, France and the United Kingdom, healthcare systems that are majority publicly funded tend to be more cost-effective than systems that rely on private funding.

Table 13.1 Expenditure on health in selected countries

	Public expenditure % of GDP	Private expenditure % of GDP	Total expenditure of GDP	Per capita expenditure $[1]	Life expectancy
France	9	2.7	11.7	4,334	82
United Kingdom	7.6	1.5	9.1	3,311	81
United States of America	8.1	9	17.1	9,146	79
South Africa	4.3	4.6	8.9	1,121	57
Norway	8.2	1.4	9.6	6,308	81
Chile	3.7	4.1	7.8	1,678	81

[1]The amounts here are in international dollars converted using 2011 purchasing power parity (PPP).

Source: All data from the World Bank, available at: http://data.worldbank.org/indicator/SH.XPD.PCAP

QUESTION

Discuss how you think health care should be funded. Given what we have discussed in other chapters on the causes of health problems, where else could money be spent in order to improve overall health and wellbeing?

Culture and history: How a nation understands itself and the values it espouses shape and influence its attitudes regarding health policy. The political battles that unfolded around President Obama's drive to introduce the Affordable Care Act (more commonly known as 'Obamacare') in the USA provide an example of the importance of the cultural dimension of policy formation. The overarching aim of the Act was to make health care affordable for the many Americans who could not afford the private or public health insurance schemes, which are the pillars of American health care. Those who opposed Obamacare did so just as much on cultural grounds as for economic or policy reasons. Sections of American society interpreted the Act as being contrary to deeply-held notions of American liberty and the individual's right to decide what is best for them (in this case, their health) without interference from the government. Some Americans regarded the increased presence of the government in health care as alien to American values and as moving the United States closer to some form of European socialism.

The attitudes displayed by certain sections of American society are in contrast with those found in the Nordic countries. Citizens in Sweden and Norway regard the state as an essential presence in their everyday lives. The state exists in order to allow them to express their individuality and to lead the types of life that they desire. Swedish academic Trägårdh refers to this cultural form as 'statist individualism'. Traditions of equality and having a society where everyone pitches in to support everyone else runs deep in their history. In Norway, cultural traditions of equality can be detected in the nineteenth century with early examples of gender equality. Legislation was passed at that time that allowed women to have a greater stake in society, especially in relation to property ownership. Norwegian experiences of Nazi occupation during the Second World War also further reinforced the collective spirit of the nation. People of all classes banded together during the occupation and that sense of unity and togetherness continued after the war.

How the Nordic countries and the United States shape their current health policy can therefore be seen as being deeply related to their history and traditions. Even after Obamacare, US health care is still modelled very much on the individual seeking their own health insurance with private firms, in line with US notions of the liberty of the individual. In Norway, health care is very much focused on state provision, again in line with their deep tradition of equality and collectivism.

QUESTION

Think about your own country. Can you identify any traditions or cultural beliefs that continue to shape how health policy is formulated?

Events: Sometimes an unforeseen event can occur that demands some form of policy response. This event can be in the form of a sudden crisis in the healthcare system or the appearance of a new disease or epidemic: essentially, a phenomenon related to health and to health care that was not expected. An example in the United Kingdom was the scandal that occurred in the mid-2000s in the Stafford Hospital run by the Mid-Staffordshire NHS Foundation Trust. The event became known as the Stafford Hospital Scandal and involved the chronic neglect and mistreatment of patients at the hospital. The examples of mistreatment ranged from patients being left unattended while covered in their own excrement, to the physical and verbal abuse of patients. It was reckoned that somewhere between 400 and 1,200 patients lost their lives unnecessarily as a consequence of the poor and sometimes abusive care that they received. A campaign led by the daughter of one elderly patient who had died at the hospital and a local newspaper brought the poor conditions to public attention. In response to the allegations being made, there was an Inquiry, led by Robert Francis QC, which resulted in the publication of 290 policy recommendations (the main aims of the Inquiry are listed in the box below). The core finding of the Inquiry was to result in a shift in the culture of the NHS towards greater transparency and accountability at all levels of the NHS. All members of staff and management are now open to scrutiny and can speak out if they feel that problems are arising, and there has been a fundamental shift towards the patient coming first at all points in their journey of care. For nurses, there is an increased emphasis on care and compassion in their professional practice and in their training.

THE RECOMMENDATIONS OF THE FRANCIS REPORT

The main recommendations of the Inquiry were summarised by Robert Francis in his report (2013: 4–5) in the introduction to the executive summary:

- Foster a common culture shared by all in the service of putting the patient first;

- Develop a set of fundamental standards, easily understood and accepted by patients, the public and healthcare staff, the breach of which should not be tolerated;

- Provide professionally endorsed and evidence-based means of compliance with these fundamental standards which can be understood and adopted by the staff who have to provide the service;

- Ensure openness, transparency and candour throughout the system about matters of concern;

- Ensure that the relentless focus of the healthcare regulator is on policing compliance with these standards;

- Make all those who provide care for patients – individuals and organisations – properly accountable for what they do and to ensure that the public is protected from those not fit to provide such a service;

- Provide for a proper degree of accountability for senior managers and leaders to place all with responsibility for protecting the interests of patients on a level playing field;

- Enhance the recruitment, education, training and support of all the key contributors to the provision of healthcare, but in particular those in nursing and leadership positions, to integrate the essential shared values of the common culture into everything they do;

- Develop and share ever improving means of measuring and understanding the performance of individual professionals, teams, units and provider organisations for the patients, the public, and all other stakeholders in the system.

Interest and pressure groups: Groups external to a government can influence the formation of policy. Interest and pressure groups comprise a wide range of actors, including bodies that represent healthcare professionals and workers, trade unions, think tanks, corporate lobbying bodies, non-governmental organisations (NGOs) or single-issue campaigns. They exist to protect and advance the position of a distinct group of people or a distinct ideological position. How effective they are depends on how much and what kind of power they can exert. For example, trade unions can exert power by calling their members out on strike, while corporate lobbying groups can exert power through their political influence and financial power.

Political ideology: Many types of political ideology exist and it can be an exhaustive process trying to outline all of them. We shall therefore explore one form of ideology, **neoliberalism**, in greater detail in the next section. We have chosen neoliberalism because of its pervasive and hegemonic influence in the world today. Broadly speaking, however, all political ideology can be distilled down to one or two very broad general forms or approaches: collectivist or individualist.

Collectivist approaches

Health is understood to be optimised by people pulling together and sharing the costs of providing health care, usually through taxation, with the government being responsible for spending that money in funding the institutional arrangements of its citizens' health. The collectivist approach is associated with the social democracies of Western Europe where the government raises taxes and then develops some form of health service (such as the NHS).

Individualist approaches

Health is understood to be optimised by individuals taking responsibility for their own health care, usually through private insurance schemes that allow them to access privately provided health care. The individualist approach is epitomised in the American model of health care, at least prior to the introduction of the Affordable Care Act in 2015.

NEOLIBERALISM

In the previous section we visited the importance of political ideology as a driver of the policy formation process. There are many different forms of political ideology, but we are going to consider only one in detail: neoliberalism. This is because neoliberalism is the political ideology that is dominant in the early twenty-first century, and to be able to capture and understand what is going on in the world today it is important that we have a grasp of this set of ideas which shape so much of global and local policy agendas.

Neoliberalism is often characterised as being primarily an economic system which emphasises the dominance of market forces and market disciplines. The central idea is that the free market offers the best mechanism to provide all that we need and desire in the most cost-effective way, so long as markets are left to compete with as little government interference as possible. How the free market is supposed to deliver those goals is illustrated in the following example.

A consumer, let us call her Sarah, has a need for a product, in this case health care. Sarah therefore requires someone to supply that need. In a free market she would be able to choose between different competitors. It is the ability of the consumer to choose within a market that, according to the neoliberal perspective, provides the motor for cost reduction, improved service and the meeting of needs and desires of society.

In our example Sarah can choose between *AceHealth* and *YourHealth*. If Sarah opts for *AceHeath* because they offer the same services but at a cheaper price than *YourHealth*, then that poses a challenge for *YourHealth*. They are not gaining custom and could therefore go out of business. To avoid that they must be able to either beat the price of their competitor *AceHealth* or offer something extra. If they decide to reduce costs, then doing so entails them to reflect on their own costs: perhaps they can make savings somewhere or they can carry out a procedure more efficiently? *YourHealth* identifies that they can save a great deal of money by switching to a new supplier of office disposables (paper and so on). They can now offer their product at a cheaper price. Sarah now opts for *YourHealth* instead as she can obtain the same healthcare package for a cheaper price. Obviously *AceHealth* does not like to lose a customer, so they in turn try to work out how they can attract Sarah back by offering her a better deal. To do so they follow *Yourhealth* and take a close look at their operation and see how they can become more efficient or offer a better overall package for the same cost to Sarah.

This process of constantly seeking an advantage over competitors is what provides the fundamental mechanism by which free markets supposedly make everything better for society. By having to compete, all waste and inefficiencies are eliminated and all needs and desires are realised. Whether it works that way in real life is another matter, but that principle of competition lies at the heart of the free-market.

Neoliberalism is also a political project on a smaller scale, at the level of micro-politics, as Foucault (2008) noted in his assessments of neoliberalism in its infancy back in the 1980s. Part of the neoliberal project is to recast people as entrepreneurs, where they, as individuals, embody the ideas and disciplines of the marketplace, are constantly on the search for the best deals while marketing themselves as if they are a brand to attract as much custom as possible.

The emphasis on individual subjects as entrepreneurs who are constantly striving to better themselves therefore places the responsibility of being healthy and fit onto the individuals. They must become the entrepreneurs of their own health. It may sound reasonable that people must take responsibility for their actions, and many health commentators concur that people do have to take some responsibility, but it is only *some* responsibility. But as Marmot (2015) has observed, not all people live in an environment where they can enact the decisions they want and they come up against many barriers that constrain their choices. Those barriers have been discussed in greater depth in Section 2 of this book. Just as a reminder, the example given in Chapter 6 of why women in a fishing community in Malawi contracted HIV identified that those women were very limited in the control they could exercise over their lives. It was that lack of control that placed them at risk of being exposed to potential infection of HIV. For some of the women, choosing not to engage in transactional sex in order to acquire fish to sell at market entailed engaging in activities that they would otherwise not wish to do, but the choice was between potential exposure to HIV or not having money to feed their families.

QUESTIONS

Discuss the issue raised above concerning individual responsibility and structural barriers. What are your thoughts on these issues? Do all groups in society share equal access to the resources required to make meaningful decisions about their lives?

There are numerous critiques of neoliberalism, but for Birch (2015) neoliberalism's claims are nothing more than a deceptive ideological manoeuvre that masks the inequalities in wealth and power of a small powerful global elite. His main criticism is that all the talk of deregulation and of spreading market efficiency is in reality just a mechanism by which additional profit can be gained at the expense both of workers and of consumers.

SHOULD HEATH POLICY ALWAYS BE ABOUT HEALTH?

Have we perhaps made a wrong turn in how we conceptualise what health policy is? Does effective policy always have to be directly about health? This is a point made by Hanlon et al. (2011): that we need to radically rethink what we mean by heath policy, and public health policy in particular. They describe 'waves of public healthcare' (see the box below) that improved the health of the United Kingdom (how these waves can be applied more globally is discussed a little later in this chapter).

THE FIVES WAVES OF PUBLIC HEALTH IN THE UK (HANLON ET AL. 2011)

First wave: 1830–1900 The provision of clean water and adequate sanitation. Bazalgette's sewage system for London is the prime example of first-wave public health. Many of the health problems traditionally faced by Londoners were caused by contaminated water and the inadequate disposal of human (and animal) waste. They were overcome by the building of 82 miles of brick-lined sewers to transport London's waste away from the city.

Second wave: 1890–1950. Scientific rationalism. In this wave of public health the discoveries made by scientists offered new insights into the causes of disease and how to treat them. The work of Louis Pasteur provides a useful example of this wave, with his setting out of the principles of vaccination and development of the germ theory of disease.

Third wave: 1940–1980. The Welfare State. In the years following the Second World War the British state oversaw the provision of health care, social security, council housing and education available to all. The National Health Service (NHS) came into being in this period.

Fourth wave: 1960–2000. This wave is marked by substantial changes that occurred in Britain and a move towards an increasingly complex and changing society. Emphasis shifts towards tackling risk behaviours (smoking, drinking and diet), alongside a concern that social inequalities lead to health inequalities.

Fifth wave: 2000 onwards. As Hanlon et al. note, we do not yet know what the fifth wave of public health should comprise. That is the challenge of our times.

The first four waves are interesting in themselves. It is evident that it has not always been biomedicine that has led to the breakthroughs in public health. The first wave of health was brought about by engineering. In Victorian Britain communicable diseases such as typhoid and cholera were big killers, transmitted through unsafe and contaminated drinking water. The vast amount of human and animal effluence, which was disposed of by dumping it onto the streets or directly and untreated into the River Thames, resulted in the perfect conditions for these diseases to break out. What solved that problem was the work of Bazalgette, an engineer who masterminded the building of the London sewage system, which safely disposed of London's waste far upstream and away from the supplies of drinking water. After the success of the London system, similar sewage schemes were rolled out across Britain, leading to the rapid reduction of deaths by communicable disease (Jackson 2014).

So, we have effectively solved the problems of ill health caused by poor sanitation, or that can be cured by a range of pharmaceuticals, or that can be treated by a health service, but, as Hanlon et al. assert, we are now facing new causes of morbidity and early mortality.

These new causes are to be found in what Hanlon terms the 'dis-eases of modernity', which are a result of the way in which we live our lives and have structured the societies in which we live. Pause for a moment and reflect on the main points in previous chapters, especially those concerned with gender, ethnicity, inequality and sexuality. What we have encountered there was the core message that it is the configuration of society that lies behind many of the health problems that are visible in high-income nations, but also increasingly in middle-income nations too. The causes of health problems today are therefore to be found in where one is located in an unequal society, in the way in which ethnic identities are racialised or how men and women perform their gendered identities. In reference to inequality, after reviewing the evidence Wilkinson and Pickett (2007: 1976) assert the following:

> Rather than providing ever more prisons, doctors, health promoters, social workers, educational psychologists, and drug rehabilitation units, in expensive and at best only partially effective attempts to offset the problems of relative deprivation, it may be cheaper and more rewarding to tackle the underlying inequalities themselves.

What they are driving at here is that it is better to focus on the deeper causes of the problems that give rise to ill health. Marmot (2015) puts it well when he says that we should be focused on the 'causes of the causes'. This is Hanlon et al.'s (2011) point too, in their call for a new form of health policy that is quite different from what we are used to thinking of as being health policy. As they say:

> In sum, public health faces a series of challenges that are not amenable to current strategies despite our best efforts, and for some of which we are ill-prepared. This suggests that a new approach is needed. (Hanlon et al. 2011: 34)

So, what is this new approach? What form would such health policies take? In Chapter 6 on gender, for example, some ideas of how to reduce health issues related to gender were outlined. The man direction of travel of those policies was not to provide clinics that would offer a service to treat the outcomes of gender-related health inequalities, but instead to tackle the social structures that gave rise to those problems in the first place. The emphasis was very much on changing the ways that men act out their roles as men and creating new, less damaging forms of masculinities.

Hanlon et al. (2011) claim that we have reached what they term the **fifth wave of public health**, where the challenges that face society in terms of health and wellbeing are quite different from the challenges that previous waves of public health had to face (see below for greater detail on the waves of public health). The first three waves of health dealt with the control and eradication of diseases such as cholera, and then the provision of universal health care. In the fifth wave, the focus shifts to what Hanlon et al. term elsewhere the 'dis-eases of modernity'. What he means here is that we are faced not with the threat of ill health caused by microbes or lack of healthcare facilities, but by the way we lead our lives in this phase of history. It is *society* that is the cause of our health problems. Modern life is increasingly complex, demanding and difficult to control and that gives rise to the challenges that can affect health.

Hanlon et al. (2011) have based their notions of waves of health very much on the British experience of public health, but their ideas are applicable elsewhere. What they are suggesting is that various issues (poor sanitation, lack of health care and the negative effects of inequality) require attention in order to improve public health. In Britain those developments unfolded in a series of waves over time, much as they did in many other high-income nations in Europe and North America. What, though, is their applicability to other places? They do not suggest that their idea can be taken into other national contexts, but what is possibly occurring in low-income and middle-income countries is that several waves are necessary at the same time. So, for example, in a middle-income country such as Ghana, the provision of a sewage system would be highly beneficial. The Water and Sanitation Program (2012) estimates that lack of adequate sanitation and clean toilet facilities lead to approximately 19,000 deaths and costs the Ghanian economy around US$290 million per year. Simultaneously, the income from expanding oil and mining sectors of Ghana's economy are beginning to increase levels of income inequality in Ghana, which brings with it a number of health and other social problems. South Africa also faces issues and challenges with sanitation and the provision of access to clean water. Therefore, Hanlon et al.'s (2011) first wave of public health – that of engineering – would greatly benefit the overall health of both Ghana and South Africa. (It should be noted, however, that a project on the scale of Bazalgette's London sewage system is perhaps not necessary today: there are many low-tech engineering solutions to poor sanitation that could be highly effective.)

As we discussed in Chapter 5 on health inequality, South Africa is beginning to encounter the health problems related to inequality. The 'dis-eases of modernity' are also prevalent there as the country as a whole becomes wealthier but more unequal. It also may require a fifth wave of public health, where the problems of inequality and modernity are dealt with alongside problems of infrastructure and communicable disease. Ghana, too, may face these challenges. So for middle-income countries the waves of public health may not be as sequential as they were in the United Kingdom. Rather, they may need to flow together, tackling different problems at the same time. The waves of public health are ultimately not a rigid step-by-step guide on how to improve a nation's health, but rather a technique for thinking about *what* is needed to improve health and wellbeing and *why* it needs to improve.

QUESTIONS

Read over the summary of Hanlon et al.'s (2011) five waves of public health once more. Try to apply it to the nation where you live. What is useful and what is not useful about this approach as a method of thinking through what is required to improve health and wellbeing in your locality? Are there other waves of public health that are necessary in the country where you live?

Marmot (2015) also offers some suggestions as to what new thinking in terms of health policy could be like. The policy suggestions he makes are applicable in a global context and draw on what has been evidenced to be effective. Again, what he highlights may not seem to be what we might first think of as being health policy, but the focus is on the deeper structural issues (the 'causes of the causes') that give rise to the social contexts that create poor health and wellbeing. In his capacity as Chair of the Commission on Social Determinants of Health at the World Health Organisation (WHO), he has co-authored the *Closing the Gap in a Generation* report that has made three broad policy recommendations (Commission on Social Determinants of Health 2008; see the box below). The report emphasises sorting out the problems in society by, for example, reshaping power relations and providing people with more control over their lives as the starting point for improving health and wellbeing. Ultimately, for Marmot (2006: 2086), all policy should be aimed at helping people lead 'lives they have reason to value'.

The three policy recommendations of the *Closing the Gap in a Generation* report (Commission on Social Determinants of Health 2008: 2)

1. *Improve Daily Living Conditions*: Improve the well-being of girls and women and the circumstances in which their children are born, put major emphasis on early child development and education for girls and boys, improve living and working conditions and create social protection policy supportive of all, and create conditions for a flourishing older life. Policies to achieve these goals will involve civil society, governments, and global institutions.

2. *Tackle the Inequitable Distribution of Power, Money, and Resources*: In order to address health inequities, and inequitable conditions of daily living, it is necessary to address inequities – such as those between men and women – in the way society is organized. This requires a strong public sector that is committed, capable, and adequately financed. To achieve that requires more than strengthened government – it requires strengthened governance: legitimacy, space and support for civil society, for an accountable private sector, and for people across society to agree public interests and reinvest in the value of collective action. In a globalized world, the need for governance dedicated to equity applies equally from the community level to global institutions.

3. *Measure and Understand the Problem and Assess the Impact of Action*: Acknowledging that there is a problem, and ensuring that health inequity is measured – within countries and globally – is a vital platform for action. National governments and international organizations, supported by WHO, should set up national and global health equity surveillance systems for routine monitoring of health inequity and the social determinants of health and should evaluate the health equity impact of policy and action.

CONCLUSION

Health policy can appear to be a challenging and esoteric subject to study, but it is essential to have an awareness of perhaps not the details of each Act or piece of legislation (though this can be useful), but rather a general understanding of some of the key processes and considerations by which health policy comes into being. Policy formation and the policy process are not neat linear events, where an idea incrementally moves through a process eventually ending up as the activities of health professionals and health workers. Instead, the formation of health policy is more complex and nuanced, with a variety of ideas, actors and other factors shaping and influencing what policies come into being.

The chapter has also drawn attention to what we might think of as being health policy. One of the key lessons of this book is that we need to appreciate how social contexts and social processes play a considerable role in shaping health and wellbeing. In the chapters on issues such as inequality, gender, ethnicity and sexuality what emerged time and again was that it was how those social phenomena are constructed that either hinders or helps people to attain good health and wellbeing. As many of the researchers and academics who have developed the research into those areas have argued, it is by focusing on those social processes that the best results can be achieved. So, trying to reduce health inequalities that exist between different social classes will involve reducing levels of income inequality.

Future health policies, then, may be centred on empowering people and creating greater equality as much as providing hospitals. This way of thinking may be different from what we are used to, but as global society advances and develops it appears that it is the problems with how we create the societies in which we live that must be the focus of our efforts to improve health and wellbeing.

SUMMARY POINTS

- It is vital to have an understanding of health policy as it influences what services and resources are available in a given nation.

- However, it is not purely health policies that affect health. All government policies (economic, housing and so on) impact to some extent on health.

- Policy is not always the outcome of a careful, considered and evidenced process. Rather, it emerges out of a complex web of influences that include politics, ideology, economics, popular opinion and national culture.

- Current thinking on health policy emphasises that a radical shift is required in how we conceptualise.

TAKING YOUR STUDIES FURTHER

This chapter will have helped you understand many of the key terms, concepts, theories and debates relating to health policy. Listed below are books and a journal article that will provide deeper and more detailed discussions of the points raised in this chapter. You will also find additional resources on the companion website, including downloads of relevant material, links to useful websites, videos and other features. Please visit the companion website at https://study.sagepub.com/barryandyuill4e

RECOMMENDED READING

Crinson, I. (2009) *Health Policy: A Critical Perspective*. London: SAGE.

Hanlon, P., Carlisle, S., Hannah, M. and Lyon, A. (2014) *The Future Public Health*. Maidenhead: Open University Press.

Kickbusch, I. (2005) 'Action on global health: addressing global health governance challenges', *Public Health*, 119(11): 969–73.

Marmot, M. (2015) *The Health Gap: The Challenge of an Unequal World*. London: Bloomsbury.

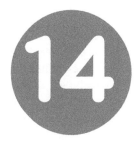

SPORT, HEALTH, EXERCISE AND WELLBEING

MAIN POINTS

- Sport and exercise are not separate from social influences and social processes.

- Sport and exercise as part of the overarching concept of leisure are complex to define and more than just forms of physical activity.

- Social inequalities such as class, gender and ethnicity exert strong influences on why people elect to become involved in particular forms of sport and exercise.

- Sport assists in the channelling of violence and similar emotions.

- Some sports, such as football, emerge as forms of social control and an expression of class identity.

- Society plays a strong role in shaping men's and women's bodies for particular forms of sport.

- Racism and discrimination influence the participation and experiences of black and ethnic minority people in sport and exercise.

INTRODUCTION

The iconic image in Figure 14.1 is from the 1968 Mexico City Olympics. In it, African-American athletes Tommie Smith and John Carlos, after receiving their winners' medals and while the American national anthem is playing, raise their fists in a Black Power salute. They took this dramatic course of action in order to protest against racism in the United States. White Australian athlete Peter Norman, also on the podium, displays solidarity with their cause by wearing the badge of the Olympic Project for Human Rights. The United States at that time was experiencing the shocks of various civil rights movements that sought to end the discrimination faced by a number of minority groups. Black civil rights was one of those social movements. Led by people such as the powerful orator Martin Luther King and the more radical and militant Malcolm X, the movement aimed to realise racial equality and to end the second-class status of African-American people, which ranged from segregation on public transport, in schools and in restaurants to denial of the freedom to exercise constitutional and political rights.

The point being made here is that sport is far more than simply an activity concerning individuals and teams competing against each other. Sport and exercise and their potentially health-giving outcomes are very much locked into society, and are subject to its norms, values, cultures, structures and inequalities.

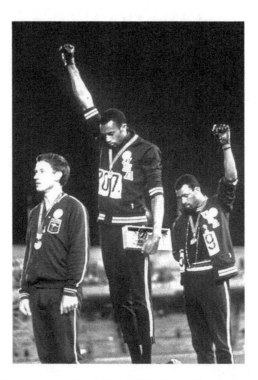

Figure 14.1 Black power salute at the 1968 Olympics: an example of where sport and wider social issues were not separate entities

© John Dominis, Getty Images

SPORT, EXERCISE AND HEALTH?

Sport and exercise are widely accepted as being important for health. There appears to be ample evidence that engaging in some form of physical activity or even purposeful leisure pursuits is associated with good health. So, for example, in reviewing a wider range of research on sport, exercise and health, Collins and Kay (2003: 28) summarise a great number of benefits. These stretch from the *personal* level (for example, individual fitness, positive mental attitude, meaning and purpose) to the *social* level (community-building, bridging with minority groups), to the *economic* level (cheap but effective health promotion, a fitter workforce), and to the *environmental* and *national* levels (improved environmental health and national pride, among others). This picture of people jogging or exercising or even, as Iso-Ahola has noted, just participating in some form of purposeful and active leisure (as opposed to passively watching the television, for example) ties in with common-sense perceptions of what it is to be healthy (Blaxter 1990).

There is a very strong sociological 'however' to be entered into the discussion at this point. Physical exercise and activity are good for health but they are *far* from being the defining criteria for good health. As we have explored in the rest of this book so far, health is multifaceted, and often social and structural mechanisms are more important for health than biological factors or risk behaviours (smoking, diet and exercise). So, staying with the exercise theme of this chapter, what makes healthy people healthy is not that they are all enthusiastic sports people or fitness fanatics, but rather their social location. This often predicts how much control they have in organising their working and home lives and in gaining a sense of reward in relation to their efforts at work – or alternatively, as Wilkinson and Pickett (2010) highlight, the levels of inequality within a society and the psycho-social impacts of that inequality. If you would like some figures to illustrate that point, Marmot (2004: 44) suggests that around *one-third* of health inequality is explicable by risk factors such as smoking, bad diet and no exercise. The rest is down to society.

QUESTION

How does the point above, that sport and exercise may not be the most successful approach to reduce health inequalities, challenge common perceptions of the causes of ill health?

So, giving everyone in the UK a free gym pass, for example, would help reduce *some* of the burden of health inequality. However, a substantial level of health inequality would still remain. To reduce that burden in any substantial amount would require deeper causes of health inequality (such as economic inequality, poverty and the negative effects of social structures) to be tackled. Indeed, it is those social structures that often prevent people from participating in sports and exercise in any meaningful way – a point considered in greater depth throughout this chapter.

The rest of this chapter focuses on the themes outlined above. It explores the interesting interrelationships between the three main social structures of class, gender and ethnicity, taking account of how those structures shape and influence people's approaches to sport and interpretations of sport. Before proceeding any further, however, and as we have done throughout this book, it is important to try to define the topic of discussion. It is on a definition of sport and exercise that attention falls next.

DEFINITIONS AND CONCEPTS

Sport and exercise are commonly perceived as being activities that occur in free time, the time after or between work, and therefore an area of life separate from work. To some extent that is true. We can, as Dumazedier (1967) has done in his classic work on the subject of leisure, define leisure activities (including sport and exercise) as being a separate sphere or area of human life, where individuals can exert more control over what they do and pursue pleasurable activities, albeit activities that are contextualised by the type of culture and society in which they live.

Substantial problems do exist, however, with the preceding definition and with considering work and leisure to be discrete and separate entities. Let us begin with the notion that leisure and work activities exist in separate domains and have nothing to do with each other. It does not take much to raise questions about whether such a clean and neat divide is actually sustainable. A recent piece of research by the hotel group Premier Inn found that for most people the weekend did not begin till 12.38 pm on Saturday and it was effectively over by 3.55 pm on Sunday, due to recovering from work in the first instance and beginning to become stressed and anxious about work in the second. The time between is not necessarily filled with relaxation and leisure, however. Smartphones and the option of having work emails 'pushed' through to us mean that work can colonise time outside the traditional nine-to-five and also outside the physical boundaries of the workplace; this tilting of the work–life balance in favour of work can have quite damaging health effects (Bryson et al. 2007). Lefebvre (2008) has also challenged the separate-domain perspective on work and leisure. He argues that leisure is freedom from work but only up to a point: the reason we need leisure is to recover from work, and people at leisure are in effect recharging themselves for work; therefore leisure should be seen not as existing separately from work, but rather as an *extension* of work.

Sport is also a reflection of the prevailing culture, norms and values of a society as opposed to a self-contained separate entity within society – a point we discuss in greater detail in the next section. The types of sport played in a society do not just rise spontaneously from nowhere; rather, they emerge from the fabric of a society and *inform* us about that society. One useful (but perhaps dramatic!) example of sport being the product of society can be found in Ancient Mayan society, which existed in Central America from *c*. 2000 BC to the arrival of the Spanish Conquistadores in the early 1500s. Their main sport was similar to a fast and furious fusion of volleyball and basketball, where teams would attempt to score points by hitting a large rubber ball through a vertical hoop inside a walled courtyard by rebounding the ball off the walls using their thighs and hips. The game itself reflected the wider tradition in Mayan society of highly ritualised human sacrifice. After the close of each game, which was attended by the high priesthood of the community, a sacrifice of prisoners, and possibly at certain times of the losing team, would take place. This ritualised killing of people was as much a part of the game as the action on the court.

There also exists the further complication that sport and exercise, like so much in a capitalist society, are subject to commoditisation and are part of some very big business indeed, where any health-giving properties and the sheer embodied pleasure of sport and exercise are lost in the cash nexus and pursuit of profit. Therefore, when one engages in sport or exercise, one is generally bound into the commercial concerns of a company and market forces. Cashmore (2005), for example, discusses the extent to which global multinationals such as Nike and business people like Rupert Murdoch can exert considerable influence and control over a wide range of sports (such as football) in terms of broadcasting rights, sponsorship, sports clothing and in some cases even outright ownership of a sporting club. Featherstone (1991: 185–6) ably summarises the intrusion of commercialism into what should be the spontaneity of exercise as follows:

> The notion of running for running's sake, purposiveness without purpose, a sensuous experience in harmony with embodied and physical nature, is completely submerged amidst the welter of benefits called up by market and health experts.

However, Moor (2007) cautions us with the interesting point that just because sport is being increasingly colonised and taken over by commercial concerns, that does not necessarily diminish the emotions and feelings of people who choose to engage in sporting practices as athletes or those of the followers of sports.

QUESTIONS

How would you define sport and leisure? Do you agree or disagree with the comments made above as to why sport and leisure are problematic to define? Try to identify other examples of where the boundaries between work and leisure are blurry and hard to define.

Trying to capture all of the above in a simple definitional schema is challenging. What we have reviewed here is that understandings of sport and exercise, or their grouping together as leisure, are open to many interpretations. The one point that is hopefully clear is that sport and leisure are elements of social life that are not separate from the fabric of the wider society of which they constitute a part. The following sociological formulation by Giulianotti (2005) goes some way to providing a definition of sport that captures both the *internal* dimensions of defining sport as it is played and something of sport's *external* relations with wider society. According to Giulianotti (2005: xii), sport is:

1. *structured* by rules and codes of conflict, spatial and temporal frameworks (playing fields and time limits on games), and instruments of government
2. *goal-oriented*, aimed at particular objectives, e.g. scoring goals, winning contests, increasing averages, and thus winners and losers are identifiable
3. *competitive* – rivals are defeated, records are broken
4. *ludic*, enabling playful experiences, generating excitement
5. *culturally situated*, in that items 1–4 correspond closely to the value systems and power relations within the relevant sport's host society.

The next section on Elias and sport further underpins how sport is tied into the deeper weave of society and culture, again demonstrating the deep interconnection between society and sport.

ELIAS AND THE SOCIOLOGY OF SPORT

Many sociological theories and perspectives seek to explain sport and investigate its role, place and purpose in the wider arc of society, but the work of Norbert Elias is, in some ways, more commonly consulted than others. What his particular writings on sport indicate is that sport is on one level about fun and excitement, but more importantly it is tied into the deeper 'building blocks' of a society; sport is more about providing a level of control and order within society, but one expressed in the control that people exert over their own aggressive and violent emotions.

The focus of the work of Elias and his colleagues on sport is therefore to provide an explanation of how society becomes less violent *internally* but yet can remain violent *externally*. What this means is that while a society can 'legitimately' engage in warfare and violence with other nation states outside its borders (for example, the current conflicts in Iraq and Afghanistan), inside those borders violence is conversely tightly controlled. This may be through coercive means, such as the police force, but much more frequently is through symbolic and ritual means (such as sport) that act by disciplining the bodily actions of people and creating a 'civilised' society within a much broader and historical **civilising process**.

This relationship between violence and civilisation is the basis of Elias's wider sociological perspective as laid out in his main theoretical framework of the civilising process. He claims that as societies develop there is an increasing and parallel emphasis and expansion on individual discipline and self-control (the rationalisation of one's body) away from external constraints in order to maintain the smooth running and ordering of society. This civilising effect operates on two different but related levels. There is a social level, whereby there is an expectation that one behaves publicly in an appropriate manner, and a psychological level, whereby our internal thoughts and ideas are reorganised to respond to the social level. Elias (1982) charts some interesting historical examples by way of illustrating his thesis in his classic work on social manners, appropriately entitled *The History of Manners*. If we take one example from that work, that of breaking wind in public, it was not a problem to do this in the Middle Ages. An

The concept of the civilising process within the work of Norbert Elias refers to the long-term tendency of the behaviour of people to become less violent and uninhibited so as to allow society to operate successfully. As a result, expressions of emotion and use of the body become increasingly controlled and refined over time, with emotions such as shame regulating social situations and violence being confined to sports as opposed to being prevalent in everyday life.

individual who broke wind at the table or in the company of others would not have been singled out as rude, and they would not have felt embarrassed or ashamed. Over time, as society develops, so too do taboos and limitations on what one can do publicly with one's body. Now the breaking of wind in public is met with disapproval and the person who has broken wind experiences shame and embarrassment. What is evident here is that as society becomes more rule-bound, this socially created framework of restraints translates into the inner psychology of the people within that society.

One note of caution is required before progressing with the discussion of Elias and sport. He uses the term 'civilising' throughout his work. He is categorically *not* referring to western civilisation as being the ultimate expression of human life, and is not suggesting that current society is somehow the height of civilisation and that civilisation has reached its end point. On the contrary, people in contemporary society may appear to be utterly barbaric and uncouth to future generations, in the same way that our medieval ancestors appear to us now. Part of the reason for being cautious is that in the original German-language publications of Elias's work, he uses the word *Zivilisation* which, though sounding like 'civilisation' in English, actually carries a slightly different meaning. It refers more to manners, etiquette and self-control rather than to notions of being superior in terms of possessing better technology, art, education and so forth.

The role of sport for Elias, then, is also to act as a method whereby the violent tensions and impulses that could otherwise destabilise and disrupt the smooth order of society are contained and controlled. Such a dynamic is evident when sport is considered historically. Over time the various activities that could be classed as being sport have become more civilised, moving away from violent contact sports that could easily result in death to sports where violence is still present but is contained and controlled by tight frameworks, rules and regulations. So, for example, in the ancient period sports were highly violent, the obvious example being Ancient Roman gladiatorial events. Though not always a fight to the death, as popularly portrayed in films, the sport could quite easily lead to the death of the combatants. The Ancient Greeks, with whom we associate the civilised Olympic sports of running, discus and javelin, also practised highly violent sports. Boxing at this time was not restricted to the use of fists; all parts of the body could be used to strike the opponent, with gouging and biting being deemed quite permissible. In the medieval period, sport also lacked the rules and restraints we associate with modern sport. Games that bear an affinity with modern-day football, in that they involved a ball of some description and had a designated place to bring the ball in order to score, were common in most villages and towns in this period. These versions of 'folk football' would involve the men of entire communities playing in teams of indeterminate numbers and guided by very few rules other than that the first team to score was the winner. Injury, sometimes death, was commonplace, with participants punching and kicking each other regardless of who was actually in possession of the ball. One of the closest surviving examples of folk football is the Kirkwall Ba' Game played in Orkney. Here two opposing teams of players, called the Uppies and the Doonies, attempt to score a single goal in order to win, with the Doonies aiming to submerge the ball in the harbour and the Uppies trying to reach the junction of Main Street with new Scapa Road. The game is played over several hours and the teams vary in size.

The transition from unbounded violence to bounded violence in sport took place in parallel with the increasing civilising and stabilising of society as a whole. In the ancient world, both Rome and Athens were highly militaristic societies with civil disputes being resolved through violence rather than through law. As society and the civilising process progressed, the requirement to internally pacify societies resulted in sports becoming considerably more rule-bound. The traditional folk games, such as the Kirkwall Ba' Game, became increasingly subject to regulation and control, a process Elias terms *sportisation*.

So, if we consider contemporary societies, we can identify the increasing rationalisation and control of the body taking place alongside the increasing regulation of games as society itself becomes more civilised. Rugby, for example, is one of the most aggressive games that are popular on a global scale in contemporary society. The playing of the game requires players to engage each other in highly aggressive physical contact in scrums, rucks and mauls, the appearance of which can seem quite chaotic to the untrained eye. It is, however, far different from the folk football games that preceded it; they were violent too but with almost no form of rules. Although rugby is still a physical and brutal pursuit, it is a highly *regulated* one: it has none of the outright violence of games of previous eras, and players are required to restrain their use of violence as opposed to acting how they would

Sportisation is another concept within the work of Elias. It is similar to the civilising process as it refers to how comparatively unregulated, chaotic and rule-free folk games become rule-bound sport. Again, this long-term process absorbs violence out of general society and places it into the safer and controllable confines of sport.

like. Certain forms of violent contact – such as the infamous 'spear tackle', which involves inverting a player, turning him upside down and effectively crashing him headfirst onto the pitch, and which can result in serious neck and spinal injuries – are forbidden, even though such tactics would be very effective for neutralising an opponent. In effect, what rugby and other games achieve for Elias is to remove the violence that could disrupt and destroy society and then to channel that violence into a ritualised format where it is contained and thereby social order is maintained.

QUESTIONS

Reflect on Elias's ideas on sport and society. Do they alter your perceptions of sport? Do you agree with him that sports are not simply 'games' but play an important role in maintaining social control? Which sports do you think exhibit the most controlled forms of violence?

SOCIAL STRUCTURE AND THE CONDITIONS OF CHOICE

As Donnelly (2005) notes, there is often an assumption that people have the agency and the free will to choose to engage or otherwise in sport and exercise. The sociological position and research on sport and exercise, he continues, strongly suggest the opposite. Why people as social agents choose to engage with certain forms of pastimes is strongly mediated by their class, ethnic and gender location in society. A useful example of how these social structures influence and shape the way people approach sport and exercise is indicated in research by Steinbach et al. (2011), who investigated the reasons why people take up cycling in London. Their research suggested that the decision to take up cycling and become what they term a 'cycling body-machine' (2011: 1129) was not accountable in terms of people wishing to exercise and be healthy, having access to resources or becoming proficient enough to cycle in such a demanding environment as London. Class, gender and ethnicity intervened as strong mediating factors. The people most likely to take up the 'active transport' of cycling were predominantly white middle-class men. As a group, cycling was an extension of both their lifestyles and their gender. They could adopt cycling as a green or an aesthetic (wearing cycling gear, for instance) lifestyle choice, while the adrenalin rush of cycling in quite aggressive circumstances appealed to their sense of masculinity. For women, the aggression of cycling could be a disincentive. In addition, the social norms of femininity (hair, make-up and clothes) constricted their choices as cycling made it difficult to perform these feminine expectations. There were also issues of childcare, with women possibly having to make longer trips to collect or drop off their children at childcare. Finally, for people from ethnic minority groups, the results of this research were less clear, but again social processes held sway. Black women could feel at odds with the white male-dominated world of London cycling, while ideas on an efficient cycling body were tied closely into white discourses of an ideal body shape that did not always culturally resonate with Asian women.

The ways these social structures intersect with sport, and how they shape individual social agents' approaches to sport and exercise, are expanded on in greater depth below. The main lesson is that there is more to sport and exercise than physical exertion alone.

QUESTIONS

Do you think everyone enjoys equal opportunities to participate in sport? How subtle are the barriers to participation mentioned in the example above?

Class and sport

Sport and class are firmly and inescapably associated with each other. Different sports appear to appeal to different social classes. In Britain, for example, and generally speaking, the working class is the mainstay of football (or soccer, as it is known in the United States), rugby by-and-large maintains middle-class support, while sports such as polo are favoured by the super-rich elite. Again, deeper currents are at play: sport throughout history has acted as a means of maintaining social control, training people for their class position, and generating differences or distinction between social classes.

First, let us investigate how sport has been a method by which to maintain social control, taking football as a useful example. Although football is often cast as possessing a long, deep history, the twentieth-century origins of many British football teams lie not with the pursuit of a pastime, or with individuals combining together for the love of kicking a ball about, but with an attempt to control and discipline working-class people in their free time, when they were away from the workplace. This concern with the moral welfare of the working class needs to be situated within the fixation in wider Victorian society on the morals and behaviours of the 'lower classes'. The sudden expansion of urbanisation throughout Britain during the 1800s had destabilised and challenged traditional conventions concerning respect and 'people knowing their place'. The newly enlarged urban environments were much freer places where people could form identities much more on their terms, free from the old restrictions (Hunt 2005). As a consequence, it was feared that the social order as a whole could collapse. Binding people, especially young men, into some form of institution and association was perceived as an effective way to prevent the further decay of society.

There was also another benefit for employers in having their employees commit their spare time to sport. This was that fit and healthy workers would make better workers, plus football acted as a mechanism to keep people out of the pubs. Manchester United FC emerged out of the Newton Heath LYR (Lancashire and Yorkshire Rail) Football Club in 1878, based, as the name so obviously suggests, on a section of workers within that rail company. The most obvious example of a football team's relationship with a workplace is probably Arsenal FC, formed out of the workforce of The Royal Arsenal, an armaments manufacturer for the British Army. The connection with the workplace is also the reason why football matches have traditionally kicked off at 3 pm on a Saturday afternoon, which was the start of the weekend for working-class men in Victorian and Edwardian Britain. An interest in sport to maintain the wellbeing of the workforce could also make the average worker fitter and more productive.

In Scotland, football also acted as a mechanism for social control, but this time based not so much on the workplace but on religion, with particular connection to the Catholic Church. Irish migration in the late 1800s had brought thousands of people from all parts of Ireland. Many of those Irish migrants were Catholic, and football was seen by the Catholic clergy and priesthood as one method whereby they could keep an eye on their flocks, so that they did not become tempted to convert to Protestantism or, even worse, become part of the increasing mass of non-religious city dwellers. The most widely known example of the relationship between football and Irish immigrant Catholics in Scotland is Glasgow Celtic, founded in 1877 by Brother Wilfred of the Marist Catholic religious order. This trend of football teams comprising Catholic Irish immigrants was also evident in Edinburgh with Hibernian, founded by Irish immigrants in 1875 (two years before their more famous Glaswegian counterparts), and in Dundee, with Dundee Hibernian (who were to change their name in 1923 to the present Dundee United) founded in 1903.

Sport has functioned for the upper classes too, but as a form of moral and physical discipline. The Duke of Wellington was supposed to have remarked at Waterloo in 1815 that the British victory over Napoleon and the French was 'won on the playing fields of Eton'. Sport provided a means of assisting the sons of the ruling classes to develop the relevant mental attitudes and prerequisite physical robustness to run the empire, display leadership, and play for the team and not for one's own personal interests. The lyrical poem *Vitaï Lampada* by Henry Newbolt (1892) – a fine example of British imperial literature – captures something of this empire-building spirit. A comparison is drawn between a schoolboy on the fields of a public school giving his all at the behest and encouragement of his captain, not for personal glory but for the greater good of the team during a cricket match (though it could be any sport played at an English public school), and the same boy as a soldier, this time fighting on a foreign field:

There's a breathless hush in the Close to-night

Ten to make and the match to win

A bumping pitch and a blinding light,

An hour to play, and the last man in.

And it's not for the sake of a ribboned coat,

Or the selfish hope of a season's fame,

But his captain's hand on his shoulder smote

'Play up! Play up! And play the game!'

The sand of the desert is sodden red –

Red with the wreck of a square that broke

The Gatling's jammed and the colonel dead,

And the regiment blind with dust and smoke.

The river of death has brimmed its banks,

And England's far, and Honour a name,

But the voice of a schoolboy rallies the ranks –

'Play up! Play up! And play the game!'

The discussion of sport so far has been historical, but it is a history that informs the present day. Football still remains a working-class activity, while the legacy of Irish immigration echoes very strongly in many local derby fixtures in Scottish football. Relationships between class and sport are perhaps a little more subtle in contemporary society but, nevertheless, are still present. The work of French sociologist Bourdieu (1984) is useful here. His sociology concentrates on how in capitalist society the distinctions between social classes are produced and reproduced using a variety of symbolic strategies and signs to denote boundaries and differences between people and their social classes. So, for example, if one considers newspapers, a different status is attached to having a copy of *The Times* tucked under one's arm rather than having *The Sun*. Buying a particular newspaper (whether the heavyweight *Times* or the tabloid *Sun*) is not purely based on what one likes to read, but also sends out a signal of social class, with certain cultural symbols indicating to which social class one belongs.

What guides social agents to particular sports is explainable by reference to what Bourdieu terms *habitus*, a concept best understood by reference to his wider sociology. Bourdieu sought to explain why people from certain class backgrounds acted in the ways that they did. What he identified was that bound up into social class were sets of practices, ways of being and doing, tastes and dispositions that guided people to behave in certain ways. These sets of practices and so forth are also learned through socialisation as we grow and mature in a particular class background, with people often carrying them out unknowingly or as if they are the 'natural thing' to do. It is these guiding practices, which we are often unaware we are following, that constitute and make up the habitus.

Earlier, when discussing cycling, we encountered an example of habitus in action. For the middle-class white men, their class habitus guided them to cycling as it was consistent with certain middle-class ideas of leisure and environmentalism. Widening the perspective, the habitus and sport can be seen in evidence on a variety of fronts. Broadly speaking, for Bourdieu, the habitus sets the scene in which people engage with a particular sport.

> In the work of Pierre Bourdieu, habitus refers to a variety of tastes, dispositions, preferences and ways of being that emerge out of the society in which we live, shaping how we act and think. The habitus often operates at a subconscious level and we do not necessarily realise that we are behaving in a way that is influenced and structured by society, as it seems a natural and normal way to be.

QUESTION

Identify other examples where society and habitus influence the choice of sport and leisure. Do you agree with Bourdieu that society subtly, and without our direct knowledge, directs our choices in sport and leisure?

Gender, body and sport

Sport is also a highly gendered landscape, where men and women traditionally play different forms of sport and exercise (see Figure 14.2). So, for example, men dominate physical contact sports such as football and rugby, and women dominate sports such as netball and field hockey, which are less physically aggressive. On a very general level this separation of sport into gender-specific activities is not wholly explicable as an accident or as a consequence of physiology. In a physiological explanation, the differences would all be seen as the result of men being naturally more muscular and therefore attracted to sports requiring a robust and strong body, while physically more diminutive women would be drawn to less demanding sports. The problem with this line of reasoning is that it runs the risk of essentialising the differences between men and women, whereby it is assumed that all differences between men and women can be understood by reference to biology alone. In such a perspective there is a rerun of the stereotypical (and sexist) notion of women being naturally and inescapably passive and men being naturally active.

Percentages

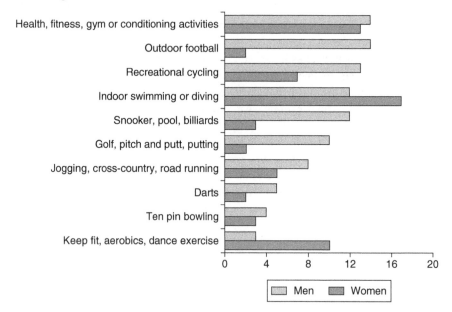

Figure 14.2 Selected sports, games and physical activities among adults, by sex, 2006–7, England

An alternative, sociological interpretation of the gendered body and sport would emphasise that the relationship between body and society is, in fact, the other way around. The actual physical dispositions of men and women, in terms of how they use their bodies and how their bodies develop a distinctive body shape (or otherwise), can be explained by how society prioritises different forms of physical being as desirable and appropriate for men and women. Socialisation and social expectation exert a strong influence in this process. Boys and girls are brought up in specific ways that help to develop their bodies in similarly specific ways. So they are directed to different types of activity, which develop their bodies in different ways. One social norm emphasises femininity, and appearing less muscular than men, a situation we touched on in the London cycling example above. In terms of a girl's social and physical development, young girls are therefore guided to less physically demanding sports and are encouraged to express their femininity by being physically less competent than boys. This sequence, which ultimately leads women to physically limit both their physical bodies and their expectations of what they capable of, is neatly summarised by Fredrickson and Harrison (2005: 93):

> Believing in their own frailty can in turn create a self-fulfilling prophecy as girls' and women's erroneous beliefs lead them to limit the effort they put into physical tasks and take the resulting handicapped performance as evidence of their low ability.

Feminist Iris Marion Young advances the above argument further in her classic essay 'Throwing like a girl' (1980), where she discusses how society is not open and equal for men and women and how women's bodies are negatively shaped by sexist and patriarchal agendas:

> Women in sexist society are physically handicapped. Insofar as we learn to live out our existence in accordance with the definition that patriarchal culture assigns to us, we are physically inhibited, confined, positioned, and objectified. As lived bodies we are not open and unambiguous transcendences that move out to master a world that belongs to us, a world constituted by our own intentions and projections. (1980: 42–3)

Sport also provides men with the means and place to perform their masculinity and to assert their male social identities (Woodward 2007). As we have discussed elsewhere in this book, masculinity and what it is to be a man are not at all monolithic. Connell (2005) usefully conceptualises masculinity as a hierarchy ranging from (a) hegemonic masculinity, which extols physical prowess, heterosexual sexual success, aggression and being the alpha male, to (b) complicit masculinity, where men may lack the resources to claim to be 'top dog' but are still heavily influenced by the ideas of hegemonic masculinity, and finally to (c) subordinate masculinity, a form for men who are gay, effeminate, bookish or physically weak. Chimot and Louveau (2010), for example, identify the problems encountered by adolescent boys who transgress and go against notions of masculinity by taking up rhythmic gymnastics, thereby placing themselves in a subordinate masculine role. Many of the boys experience some form of stigma for participating in what is perceived as a women's sport. As they report of two boys who had decided to give up rhythmic gymnastics:

> When we interviewed them, they had stopped this sport to play a sport considered 'more masculine' like football or rugby. When they were performing rhythmic gymnastics they were not encouraged by the men of the family and were stigmatized by other boys. This 'feminine' practice became too costly for them within the framework of the construction of their gender identity at adolescence. (2010: 454)

One further example of the influence of hegemonic masculinity in sport can be found in the paucity of openly gay professional football players. There is currently only *one* professional football player who has come out publicly as being gay. Twenty-year-old Anton Hysén, who plays in the fourth tier of Swedish football, came out as gay in March 2011. His decision to come out has received mixed responses.

LINK

See Chapter 6 on gender and health for more detail on Connell's theory of hegemonic masculinity.

His team-mates have been supportive, while some sections of his club's supporters have been hostile. Considering how much homophobia as a negative undercurrent and form of discrimination in society has been challenged and its prominence reduced in European society since the 1960s, it is surprising that such a development nearly 50 years later has taken so long to emerge. The continuing presence of homophobia is also surprising considering that one of football's main celebrities, David Beckham, is also a gay icon and often presents a very feminine dress sense (the sarong episode in 1998, for example) (Cashmore 2002). Even though one can point to figures like David Beckham within football and broader developments against homophobia, the continuing suppression of openly gay footballers perhaps indicates just how deeply the dominant forms of masculinity are entrenched within football.

In addition to marginalising the participation of gay men and women in sport, prevailing norms of gender hierarchy also carry 'health risks'. As Fogel (2011) notes, dominant forms of masculinity encourage professional sportsmen to endure high levels of injury and pain for fear of being castigated as weak or letting the side down. Among the Canadian football (American gridiron football, this time) players he interviewed, Fogel found that some injuries were considered to be more 'manly' than others. If there was blood or broken bones, then that was considered an acceptable and legitimate injury to receive. If the injury lacked those more dramatic physical signs of pain, then the injury lacked legitimacy. This situation was especially relevant for concussion injuries, where players stayed on the field of play after being concussed because of the hidden nature of the injury, leaving them open to the accusation of faking it or being soft.

QUESTION

In Chapter 6 on gender, we discussed how hegemonic masculinity could actually work against the health of men. Reflect on why this may also be the case with sport. In what ways does performing traditional ideas of masculinity actually harm your health?

Ethnicity and sport

Chapter 7, on ethnicity and race, outlined the various modalities and routes by which stereotypes and out-and-out racism negatively affect the health of black and other ethnic minority people. Those same processes shape black and ethnic minority experiences of sport and exercise. One obvious example of how racism affects sport is evident in the over-representation of black people in various sports at a field level, but the under-representation of black people at higher governing levels of sport. English football provides a useful example. Approximately one in five players have a black Caribbean heritage, yet only 3% of the English population are from that ethnic group (Cashmore 2005). If we examine the other end of football and look at the number of officials, managers and executives, the overall picture becomes almost exclusively white. In the 2010–11 season there were no black managers in the English Premier League, and only two black managers in the top four divisions of English football (Paul Ince at Notts County and Chris Powell at Charlton Athletic). Given the numbers of English black players that came into English football in the 1980s, there should be a much higher number of English black managers in all four divisions. At the executive level of English football, the Football Association (FA), none of the main board members of the FA is black (and none is a woman). A similar situation exists in the United States, where African-American players are over-represented on the field in sports such as American football and basketball (Cashmore 2005).

QUESTION

Can you identify certain sports where there is an over-representation of a particular ethnic group? Think about the reasons why that may be the case in the sports you have considered.

Very clear patterns of variance in ethnic levels of participation on the field and exclusion from powerful positions across different sports do exist, but the interesting point is to try to explain why these patterns exist in the first place. Various reasons are put forward to explain why this should be so (Giulianotti 2005; Sailes 1998). Some, for example, focus on supposed physical reasons, such as that the physiology of black people provides them with an edge at sport. Others focus on cultural reasons, such as that the high rate of absent fathers prompts young black men to seek a father figure in sports coaches. There is no convincing evidence to support either of these explanations. In addition, reasons put forward for black sporting superiority may lapse into racist stereotypes which recall older forms of racism, such as that black people are physical superior but intellectually inferior or that they create cultures with unstable families and welfare dependency.

It is therefore to how racism plays out in society that we must turn in order to provide the most convincing explanations. The main reason – historically at least – is that sport was one of the few social milieux where black people were allowed to be successful. Entrance to high office in either the public realm or the corporate boardroom was always difficult, but access to the sporting arena was much easier, especially in overtly physical and muscular sports such as boxing or football (both soccer and American gridiron), but less so in the more 'genteel' sports, such as tennis and golf.

This interpretation of black sporting success as being a product of racism may seem hard to sustain now, given the high number of black athletes and sportsmen and sportswomen competing globally – and often very successfully. As Carrington (2010) argues, however, perhaps black sports have left the downtown ghetto but only to have entered what he terms the 'Golden Ghetto'. In this new ghetto black sportsmen and sportswomen have the opportunities to become successful and very rich, but the wealth and success do not fundamentally challenge existing (white) power structures. Cashmore (2008) discusses the emergence of golfer Tiger Woods, who has managed to breach the barriers around ethnic minority participation in golf, but whose individual success has not translated into wider changes for ethnic minority people in that sport or across wider society.

This point takes us back to where we started in this section on ethnicity in sport (and indeed to the opening image from the 1968 Olympics) and helps to explain why British football may have many black players but very few black managers. Black people and people from other ethnic minorities have the ability to lead but are prevented from doing so by a range of often quite subtle mechanisms that exclude them from reaching positions of leadership.

CONCLUSION

In this chapter we have sought to explore sport and exercise in relation to health. What we identified was that sport and leisure are not simply separate entities in society that exist on their own terms. Accepting such an interpretation of sport and exercise in turn leads us to question the 'neutrality' of sport and exercise and their existence as pure forms of physically and mentally healthy exertion. They are, instead, bound into broader society, reflecting the various social structures, inequalities and cultures of that society. There is also a more fundamental lesson: that while sport and exercise definitely do make a difference to individual health, at a population level they are not enough to reverse the various health inequalities that we have explored in previous chapters.

SUMMARY POINTS

- Sport is not simply about health and exercise, and particular sports can only be understood by reference to the society in which they are played.

- For sociologist Elias, sport plays a significant role in bringing about greater degrees of social control in society as violence is displaced from everyday life and into the 'safer' arena of sports, where it can be regulated and confined.

- Sport is highly gendered in that it acts as a way for people to perform their gender identities, but also acts in shaping those gender identities by influencing the physical development of men's and women's bodies.

- Sport also displays other social inequalities in relation to ethnicity and class.

- In relation to ethnicity, sport can be a contradictory place where people from ethnic minority groups can tackle and overcome the barriers of racism, while simultaneously being a place where racism is experienced.

- In relation to class, sport acts as a symbol of distinction between different class groups and can assist in reproducing wider class identities and inequalities.

CASE STUDY

Richie has been suffering pain in his leg for several weeks now. He can walk and jog without difficulty, but it is when he picks up the pace a little more, approaching a run, that the problems really begin. The pain starts in his knee and then quickly spreads down his leg towards his calf muscle. If he focuses hard he can ignore the pain for a while but after perhaps twenty minutes or so the pain saps his energy and focus. The cause of the pain in his knee is easy enough for him to identify – a big crushing tackle in that away game where he found himself upended into the air before being brought down heavily to the ground, his knee being the principal point of contact between him and the pitch. He had been so close, just two more metres and that would have been an excellent try – one to remember. The ball had broken loose after a botched pass back from a maul, the opposing team's scrum-half somehow fumbling a relatively simple catch. Richie was first to react, breaking forward and scooping up the loose ball, before stepping inside their full back (who really should have nailed him then and there as he was still picking up speed) and then opening up his pace as he sprinted towards the line. Big mistake, 'white line fever' as the coach calls it; all you see is the glory of a score and not the massive wing-forward coming at you with the simple task of stopping you at all costs. It wasn't until about five minutes after his moment of glory had terminated into a messy heap of bodies, with him dropping the ball forwards that Richie realised he was in agony. He kept playing, though, as there was no obvious sign of injury – no blood or swelling or anything obviously broken; it was just intensely sore.

He really should tell someone about it. He's sure the coach would like to know or the team physio, after all he could be making things worse for himself, but somehow he just can't bring himself to do it. Perhaps if he keeps playing and training the pain will just simply go away …

Before exploring the more health-orientated questions below, discuss the role of physical sports such as rugby, featured in this case study, in society. You should discuss your answer in relation to:

(a) class (in what ways does rugby differ from other physical sports, such as football, for instance?)

(b) Elias's theory of the 'civilising process'.

QUESTIONS

1. Identify and discuss the wider discourses of gender that may be influencing Richie in not seeking help for his injured knee.
2. How could you change the culture in a sports team to make it easier for injured players to seek assistance for their injuries?
3. Can such a change be achieved solely in one team or do you think that it may require changes on a larger societal scale?

TAKING YOUR STUDIES FURTHER

This chapter will have helped you understand many of the key terms, concepts, theories and debates relating to sport, exercise and the body. Listed below are books that will provide deeper and more detailed discussions of the points raised in this chapter. You will also find additional resources on the companion website, including downloads of relevant material, links to useful websites, videos and other features. Please visit the companion website at https://study.sagepub.com/barryandyuill4e

RECOMMENDED READING

Andrews, D.L. and Carrington, B. (eds) (2013) *The Blackwell Companion to Sport*. London: Wiley.

Carrington, B. (2010) *Race, Sport and Politics: The Sporting Black Diaspora*. London: SAGE.

Giulianotti, R. (2015) *Sport: A Critical Sociology*, 2nd edn. Cambridge: Polity Press.

DEATH AND DYING

MAIN POINTS

- Death is inevitable for human beings and an inescapable element of the life course.

- Death as a definite and incontestable state can be difficult to identify and define, being dependent on social and historical contexts as much as medical classifications.

- Causes of death, and experiences of death and dying, vary considerably across different cultures and throughout history.

- Contemporary society in high-income nations, such as the United Kingdom, displays complex and contradictory attitudes to death and dying, being simultaneously death denying and death aware.

- Sacral or secular ceremonies are important for assisting in social and individual transitions following death.

- Psychological and sociological explanations and interpretations of the processes and experiences of dying offer different but also incompatible insights.

- Health workers and health professionals working with people who are dying can be required to engage in demanding forms of emotional labour.

INTRODUCTION

Quite simply, death is unavoidable and an inevitable feature of human existence. As corporeal biological and embodied beings, humans are locked into an inescapable sequence of birth, life and death: cells wear out, core vital organs shut down, and the biological body ceases to function. Regardless of all humanity's achievements in altering and controlling for its own benefit many of the challenges posed by nature, death remains as a place and part of existence beyond our complete control. Humans can definitely alter and condition the cultural practices surrounding dying and the causes of death, but the actuality of death occurring cannot be transcended. A wider study of death and dying, and the rituals and representations that surround death, reveals the impulses and motivations behind many human activities and cultural practices involving death, whether in commemorating the passing of loved ones or in dealing with the existential anxiety of one's own demise. In the British Isles, for example, many of the significant structures that mark the rural landscape or punctuate the urban skyline involve death to some extent. The oldest surviving structures, megaliths (more commonly referred to as standing stones) and chambered tombs from the Neolithic period, involve some form of engagement with death, dying and the cycles of life, while even in the increasingly busy and high-rise profile of many urban environments it is still spires and steeples that rise above the rooftops, again structures whose rationale was in part to engage with the dramas of life and death.

Secularisation refers to the process whereby society becomes increasingly less religious. Secular refers to a non-religious society or non-religious ways of understanding society. Sacral refers to religion and religious understandings of the world.

The main lesson to be found in this chapter is that for all that death may be regarded as the ultimate 'victory' of biology and nature over all the abilities of humanity, the process of dying and the moment of death are as profoundly social as they are natural – and it is this theme that is explored in greater depth in the six main sections below. First, in keeping with the practice throughout this book, we scrutinise the actual concept of death in order to open up and query basic assumptions of what constitutes death and how it can be defined. What is important here is that defining death is far from easy and without dispute, and is strongly bound into social and cultural norms and traditions. Attention then moves to discussing how the causes of death vary between nations and within nations. What becomes evident is that what leads to one's death depends on the society in which one lives. Dying of natural causes after a long life, for instance, may be the preserve of a select section of relatively wealthy people living in high-income nations like the United Kingdom, whereas other poorer members of that same society can die much younger. When we open a wider global perspective, it becomes obvious that causes of death and age at death are once more heavily dependent on the society in which one lives. The third section considers a topic of considerable debate in sociological assessments of death: whether or not contemporary western society has become increasingly death denying, in that death as the inevitable end of human life is a taboo topic. The final two sections focus on the parallel experiences of those who are dying and those health workers and health professionals who work with the dying and the dead.

WHAT IS 'DEATH'? CONCEPTUALISING AND DEFINING THE END OF LIFE

One important function of the sociological imagination is not to accept any social phenomena at face or surface value. What people encounter on a daily basis is always open to further question and deeper investigation; that is the purpose and promise of the sociological imagination. As has been explored in relation to class, gender and ethnicity, new insights into what we are studying can be gained by questioning what the concepts of, for instance, class, gender and ethnicity actually mean and how they relate to events and patterns in wider society. So, when discussing death (and we shall return to defining dying later), what do we mean by death? A review of the main debates and arguments reveals that it is more complex than first inspection would indicate.

French poststructuralist philosopher Derrida (1993), in his deconstruction of popular and scholarly ideas, has questioned the existence of a tight and clear delineation and border between life and death. Instead, he draws attention to how mutable and fluid ideas of death are bound into different cultures and are variable and changing across time and history. Death is also, he notes, a state of being that is neither fully social nor fully biological but exists in the fusion and interrelationship of the two. This highlighting of issues relating to defining and conceptualising death and dying is highly useful as it guides us to thinking of death not just as a simple state of 'non-life' or the non-functioning of core bodily processes and no brain activity, but rather as a process which exists in the midst of other processes, bound into culture, society, history and biology.

Let us focus a little more on the biological aspects of death briefly mentioned above. In many popular hospital-based dramas, the iconic image of a heart monitor flatlining while emitting a high-pitched monotone is used to signal the death of a patient. Such an image informs lay perceptions concerning the finality of death, that death is an unambiguous and definite state: the person alive is now dead, and the two are very clear and distinct separate states. A great many complications exist, however, that question and challenge this straightforward understanding of death. Philosophically, it can be asked: what is death? Such a question raises thorny issues about the relationship between mind, body and self-identity, or more broadly put: what is it to be alive? This question is very difficult to answer succinctly. Is life purely a biological function? Is life the ability to interact with other human beings? Is it a combination of both? And, if so, is one more powerful than the other?

Kellehear (2008) has identified how the criteria used to pronounce death have changed over historical time. In the Middle Ages, the signs that were sought out to establish death were *external*: the body was examined for stiffness of the muscles, discoloration of the skin, or putrefaction and decay. In modernity, the focus has become increasingly *internal*, with an emphasis on cardiovascular and brain activity. The change as to what constitutes death parallels, in certain regards, the wider historical trend of the increasing rationalisation and advance of technological scientific perspectives, in that designating someone as being dead is made in the context of what a piece of technology (what Latour (1992) would term a 'non-human actor' in a wider network of activity and decision making) records as being patterns of a particular electrical or neural activity that are interpreted as being significant of a change in status, in this case, from being alive to being dead. As has been raised in Chapter 2 in a discussion on medical technology and the wider medical model, just because a particular event or interaction between people is mediated by scientific principles does not necessarily entail that scientific medicine provides any definitive answers. There are cases, as Kellehear (2008) notes, where people who may be classifiable as 'brain dead' and therefore technically dead, but who are kept going only with the support of technology, are still capable of conceiving or giving birth – two qualities that for many people would signify life not death.

The inverse of the above may also be true, because the body may remain clinically alive in that the heart beats and the various biological organs function perfectly well, but that does not necessarily entail that the person is alive. After all, sociologically speaking, being an active human agent usually implies some form of interaction with others. So the body can be alive, but what makes the individual a particular person is no longer present. Such a state can be evident in cases of dementia and allied conditions that affect the memory of an individual, where what is termed a 'social death' can occur. The body is physically present but the person who was known by their friends and family has, to all intents and purposes, passed away. Defining death is made even more complex with current technological developments. Stem-cell technology, and the ability of science to operate on a molecular level, opens up a range of debates as to what is alive and what is dead, given that the lifetime of human cells can be prolonged almost indefinitely, which again raises the question: when is someone truly dead?

MORTALITY AND THE GLOBAL CAUSES OF DEATH

Seale (2000) has mapped out the main coordinates of death in contemporary global society, and what his work reveals is that death is far from a unitary phenomenon and experience across all societies. Death rates, trajectories of dying, causes of death and age at death (see Figure 15.1) vary markedly from country to country. What passes as being a 'normal' way to die in a high-income western nation is notably different from what is normal in a low-income sub-Saharan nation. Comparing deaths due to HIV/AIDS and cancers provides a useful illustration of these differences between global regions (see Figure 15.2 for other selected causes of death). According to the World Health Organisation (2011: 74), the mortality rate for HIV/AIDS in 2009 in the Africa region was 117 per 100,000 in comparison to 19 per 100,000 in the Europe region, a rate that is just over six times higher. In comparing cancer (or malignant neoplasms), the differences in mortality between regions are less stark, but they are still quite pronounced. It is the Europe region this time that exhibits the higher number of deaths, with a mortality ratio of *c*. 350 per 100,000 in comparison to a

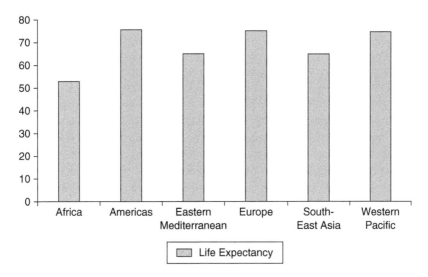

Figure 15.1 Average life expectancy by WHO global region for both sexes, in 2008

Source: WHO (2011) *World Health Statistics*. Geneva: World Health Organisation.

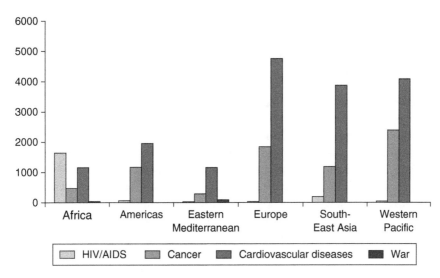

Figure 15.2 Deaths (000s) in WHO regions, estimates for 2004

Source: WHO (2008) *Global Burden of Disease: 2004 Update*. Geneva: World Health Organisation.

mortality ratio of *c*. 160 per 100,000 in the Africa region (WHO 2010: 14). These statistics reveal a number of interesting insights into just how experiences and contexts differ globally. First, the leading causes of death are quite different: HIV/AIDS in Africa and cancer in Europe, with each cause of death accounting for quite high numbers of people. However, one should take care not to lapse into some form of equivalence – into thinking that the two causes of death are essentially similar in that they are both likely to lead to illness with the strong possibility of death. How those causes of death are socially situated, and what the contexts are in which death occurs, are decidedly and critically different.

HIV/AIDS in the Africa region is more likely to kill younger people in their teens and twenties, thus reducing the numbers of economically active people, and also creating a crisis with the number of children who are orphaned after their parents die of AIDS. There may also be a lack of medication and appropriate hospital services, which means that the process of dying (of which more later) is marked by higher levels of discomfort and pain, plus a reduction in the time available in which to live out an already shorter life. Cancer deaths typically (though not in every instance) generally affect older people who have been economically active, but more importantly the European person dying of cancer will have led a longer life, with the advantages of being able to achieve life goals and engage in the various activities that are important and meaningful to someone across their life course.

Considerable and substantial differences are also present *within* countries just as much as *between* countries. Section 2 of this book focuses on health inequalities that emerge out of wider social inequalities, and these wider social inequalities also apply to death. What is evident is that death is not due to random chance, an unlucky roll of destiny's dice, but is found in one's class, ethnicity and gender location. So, a person from a working-class background will live on average seven years less than someone from a middle-class background; and in some cases, as was discussed in relation to areas in Glasgow, the mortality difference can be up to 30 years. In terms of gender, even though the gap is closing, women still outlive men by five or so years. And in regard to ethnicity, people from ethnic minority backgrounds will on average die earlier than those from ethnic majority backgrounds. Remember that these inequalities often run together, and people who are at the intersection of inequalities will experience increased chances of early mortality. Death, as with so much in life, is therefore to do with social structures rather than chance, biology or individual agency.

War as a cause of death is included among the more expected 'medical' conditions in Figure 15.2. It is included to highlight that when seeking to understand death it is important to situate death in its fullest context, and that considerable numbers of people die of a cause that is purely the outcome of human intervention in the form of particular (and failed) social and political processes. Medical sociology as a sub-discipline has, as Williams (2004) notes, been silent on the issue of war and health, which is surprising given that war is fundamentally concerned with the negation of human life and bringing harm to embodied human beings. The actual numbers of people killed in the recent wars in the Middle East, for example, are hard to identify. Estimates of deaths attributable to war-related violence in Iraq have ranged from 151,000 in a survey for the World Health

Organisation (Alkhuzai et al. 2008) to 607,207 in a survey published by *The Lancet* journal (Burnham et al. 2006). Regardless of the exact numbers of civilians who have died as a direct and indirect consequence of conflict, the point here is that death for many is the result not of ill health but of violent human action.

MODERN SOCIETY: 'DEATH DENYING' OR 'DEATH AWARE'?

Since the publication in English of the highly influential and stimulating work of Philippe Ariès on death, *The Hour of Our Death* (1982) and *Western Attitudes toward Death: From the Middle Ages to the Present* (1974), modern European society has been characterised as being *death denying*. This particular concept implies that modern society silences discussion of death, forbids the topic of death and dying in everyday conversation, and excludes and isolates the dead and dying to the physical and symbolic outer regions and limits of society. In effect, a taboo surrounds death and modern society denies its existence, to a similar degree that sex was taboo in Victorian society. Ariès' thesis is based upon his empirical study of cultural, literary and artistic representations of death and dying. From his study he contends that practices and rituals surrounding death have changed over time in parallel with how society understands and creates death. He offers a periodisation (Small 1997) of death in which it moves from being seen as an inevitable experience towards being an experience that can be tamed, where the dying person can focus on sorting out their affairs with the full involvement of their family and friends so as to lead to a good death. In the eighteenth century, death was romanticised as being almost a beautiful experience, but one bathed in pathos and ideas of personal tragedy. The one main arc of historical change he notes is the move away from public recognition – if not the very public display – of the dead and the dying to a privatised and hidden death, where death becomes dirty and an event to be shunned and relegated to the margins of conversation.

It is useful to consult the historical record again, briefly, in order to indicate just how much has changed in terms of our relationships with both death and the dead. At other points in history death was all-pervasive, experienced by having dead family members in the household, seeing the dead in the streets and observing the dead represented in art forms. The Black Death that raged across Europe in the mid-1300s claimed the lives of somewhere in the region of 375 million people, one of the most devastating pandemics in human history. The sheer scale of the disease challenged and reshaped society on myriad levels. The power and social role of the Church was questioned, for example, but one of the more visual manifestations of death in this period was the frequent use of death images in

Death denying implies that a society and the individuals who are part of that society attempt to ignore the subject of death in conversation and generally behave as if death does not exist. Death aware is the reverse of death denying, where death is acknowledged and accepted but not necessarily in a way that is consistent and without contradictions.

art. This tradition was most evident in the medieval period in the various images of the *Danse Macabre* (Figure 15.3), where skeletons engaged in a wild dance with each other or mischievously taunted the living that their own death could happen without warning at any moment.

The possible reasons for the movement from an open and accepting culture of death to a denial of death can be traced to distinct social developments within the twentieth century. Walter (2004: Chapter 1) advances the following reasons why contemporary society can be perceived to be death denying, a state in which the often interrelated processes inherent in modernity lead to the depersonalisation of death and the repression of emotion and grief. The end result of all these processes acting on and shaping societal and individual beliefs is that death becomes a taboo subject, an off-limits area of conversation, blanked out as an issue for personal reflection on one's life and its future:

- *Rationalisation.* Like so much of modern life, death has become the object of the various forces and processes of rationalisation, where the very intimate moments of death become subject to timetables, bureaucracy and categorisation. Death is not just the ending of someone's life, but an element of the great paper trail of modernity, where every aspect of life is recorded and filed. The end result is that death becomes disconnected from private emotional reference points, grief in particular, and attached to the cold emotionless framework of the public office and public official. The death certificate is an example. As a document, the death certificate records very objective information, such as date of birth, the cause of death and the name of the recording

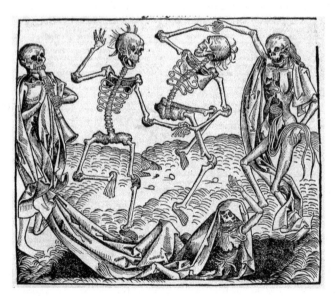

Figure 15.3 The Danse Macabre

Source: Wolgemut (1493) 'Dance of Death'. Available at en.wikipedia.org/wiki/File:Holbein-death.png

officer. Subjective and affective information, such as the emotions of the surviving relatives, go unrecorded. This is all very useful for the running of a large bureaucratic state, which requires information on its citizens, but is not very effective at dealing with the issues of loss and grieving.

- *Medicalisation.* Discussed earlier in this book, medicalisation involves the colonisation (the 'taking over') of an increasing number of areas of life that were once regarded as existing outside the medical gaze. The same applies to death and dying. Death for most of human history was explicable in religious terms; it was God's will that people should die, and therefore religion was the only source of insights into and understandings of death. As medical technology has developed, however, death has become framed less as a moment defined by the divine and increasingly as a medical event, with death resulting out of a distinct sequence of biological stages. Walter (2004) also notes one further way in which death has become medicalised: the change in the location of dying. In western high-income countries the place of death is now more likely to be in the hospital under the auspices of the medical profession than in the home supported by friends and family.

- *Secularisation.* Allied to the point above, one other development within modernity is the decline of sacral or religious belief. Modern society has become increasingly secular, which means that people do not interpret their lives within the symbolic framework of religion. Previously, in a Judeo-Christian context at least, images of death, resurrection and redemption informed the minds and actions of people. Without the presence of such imagery, death becomes less a feature of life. Walter (2004) points to the First World War as a turning point in religious belief in Western Europe, where the idea of a loving God became increasingly untenable given the mass death and suffering of the conflict. However, as both Hunt (2005) and Bruce and Glendinning (2010) maintain, secularisation begins much earlier in the eighteenth century, when the new urbanisation brought about by the industrial revolution removed ordinary people from the control and teachings of the church.

- *Individualisation.* One debated trend within contemporary society is the move away from community to a life based more on individualism. Such a trend may sound appealing in that we now possess the potential to make more of our lives as and how we wish, unbidden by pressures from the wider community. Walter (2004) notes, however, that one rather demanding cost of being individual is that one lacks the ties to other people who could provide emotional support in times of crisis, such as when facing death. The upshot is that it is better to ignore rather than embrace death.

Rationalisation is where society becomes more controlled, governed and ordered but at the expense of spontaneity and human emotion.

Medicalisation is where the medical profession increasingly colonises more aspects of everyday life, and what were once regarded as normal social problems (shyness, for instance) are recast as medical problems.

Secularisation is where society becomes less religious and more inclined to humanistic or scientific understandings of social and natural events.

Individualisation is where people focus less on the wider community and more on themselves, with their actions being self-directed rather than other-directed.

Walter (2004) does not include *consumerism* in his summary of why today's society might be death denying, but the various characteristics of consumer culture could also contribute to a death denying culture, extolling as it does the perfect, young but crucially *living* body. The number of facial cosmetics and the ease of access to cosmetic surgery could be cited as further evidence of death denial, since the purpose of such products (and here surgery is as much a product as an anti-ageing cream) is to deny the passing of time and ageing, let alone the very real finality of death.

QUESTION

In what way are the processes that have, arguably, led to a denying of death unique to modernity as a historical epoch? Identify further examples of how each process could influence how we approach and understand issues of death and dying.

This perception of modern society being death denying has been challenged by a number of sociologists (such as Seale 2000), and the work of Ariès and others who have advanced the death denying thesis has been critiqued. One of the main objections to Ariès' analysis of death, for example, parallels that of critiques of his work on childhood: that by drawing ostensibly on artistic and literary sources for his empirical data, he does not allow for those sources to be contextualised as idealised versions of death and dying at a particular point in history rather than as how death and dying were actually experienced and understood at that time. What Ariès presents, in effect, is an overly romanticised view of death and dying that is nostalgic for a past that never was, as opposed to an accurate recreation of the place of death and dying in the past and over time.

The main thrust of the counter-argument is that contemporary society is not death denying but is just as *death aware* as in previous times, only in a way that is more fluid, complex and contradictory. On the one hand, unlike Victorian society, contemporary society denies death; it is a topic shunned in conversation, and issues of dying, such as the ageing process, have become almost a taboo subject. On the other hand, death is frequently depicted in many mainstream cultural products, where the subject of death and what it is to be dead form the basis of plotlines in films and television serials. Death and what the dead are like are very distinct and idiosyncratic in such media. In many contemporary films and TV shows, such as the *Twilight* trilogy or *Buffy the Vampire Slayer*, to be dead is to be reborn in the afterlife as an emotionally complex but still very sexy American teenager, where death is not about bodily decay or the end of self but instead is a continuation of self at the peak of one's young powers. One could claim, as Gorer (1965) did back in the 1960s, that this form of death awareness is 'pornography' and does not really deal with death; yet these depictions of the dead and death are often more nuanced and subtle than the traditional blood-'n'-gore movies of that period.

Throughout popular culture there is other ample evidence of engagement with death. In addition to the new wave of vampire movies, one could point to *The Time Traveller's Wife* (both the novel and the film), which focuses on memory of a loved one and dealing with loss, as does the book *The Finkler Question*, and to the various geographic variations of the American crime series *CSI*, where death and the dead are treated and portrayed in computer-generated high detail. In popular music there is the subgenre of death metal, where fast and furious bass-heavy songs in doom-laden minor keys celebrate motifs of death and dying, and where bands refer to death in their names, such as Korpse, Entombed and (the not so subtle) Death. There is also, of course, the Goth subculture (Hodkinson 2002), in which adherents also, albeit probably more playfully and elegantly than in death metal, adopt imagery and symbols associated with death.

It is, overall, difficult to sustain a perspective that claims that modern society is exclusively death denying. A quick survey of popular culture, as revealed above, finds plenty of evidence to the contrary. Seymour (2001), though, cautions against such a simplistic 'either/or' dichotomy of society being either death denying or death aware. The actuality, she argues, is much more complex, but then again so is the phase of modernity. As Kellehear (2007) maintains, the practices and understandings of death and dying parallel the norms and cultures of a given society; so as society becomes much more complex, an equally complex approach to death and dying develops. Walter (2004) characterises this complexity towards death and dying as being consistent with postmodern trends in society. As with other postmodern trends there is a rejection of a simple 'one-size-fits-all' approach, with its implication of everyone acting uniformly, and instead an acceptance that everyone follows a path that is much more of their own making, drawing on whichever elements of social culture and social symbols they choose. Seale (2000) notes something similar: that in late modernity a greater reflexivity exists in how people approach various aspects of their life course, in that they are frequently engaged in working out how they make *their* lives meaningful, in a context that is most appropriate to them. So, what we can see today is not one mass society-wide approach to death but myriad individual approaches. However, one must be careful to acknowledge that these choices are not open to all. As Kellehear (2004) reminds us, not everyone possesses the power to choose exactly how they live and how they die, depending on class, gender and ethnic differences.

RITES, RITUALS AND CEREMONIES: DEALING WITH DEATH

Regardless of how a society defines death, when it does occur it can lead to a traumatic and significantly upsetting period both in the lives of friends and relatives and also in wider society. The various bonds that link a person to others and to wider society are, for a time at least, broken and damaged. A phase of uncertainty and change follows, where people need time to make adjustments and hopefully re-establish their own personal and social narratives. That is why so many rites and rituals surround death, the purpose of which is to repair and heal those social and individual bonds so as to allow for the return of some form of 'normal' functioning.

Religious narratives and symbols were the traditional discourse that people deployed to deal with and assist in either their own dying or the death of a loved one. All religions, whether historic or contemporary, offer a core set of symbolic beliefs concerning death and dying. Historically, for example, in Neolithic (Stone Age) and Iron Age Britain the dead were not separate from the living. As archaeologist Francis Prior (2004) has discerned about Neolithic society and its religious affirmations, death and life were firmly enmeshed together both physically and symbolically. It was common in that period for burials, for example, to be close to human habitation. In some instances, the dead were buried beneath the floors of roundhouses to indicate a connection with their ancestors and the great cycles of life and death, the moon and the sun; while the landscape itself would be altered to symbolically record the dead with burial mounds and standing stone circles marking the horizon (see Figure 15.4). Neolithic social ceremonies also involved a close physical and symbolic relationship with the dead. The placement of human remains found

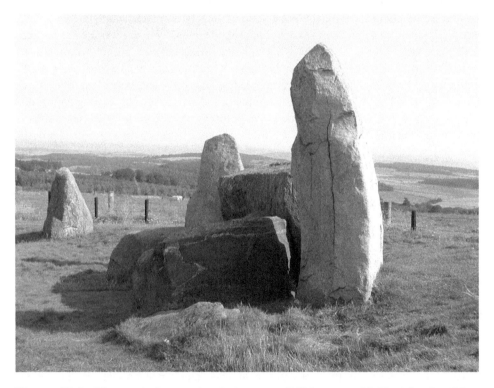

Figure 15.4 The central recumbent stones, *c.* 5000 years old, East Aquhorthies Neolithic standing stone circle, near Inverurie in Scotland

in chambered tombs, such as the West Kennet Long Barrow near Silbury Hill in Wiltshire, strongly suggests that the disarticulated bones of deceased relatives of ancestors were regularly moved around, taken out from the tomb and used in ceremonies that were important and significant for the people of that time.

In western Judeo-Christianity the central symbolic narrative and mythology concern resurrection: that by believing in God, not committing sin and acting in a compassionate and caring manner, your soul will be saved and you will be granted eternal life in paradise. Other religious faiths and belief systems offer different interpretations as to what happens after death. Hinduism and Sikhism, for instance, have reincarnation as their understanding, while Buddhism reveals rebirth, in some respects similar to reincarnation. There may be some quite different ideas as to what happens after death throughout the world's religions, but the fact that they all deal with issues of death is what is important. The world's religions also provide various ceremonies and rituals to structure and provide focus for those who have lost someone. As Durkheim highlighted in his functionalist sociology, humans require and develop rituals and ceremonies to mark all the important transitions in their lives, and death is no exception. The traditional Christian funeral in western high-income nations involves either a burial or a cremation, preceded by a ceremony that focuses on how the departed individual is now in a better place, involving prayers and hymns and reference to God and an afterlife. The ceremony also allows relatives and friends an acceptable place and appropriate occasion in which to grieve, although, as Elias has argued, grieving is not always a spontaneous outburst of emotion, and the various civilising processes present set parameters, especially for men, as to what is appropriate or dignified.

One current social trend, however, is the increasing secularisation of society, principally within the United Kingdom and other European states, where belief in organised Christian religion is in considerable decline. This development does pose a question: how do non-religious societies deal with death? If Durkheim is correct in claiming that humans require ritual to mark and make sense of important stages in the life course, then what ceremonies do secular societies provide to endure the challenges posed by death? In fact, there has been a proliferation of different forms of funerary practice. Humanist funerals have become increasingly popular. As a ceremony they may resemble conventional Christian funerals in so far as there will be a burial or a cremation, with the ceremony led by a specially designated individual, accompanied by songs and readings. There are crucial differences, however. The focus of the ceremony is not on an afterlife or a supernatural being (or God) but entirely on the deceased, celebrating their life and recording their favourite experiences and music. One of the more colourful practices that can be used in secular funerals is the balloon release. Here mourners gather together, each holding a balloon. Once they have reflected on the life of the deceased, and they feel at some form of peace, they release the balloons, symbolising a letting go of grief.

In addition to the secular ceremonies and belief structures discussed above, Lee (2008) notes that various developments concerning New Age religion and beliefs offer a re-enchantment of society. He makes this point in reference to Weber's key criticism of capitalist society: that it robs the world of enchantment and the 'magic' of life and replaces all that is special and unique in a process of disenchantment that leads to modern life being similar to living in an 'iron cage'. Finally, one other recent trend in memorialisation of those who have died is evident in the increase of roadside memorials, usually in the form of flowers, but also including poems, stuffed toys, football shirts, or other objects that were meaningful for the deceased. So, even if the traditional forms of funeral and memorialisation are on the wane, new forms are beginning to appear that could become how future societies celebrate the life of a deceased friend or family member.

DYING AND THE ANTICIPATION OF DEATH

It is useful once more to highlight that death and dying are not solely biological events, but are crucially bound and interwoven into social relationships and the culture of a particular society. What counts as being dead, and the experience and process of dying, are defined and set by the context and society in which someone lives (and of course dies!). In this section on dying – about the anticipation of death and how both the individual and society make adjustments to the end of life – it is vital to bear in mind that dying here is not limited exclusively to the biological experience of dying. What is under discussion is how that biological (or embodied) element of the process is prefigured and contextualised into an array of social relationships that vary by society and by historical period.

Before any further discussion it would be helpful to tie down what is meant by dying, as was carried out earlier in this chapter when defining death. As Kellehear (2007) notes, death is a very particular biological point when nerves and tissue irreversibly cease to function; but as humans are emotional beings, their experience of dying is not just limited to the biological horizon but is, instead, tied into existential reflection, social norms and personal relationships. Kellehear also usefully defines the process and anticipation of dying in the following more sociologically nuanced manner, where emphasis is placed on wider social relationships, and dying is seen as a social process but one which is also animated by individual desire and agency:

> I speak here of dying as a self-conscious anticipation of impending death and the social alterations in one's lifestyle prompted by ourselves and others that are based upon that awareness. This is the conscious living part of dying rather than the dying we observe as the final collapsing of a failing biological machine. (Kellehear 2007: 2)

For people living in contemporary high-income nations, the idea of dying, or the anticipation of dying and their own death, exists in the distance of time, a process to be encountered and endured towards the end of up to eight or more decades of life, probably following a lengthy debilitating illness or the slow natural demise of the body. During the intervening years the focus is on life and living rather than on dying. This distancing of dying is a comparatively recent development in experiencing the life course brought about by the extension of life expectancy through the twentieth century. In previous epochs, the distinction between life, dying and death would not have been so marked. There would have been greater awareness of the inescapable fact that life is short and death can happen much sooner than one would wish. Indeed, given how rapid death could be in historical times (due to an accident or aggressive infectious disease), dying as both a social activity and a social relationship may have been quite different from how dying is thought of today. In the Neolithic era, death was, for example, a very sudden event, and there simply would not have been an extended period for the dying person to reflect on their life and the big change that was happening to them. Instead, the process of dying would begin well *within* life, but essentially as a *symbolic* activity, with people making preparations for their death by making sure that their journey through the afterlife was well stocked with appropriate weapons, for a man, or food supplies, for a woman. These preparations could have involved planting a certain type of tree that was symbolically rich for the tribe, for example, or by storing an axe to be collected in the afterlife. Once someone had died, let us say, of an accident while out hunting or gathering food, it was the surrounding members of the tribe who would 'do' the dying, engaging in ceremonies that would ease the journey from this world into the next world for the recently deceased member of their tribe and community (Kellehear 2007).

As human society develops and changes over time so does the process of dying and how people go about the business of dying. One advantage that humans gained from establishing settled farming communities is that they could begin to develop the basics (steady food supply, shelter and safety) that would allow them to live longer. By living longer, time for dying and a space for personal reflection were created, as death would become less of a random, swift and unexpected event. Again, how people approach dying alters across time as society develops.

The best-known interpretation of what a dying person undergoes is provided by Elisabeth Kübler-Ross. Her work emerges out of her reaction against what she perceived to be the increasingly inhuman and cold treatment of dying people in modern society. In her landmark and highly influential work *On Death and Dying* (1969) she presents a stage model consisting of what Walter (2004) terms the 'famous five' stages that dying people pass through as they die and move from denying to accepting that they are dying:

- *Denial*. This is a phase of the person not believing what they have been told by the doctor or specialist, that the terrible news they have been given must be the result of an incorrect test, that someone has made a mistake in the lab, and that if the results were to be rechecked then all would be well and they would not be dying. The related reaction of *isolation* can also occur here, where the dying person withdraws from the world about them, seeking their own company and avoiding the company of others.
- *Anger*. Denial may be impossible to maintain and the initial feelings of rejecting what they have been told transmute into anger and rage. The target of this anger can be

people they know who are healthy despite having engaged in much less healthy life-styles than they have, but more likely the anger will be funnelled towards the medical staff and health professionals around them.

- *Bargaining*. Here the dying person attempts to gain more time in which to live. Bargaining can be with God or the medical staff, running on the lines of, 'If you give me more time, then I'll do something for you in return'.
- *Depression*. As the realisation sinks in that bargaining leads nowhere, due to ongoing and increasingly debilitating medical and surgical procedures, for example, the dying patient can experience loss of role and an awareness that the end is near. They can remain in this stage for quite some time.
- *Acceptance*. This is the last stop on the journey of dying and accepting that death is now inevitable.

This five-stage model may read quite neatly and provide a nice and ordered approach to the no doubt highly traumatic and difficult experience of dying, but it is not without its shortcomings, which throw into question the actual usefulness and accuracy of its basic precepts. Walter (2004) provides a useful summary of the problems that have been identified with the Kübler-Ross model of dying, and the key ones are as follows:

- Doctors and health professionals may misinterpret the patient's actions and behaviours, incorrectly assigning them to the denial or anger stage. Doing so can give rise to miscommunication and misunderstandings, resulting in negative impacts on the patient's health and care in the ward.
- Very little empirical research has been carried out on the five-stage approach in order to assess how accurate it is. This lack of rigour has potentially allowed the stage model of dying to gain a credibility that is perhaps questionable.
- It is *too* neat and tidy. The concept of such a linear approach to death is not necessarily reflective of reality; approaches, adjustments and interpretations of death and dying (as discussed in the previous section) are more fluid.
- The whole model is very American in its orientation, reflecting American cultural values of individualism, with the emphasis being on the person and not the wider social context in which they live.
- Finally, Kübler-Ross' work is perhaps less an academic thesis and more a personal vision of how dying could and should be.

QUESTION

Assess the disadvantages and advantages of the Kübler-Ross approach to dying. Do you agree or disagree with the criticisms listed above? Provide reasons for your answers.

THE EMOTIONAL LABOUR OF WORKING WITH THE DEAD AND DYING

As indicated earlier in this chapter, the majority of people in contemporary high-income nations such as Britain die in a hospital. In such locations a whole array of health professionals and health workers will obviously be found, and part of their daily labour and practice will involve working with people who are dying and with those who have died. One sub-theme of this chapter has been that death involves a certain emotional cost for those who are connected in some way with the dying and the dead. If that is the case – and here the more 'negative' and troubling emotions of grief are the focus – how are those workers and professionals affected?

The theory of *emotional labour*, as developed by Arlie Hochschild (1983), provides a useful starting point in exploring and answering the question just set. Her theory centres on one particular development in the field of work in late modernity: the shift away from work requiring a set of skills to do with the physical movement of the body (such as being able to turn a lathe or operate machinery) to work involving the emotions of the body, where as part of the working day (or night) enacting and performing appropriate emotional displays are the core requirement of the job (hence *emotional* labour). Emotional labour can therefore require the suppression of how one is really feeling and the simultaneous performance of emotions that one is not really experiencing. So, for example, when working with a client, the health professional may have to refrain from displaying feelings of boredom and frustration with that client and instead perform or enact an outward display of care and interest.

> Emotional labour refers to the performance, suppression or drawing upon of emotions as required of an individual person by an institution (usually the workplace). As a form of work emotional labour – using one's emotions to work – is increasing in the modern workplace, replacing older manual skills. Emotional labour can exert a cost on the worker as they may feel emotionally burned out or that they are emotional fakes.

The original focus of Hochschild's research fell on female airline stewardesses, who as part of their job were obliged by the organisation they worked for to create a certain emotional environment for the airline passengers, involving making them feel welcome. The creation of a relaxed and welcoming ambience relied on the ability of the stewardesses to act enthusiastically in response to the passengers' needs and demands. On first inspection, having a job that involves only flashing a few smiles and being 'nice' to people may appear to be relatively undemanding and perhaps even enjoyable. Hochschild's (1983) findings, however, pointed to a quite different reality. The stewardesses reported that they were alienated from their emotions, they felt that their smiles were no longer their own, their emotional display and feeling were somehow 'false' and synthetic, and they had an overall feeling of being 'burnt out'. The reason for the stewardesses reporting emotional exhaustion and damage to their emotional self was that the surface acting of emotions (that is, smiling to welcome a passenger) can require the manufacture of emotion and also a drawing upon real, deep and core emotions, which were not an infinite resource and whose reserves could be depleted over time – in effect, using up all their emotions.

A parallel situation can be seen to exist for health workers and health professionals in working with the dying and the dead. Contemporary health care requires a combination of professional, instrumental skills and, just as importantly, the emotional skills necessary to engage with the emotional aspects of care and the patient experience. There are distinct occasions in health care where emotional skills play an important role in assuring both patient dignity and the success of care and treatment. Nurses working in intensive care, for example, may engage in emotion work in order to provide a more human environment for patients who are dying in a place that is cold and filled with cold technology, and to assist in the development of good relations between the patient, clinical staff and family members (Seymour 2001). Emotional labour, as Hochschild strongly suggests, often comes at a cost, as indicated in the discussion above concerning airline stewardesses. A variety of research has identified that the emotional labour costs associated with the care of dying people are multiple, and include burnout, feelings of aggression, alcohol or substance (mis)use, and suicidal ideation. As Sorensen and Iedema (2009) argue, the problem with the stresses and anxieties that emerge from emotional labour in a hospital or healthcare setting is that they are less well understood than the normal stresses and anxieties (such as the number of hours worked and the amount of task-centred labour) associated with organisational and institutional demands. They are less obvious and therefore harder to identify and quantify, which makes taking any ameliorative action quite problematic. The negative consequences of emotional labour therefore remain unchallenged, creating further and deeper issues of wellbeing for health workers and health professionals.

QUESTIONS

Reflect on the concept of emotional labour in relation to your own experiences of work (this does not necessarily have to be in the health field). Can you identify how important certain emotional performances are in the modern working environment and what effect they can have on the person doing the performing?

CONCLUSION

Death will, unfortunately, come to us all; that is an inescapable part of being human. However, our experiences of dying and our understandings of death will differ greatly by social class, gender and ethnicity, on the one hand, and by wider social, global and historical developments on the other. So, we will all die but that final stage of existence is also cut across by the various inequalities that structured and conditioned the life we had before our death. By also discussing those social differences, another point is made about death and dying: as moments in our life, they are not solely explicable in biological terms. Biology is a very important element in relation to the terminal changes that occur in the body, but these biological events are woven into the wider social and cultural contexts that can be both the cause of death and the provider of the symbols and rituals that help to make sense of death and dying.

So, once again, we can see how sociology and the sociological imagination provide insights into a very intimate and difficult part of our life and our health, and how essential an appreciation of social processes is in order to gain a fuller and deeper understanding of death and dying.

SUMMARY POINTS

- Human beings have always sought to deal and cope with death and dying.

- Death is not necessarily an unambiguous state, and what counts as being dead changes across time and across cultures.

- The reasons why people die are highly variable and depend on the part of the world in which you live.

- There is a debate as to how much contemporary western societies deny death. There may not be the same direct openness about death that existed in Victorian times, for example, but perhaps a more subtle and nuanced acceptance of death has developed which does not necessarily rely upon public display.

- New forms of funerary rites are beginning to emerge that are replacing older and traditional religious approaches as society becomes increasingly secular.

- Health professionals require a certain level of emotional labour when working with people who are dying.

CASE STUDY

What some people noticed at Jamie's funeral, especially the older people who had a little more acquaintance with death and what must be done when someone passes away, was that even though it was in the city crematorium it wasn't a minister or a priest who conducted the service. Instead, there was a man who, in very dignified tones, informed the packed room that he was a humanist celebrant and would be leading not a funeral service but instead a celebration of Jamie's life. Jamie was nineteen when he died, a silly and pointless accident where a second's inattention had made the difference between life and death. Out camping with friends he had walked to some nearby cliffs. The long coastal grass had overgrown the cliff top, giving a false impression that the edge was a little further away than it actually was. He had stepped forward not realising where the true edge was. Both he and his family were not religious and it just seemed inappropriate to involve someone from the church – plus the last thing Jamie would have wanted was for his farewell to be anything but a big joyous party! So, no one was to wear anything associated with mourning, and the music that was played between the various speeches made by friends and family were his favourite songs and some of the demo tracks he had recorded with his band.

QUESTIONS

1. The above case study may seem to portray a very modern way of managing death and conducting a ritual for someone who has died, but try to detect and identify themes that could be found in other historical times or even in other societies.
2. Jamie's funeral was a humanist service. How does this choice of ceremony reflect wider changes in society in relation to organised religion?
3. Why do you think humans need to mark key moments across the life course (think of other events as well as death)? Try to relate your discussion to socio-logical theories and concepts.

TAKING YOUR STUDIES FURTHER

This chapter will have helped you understand many of the key terms, concepts, theories and debates relating to death and dying. Listed below are books that will provide deeper and more detailed discussions of the points raised in this chapter. You will also find additional resources on the companion website, including downloads of relevant material, links to useful websites, videos and other features. Please visit the companion website at https://study.sagepub.com/barryandyuill4e

RECOMMENDED READING

Kellehear, A. (2007) *A Social History of Dying*. Cambridge: Cambridge University Press.

Seale, C. (1998) *Constructing Death: The Sociology of Dying and Bereavement*. Cambridge: Cambridge University Press.

Walter, T. (2004) *The Revival of Death*, 2nd edn. London: Routledge.

HEALTH TECHNOLOGIES

MAIN POINTS

- Societies have always used and developed some form of technology to improve health and wellbeing.

- Health technologies are an increasing presence within health and social care.

- Health technologies are not separate from society, but firmly part of the social.

- Health technologies should not be thought of as inanimate machines but as also possessing the agency to alter and transform social agents who interact with them.

- Theories such as Actor-Network Theory assist in understanding how humans and technology exist with networks.

- A level of critical sociological enquiry is necessary to counter popular perceptions that the use of technology is inherently good, useful or effective.

INTRODUCTION

As humans we have always relied on technology in some form or other to make our lives easier. The archaeological record is replete with examples of very early technology, usually in the forms of flint or stone tools, that humans have crafted, developed and constantly reinvented to meet their needs for food, clothing and social interaction. Some of those tools in the Neolithic era (as we discuss in Chapter 3 on the history of healing) were deployed in the undertaking of quite challenging surgery. Two Neolithic skulls excavated in Germany in 1990 and 1993 exhibited the signs of cranial surgery, or trepanning, where the bone of the skull was scrapped away using highly specialised flint (or sometimes obsidian) tools specially created for that task (Weber and Wahl 2006). A contemporary analysis of the bone indicates that both individuals survived for some months following surgery.

Health technologies need not always be cutting-edge pieces of tech driven by high-end computers that exist in present-day society. Some of the most effective and commonplace health technologies are so simple we might not even consider them to be technology. Two examples of simple everyday technologies are the toothbrush and the flushing toilet. So, when we use the term 'technology' it does not only apply to high-tech pieces of equipment or to a range of pharmaceuticals, but to a variety of implements and drugs. The simple stethoscope, invented in 1816 by Frenchman René Laennec, is another piece of technology that many of us take for granted, but it is an essential non-invasive piece of technology that forms the bedrock of many medical diagnoses.

Since 1816 health technologies have become more complex. We can think of innovations such as Magnetic Resonance Imaging (MRI) scanners that make the interior of the body visible, personal wearable health technologies produced by commercial companies, such as the Apple watch or the Fitbit that can monitor the body, or digital web-based health technologies, including social networking sites where all sorts of information can be exchanged. The increasing use and presence of health technologies need to be factored into how sociologists analyse health. These technologies have not, as yet, totally disrupted how we approach health in the way that other new technologies have totally disrupted other aspects of life (think about how Uber has disrupted the taxi industry, for example), but they have definitely altered and reconfigured our understandings of health and how we can create relationships between health professionals and wider publics.

This chapter begins by tackling a critical question: Why should sociologists be interested in technology? That question is answered by discussing how technology is not at all separate from society, but rather is fully part of society, and an outcome of social processes and social interactions.

WHY IS TECHNOLOGY A SUBJECT FOR SOCIOLOGY?

A very reasonable question to ask is why health technology is of interest to sociologists. After all, sociologists are interested in the relationships between people and the various social structures (class, gender and ethnicity, for example) in which they live. Technology is not a living entity as such; it is a mere 'thing' that people use as and how they want. If we deploy the sociological imagination and step back from how we might normally understand technology, and think a little deeper about the world around us, we can find a different picture, where technology is very much bound into social relations and plays an important role in producing and reproducing those relations.

In one of the earlier pieces of research into technology and health, Prout (1996) makes the following observation concerning technology in his research on Metered Dose Inhalers (MDIs):

> As a device it did not simply 'impact' on social relations nor was it passively shaped by them. It was socio-technically embedded from the first instant. It acted and interacted with various kinds of entity (including other devices and humans) to create and distribute novel competencies. These interactive processes gave rise both to attempts at reconfiguring human beings in line with the competencies the MDI. (Prout 1996: 214)

The point he is making is that technology does not sit on the side, existing in its own world, but is rather part and parcel of social relations. It plays an interactive role in human relations: it is simultaneously created by human interaction and creates human interaction. Faulkner (2009: 17) also points to this 'co-creationist' approach to technology. As he pithily puts it: 'Society shapes technology; technology shapes society; the components of each interact with the others.' That, as he cautions, does not entail accepting that all things are equal, that the interactions between technology and society are on an even footing with each other. It is likely that on all occasions the relationship between the two will be asymmetrical, with one exerting more power than the other. Faulkner suggests that a better approach to adopt is through empirical engagement and research with the particular circumstances in which the technology is located and in that way to work out the various powers relations. As this chapter progresses, research on health technologies is discussed that expands on what Faulkner is advising: that we must engage with the particular and specific situations of health technologies in order to understand what is happening in that context.

The idea of technology and social agents being involved in co-creative relations with each other is a feature of one of the main theories that is frequently called on by researchers working in the field of health technologies: **Actor-Network Theory** (ANT), a theory associated with Latour (1979). As with other subjects in this book, the application of a sociological theory is invaluable in thinking through quite complex issues in a clearer and more ordered way. The basic premise of ANT, as Prout (1996) notes, is that technology does not appear from nowhere; it is not something that mysteriously arrives amid people, almost imposing itself on society. We must instead understand technology as emerging from *within* society. Technology, after all, must be invented by someone and, as Bhaskar (2007) points out, science is a social activity with myriad social processes required for any invention and innovation to take place. Critically, though, for ANT, technology and social agents co-create each other, pretty much as we discuss each other. What that means is that people have an effect on technologies and technologies have an effect on people; they shape and reshape each other. What ANT encourages us to do is to seek out the various **actants** in the network and work out what they do, how they relate to other actants, how they co-create, change and transform each other, and to clearly identify how power relationships emerge out of those relationships. An actant in ANT can be human (that is, a person) or non-human (that is, a technology). The point is that neither holds primacy over, or is more important than, the other.

One example is to think of your mobile phone (or cell phone). It no doubt plays an important role in your personal life, acting as the main piece of technology by which you maintain contact with friends and family (these are human actants). But it is more than just a thin sliver of plastic and metal. The phone has the capacity to receive texts, take photographs, make calls or connect to the internet, and actually structures *how* you have a relationship with your friends and family. The most obvious instance of this is that we do not have to be physically near someone to interact with them, yet we maintain a relationship with that person. Mobile technologies therefore allow us to have a continuing relationship with someone we may never actually see or meet that often. It is a form of relationship that would have been impossible perhaps twenty years ago, prior to such technologies becoming widely available.

The main tenet of Actor-Network Theory is that technology is not passive but plays an active role in shaping networks, relationships and power between humans and technology. All entities within a network (or assemblage) are accorded equal status and are referred to as actants.

An actant can be a human or a piece of technology, or indeed anything that is part of the network. Sometimes the terms human actant and non-human actant are used to help differentiate between actants (although this is not always the case and sometimes the term 'actant' is used to refer to both).

QUESTIONS

Following on from the above discussion of mobile phones and how they weave into our everyday lives, try to live a week without using your mobile – if you have one. How long can you do that for? Then reflect on how it is a non-human actant, in Latour's words, within your own personal network.

Returning to Prout's (1996) classic work on MDIs, he used ANT to help make sense of what he found in his research. What he found was that both technology and the people who used it exerted an influence on each other, as one would expect with ANT. The original MDI (the non-human actant), while perfectly functional as a device to deliver a dose of inhalant, when it left the test conditions of the laboratory did not fair in real-life situations as well as had been anticipated. Actual users (the human actants) found it difficult to use in ways that the designers had not considered, or were resistant to using it at all and created various ways to misuse the device. This misuse led to the device being continually altered and updated by the developers, with the social use of the MDI shaping those changes and revisions. The MDI in turn affected and shaped the subjectivities of the people who used it. One change was that for those who used the technology as directed, it lead to a new way of relating to their bodies. They found themselves developing a more disciplined approach to their bodies in order to administer the correct dosage as and when instructed. For those who misused the inhaler, and for children in particular, one change in their lives that was introduced by the technology was increased surveillance, by either other family members or by health professionals, to make sure they were using the inhaler correctly.

In addition to possessing an awareness of the fundamental connectivity between humans and technology, Timmermans and Berg (2003) also note that care must be taken not to fall into one of two traps: social essentialism and technological determinism, where either the social or technological aspects of a situation are overemphasised in an analysis of medical technologies.

Technological determinism refers to thinking that whatever you are studying or researching is explained (or determined) solely by technology. The drawback with taking this approach is that it grants technology powers above and beyond what it actually possesses, or what can be empirically verified. This rather blunt perspective on technology can therefore obscure and occlude many of the subtleties of how technology exists within a specific context. Research that overemphasises the powers of technology, as Timmermans and Berg (2003) argue, tends to be critical and suspicious of technology, depicting it as a negative development that advances a regressive, if not repressive, social agenda.

The opposite of technological determinism is social essentialism. Research that slips into social essentialism typically omits any real engagement with what the technology does and instead focuses on what social agents do with the technology. So, as with the technological determinist, the properties and abilities of technology are not fully engaged with, and how they alter and change the social agents using that technology is not taken into account.

> Technological determinism and social essentialism are both instances of reductionism, where either technology or society is privileged as the main reason why something happens. Technological determinism refers to explanations where technology is credited as causing change, while social essentialism favours social and cultural processes. With reference to health technologies, both approaches miss the nuances of how human social agents and technology interact.

A study by Griffiths et al. (2010) brings out the specific functions of a health technology and its relation to the people who use it. Their research focused on midlife women's experiences of screening technology for breast cancer. Mammography is used to detect signs of cancer through a process of visualising the internal body. It is the capacity of the technology to see into the body and then to provide a representation of the body that is important here. Notable in the accounts given by the women in the research was a sense that their breasts became an object that were to be looked at as an external object, an image present in a mammogram, rather than as an integral part of their own bodies. The mammogram altered how they understood and experienced their own subjective embodiment, resulting in them feeling disembodied from their breasts.

The women also felt that the technology undermined their own agency in checking their health and wellbeing. In comparison to the colourful imaging that the mammogram provided, other approaches, such as self-examination or bodily awareness, seemed inferior. The consequence of devaluing their abilities to monitor their own health was that self-examination was not routinely followed. Instead, the women found themselves trusting the experts and technology rather than their own abilities, and waiting every three years for the next check-up as opposed to engaging in their own self-care.

DIGITAL HEALTH TECHNOLOGIES

In addition to technologies that are physical objects, such as an MRI scanner or the MDI mentioned earlier in this chapter, another group of health technologies exists in digital forms. The development of Web 2.0 and the increasing shift to what is termed the 'internet of things' allows for the gathering and exchange of data between people and technologies in a way that opens up new modalities through which health can be experienced. In a critical review of **digital health technologies**, Lupton (2014) notes that, given just how recent the arrival of digital technologies are within health care, a great deal of research, both theoretical and empirical, is required to sociologically understand these proliferating technologies. She urges us to note that from the evidence so far we must not think of such technologies as inherently benign and a magic panacea to the health problems that we face. The reality is much more complex, with the effects and outcomes of digital health technologies likely to be highly uneven. For example, personal health technologies may give people more individual control over their health and exercise, but, at the same time, open up the possibility that it may place them under greater levels of surveillance – insurers and employers may be interested in gathering fitness and health data on those they insure and those they employ in order to reduce costs, for example.

QUESTIONS

Do you agree with Lupton (2014) that we must take care in not expecting technology to be the answer to all our problems? Think about how new health technologies are presented in popular media. What kinds of words are used to describe what they can do?

Lupton (2014: 1345) provides a useful typology of digital health technologies (see the box below). This chapter will not discuss each one in turn but will instead focus on three key areas: telemedicine, digital health promotion and self-care monitoring devices. (You may notice that sometimes slightly different terms for the same technology are used by different authors, but this just reflects how new the area is and that all is yet to be agreed.)

TYPOLOGY OF DIGITAL HEALTH TECHNOLOGIES

Telemedicine and telehealth: medical consultations, clinical diagnosis and health-care delivery offered remotely via digital technologies

Medical education, training and exchange of information between doctors and other healthcare providers using digital technologies

Digital diagnostic, genomic, risk-assessment and decision-making technologies, including apps, online tools and add-on technologies to smartphones for use by doctors

Digitised devices for delivering medicine or regulating/enhancing bodily functions (cochlear implants, cardiac monitors, insulin pumps, digital pills, and so on)

Health informatics, such as electronic patient records and other online health information, triage and appointment booking systems

Digital health promotion: disseminating health education messages via digital technologies

Biometric tracking, patient self-care and monitoring devices: apps, smartphones, smart objects and wearable technologies for monitoring and tracking bodily functions and activities

Patient blogs, social media sites and dedicated platforms for exchange of information by patients, enrolment into drug trials and crowd funding for medical research

Digital epidemiology: tracking disease outbreaks and spread using digital media

Sensor-based environmental monitoring, community development and citizen science initiatives

Digital health games: console, online and app games designed for fitness, tracking biometrics, health promotion and health education

Telemedicine (or telecare or telehealth) is an increasingly common approach in providing health care to certain groups in society. This technology purports to either offer diagnosis or provide support and care at a distance without the need of the presence of health professionals. The maintenance of independence for service users is often identified as an advantage of telemedicine, as people can continue to live in their own homes, or if they are in an institutional setting they can live more independently in that setting. Older people are a prime user group for this technology as telecare technologies offer the potential to provide a greater degree of autonomy and personal safety.

Wigg (2010) provides a useful insight into how telecare technologies can benefit older people with dementia, but only if the technologies are embedded within a distinct approach to caring for older people with dementia. Researching in America, the main focus of her research was on how technologies are used in managing wandering, a common feature of dementia where people with dementia feel a compulsion to walk or roam about.

> Telemedicine or telecare are technologies that allow people to live with greater independence or at a distance from a healthcare provider.

There are many reasons why wandering among people with dementia may occur and they include the need to relieve boredom, to reduce anxiety, to take exercise or to continue a part of their life that they enjoyed pre-onset to the disease. Often that compulsion is interpreted and defined as a risk, where the person with dementia can become lost or put themselves, or others, in danger. Responses to wandering have traditionally focused on risk reduction, which means effectively curtailing the opportunities for someone to wander. Locking doors and prohibiting access to the outside world are preferred methods. One of the downsides of that approach is that it limits freedom and the opportunity to take exercise. It can also create additional stress and anxiety as the person with dementia may attempt to unlock doors and become agitated and frustrated at not being able to do so.

Wigg (2010) compared two different residential care homes. In one home, wandering was pathologised and considered to be dangerous. The technology deployed there was the traditional locked door approach that prevented the residents from accessing the outside of the home. In the second home, wandering was regarded to be a normal activity, so long as some form of monitoring was in place to check that a person with dementia did not place themselves at risk. The technology used was motion detectors, but in this particular assemblage, the surveillance capacity of the detectors was deployed to support and facilitate movement rather than confine and limit movement. If the monitor was activated, a care provider would find the resident and then accompany them on a walk around the care home.

In a study by Mort et al. (2013) of older people using telecare in England and Spain, similar complexities to those identified in the previous example can also be found. For some of the older people in this study the technology was liberating, assisting them to gain the confidence to lead an active life. For example, the wearing of pendant alarms facilitated some older people to move around their house or visit friends, safe in the knowledge that if there was an accident they would have the means to call for help. However, for others in the study, the telecare technology was not interpreted as being liberating. Instead, it was interpreted as coercion and a threat to their identity as they felt they were forced to use the technology.

The study also picked up that the participants would, from the perspective of the telecare providers and social services, use the technology in an inappropriate manner. Such 'inappropriate' use could include an older person triggering devices not because they had fallen or were in danger, but because they sought social interaction. When a device was triggered the older person could speak with a tele-operator even if only for a short while. What we can observe here are the multiple, if not competing, ways that technology can be used and understood by the users of that technology.

Social networking

Social networking technologies, such as Facebook or Twitter, are a familiar and, in many respects, an unspectacular aspect of our daily life, unquestionably embedded in how we live and conduct our friendships. Through those platforms myriad information, images, opinions and updates are posted, read and exchanged. Given the ubiquity and density of social media, they exert an appeal for health professionals, who believe the power of social media can be harnessed to not only disseminate positive health messages across the general population, but also to contact difficult-to-reach groups and create more participative two-way relationships with health service users.

Koteyko et al. (2015) encountered that optimism and a celebratory tone in much of the clinical literature when they undertook a review of how clinicians perceived social media. They observed that clinicians were typically uncritical in how they approached social media, welcoming it as a tool they could employ in pursuit of their own ends. Some clinicians, though, were wary that social media sites could be routes through which false or misleading information could be disseminated.

That enthusiasm, Koteyko et al. argue, must be tempered. The literature that extolled the benefits of social media typically made one error – that it decontextualised the use of social media. One theme that runs throughout this book is that people and their health exist in particular contexts that are shaped by social and historical processes that are often beyond their immediate control. Those contexts can be social structures such as gender or class. What that entails is that not everyone possesses the same opportunities or resources to enact the information that they receive. So, someone may receive information via Facebook or Twitter outlining how to eat healthily and what foods to avoid, but that information presupposes that they can access certain resources to realise that advice and put it into practice. Those resources include having the money to afford the food in the first place, or being able to physically access places where what is classed as healthier food can be purchased. The point is that it takes more than simply information to make a difference in someone's life. Lupton (2012b: 239), in a similar vein, also points to the way in which targeted individual messages sent through social networking site are problematic:

> … the individualistic, targeted approach that appears such an enticing aspect of social media is also its disturbing property. By focusing on the individual, sending regular messages to encourage that person to exercise or eat well, these technologies reduce health problems to the micro, individual level. Such approaches do little, therefore, to identify the broader social, cultural and political dimensions of ill-health and the reasons why people may find it difficult to respond to such messages.

Therefore, as Koteyko et al. (2015) argue, it is perhaps better to regard social networking not as a means that sees a complete transformation of how health professionals interact with service users, but rather a way of reconfiguring that relationship by providing another option amid other contemporary and traditional approaches by which information can be shared with target groups.

Self-care monitoring packages (or personal health technologies)

We are familiar with technologies such as smartphones and devices such as Fitbit or the Apple watch where various elements of our health can be monitored, tracked and presented to us. Such technologies, for example, can count the number of steps taken in a day and then display how many calories were burned, how far we walked and how well we have slept.

Just in terms of their technical capabilities they can be quite powerful. The new Apple watch, for example, offers the ability to differentiate between the heartbeats of a mother and her unborn, but not only that: it can record the baby's heartbeat and send it to other Apple watch wearers who can then actually *feel* the baby's heart beating through the watch that they are wearing.

As Fox (2015) notes, what makes these technologies sociologically of interest is not only that the clinic is extended out into the homes and bodies of people, but that personal health technologies also operate on a level of micropolitics. What Fox implies by the term '**micropolitics**' is how individuals or organisations can exert their influence to realise their goals in a specific area. The 'micro' element of micropolitics refers to the politics of everyday life and is removed from the large-scale politics of political parties and government.

> Micropolitics is how individuals or organisations can realise their aims or exert their power in a specific defined context.

How the micropolitics of personal health technologies (PHTs) play out depends on which organisations or individuals develop the technology. Fox (2015) identifies four different groups and how each may have a different perspective on personal health technologies: public health organisations, corporations, patients, and what he terms a 'resistance perspective'. The basic run of his argument is that for the first three perspectives a variety of negative outcomes of the use of PHTs may emerge. For example, the patient perspective and the public health organisation perspective may result in health care becoming increasingly individualised and centred on a medical model approach, where the physiological aspects of someone's health gain a prominence over their social situation. We encountered a similar criticism made by Lupton (2014) that social media runs this risk too. One further potential negative, for Fox (2015), is that PHTs allow commercial corporations to further commodify health, where well-being can be supposedly purchased through the acquisition of technology. These perspectives are contrasted with a resistance perspective that Fox claims could allow marginalised groups (he mentions LGBT and teenage parents) to collectively organise against discrimination and against the commercialisation of health care as a form of critical public health.

QUESTION

Discuss what you think are the advantages and disadvantages of using digital health technologies. Do you agree with Lupton (2014) that a certain level of caution must be exercised when using such technologies?

THE LIMITS OF TECHNOLOGY?

The main argument in this chapter has been that technology is playing an ever increasing role in health and medicine, whether it is the simple technologies of dental care, or health technologies embedded in apps on smartphones, or technologies that can hold the promise of counteracting the worst effects of chronic illness. One current fear that contemporary societies exhibit is that some form of technology will one day replace or supersede humanity (the staple diet of much science fiction writing and films). That scenario is highly questionable. Technology is capable of the wholesale transformation of our lives. In health and in health care, technology may be beginning to absorb many routine and advanced functions currently performed by people. It seems only a short leap to think that all functions of health care could fall into the orbit of technology. As x and x point out, that makes a mistake about what technology is capable of. Technology may be able to excel in the technical functions of humanity, in areas such as, let us say, monitoring vital signs and so on, but technology at the moment cannot match the empathetic and emotional capacities of people. So what we could encounter in the future is a world where health providers are freed from mundane and time-consuming tasks, and can instead devote more time to the emotional and compassionate aspects of care.

Frey and Osborne (2013) have recently researched what occupations are most at risk from computerisation or automation. There are some occupations that are at very high risk of being automated. Jobs in manufacturing that are characterised by routine tasks are especially susceptible to automation, while those employed in occupations that involve human interaction and caring are at very low risk of automation. In a BBC (2015) online article, readers were invited to submit their line of work to assess the chances of their job being taken over by a robot or some other form of automation. Professions such as nursing, occupational therapy and physiotherapy came out with a very low 5% or less chance of that happening.

QUESTION

If you are a health professional or studying to be one, what aspects of your practice would be difficult for a machine to replicate or take over from you?

CONCLUSION

In this chapter we have surveyed an important aspect of health: the increasing presence of technology, whether that be in the form of an app on your smartphone or a high-technology scanner that is capable of generating images of the internal body. Two main lessons are suggested in this chapter. First, we must understand technology as a part of society, woven into a network of relations where humans and technology co-create, shape and re-shape each other. Second, technology is often presented as being inherently benign or positive. New health technologies will undoubtedly bring many useful changes, but that does not mean abandoning one's critical faculties and accepting technologies at face value. We need to research and analyse what makes them good. As Pols and Willems (2011: 495) point out, 'To say that a technology is good does not merely point to a characteristic of the technology, as most evaluation studies seem to take for granted. Rather, this "good" emerges when users and devices develop relationships'. Over the next few years it will be interesting to explore and research how such technologies intersect with other health issues, such as the various forms of inequality that we have explored in this book.

SUMMARY POINTS

- Technology is playing an increasing role in health and health care.

- Technology should be understood as occupying an active role in human relationships, shaping and forming those relationships.

- Sociologists point out that we should be cautious in seeing health technologies as being inherently an advancement or good. Their success depends very much on how they are used and the contexts in which they are used.

- It seems unlikely that health technologies can replace all human involvement in healthcare. Attributes such as compassion are hard to replace. It is also unlikely that health technologies will be able to challenge and transform the deeper underlying structural causes of poor health.

CASE STUDY

John and his partner Thomas have both downloaded the Fitbod app on their smartphones. The app monitors many aspects of their health and wellbeing. Everything from how many steps they take, how fast they move, what they eat, their heart rate and even how they feel emotionally can be accessed by the app. The two of them, plus a few friends, have synchronised their apps so that they can participate in a fitness league, each competing with the others to see who can be the healthiest that day. John is currently leading by some distance; Thomas's job requires him to work late most nights and he finds it hard to find the time to walk the recommended

10,000 paces a day. Also, when he gets home, John can be out notching up a few hundred more paces to ensure his lead in their league.

At John's work the new head of Human Resources has thought that it would be good idea to encourage better health in the workplace as he is worried about the high sickness rates due to stress. He is thinking of requiring all staff members to use the app. He has been in touch with the app's developers, Well-B tech, to see if they can supply a slightly modified version of the app for use by the company. John thinks this a great idea.

QUESTIONS

1. Using Actor-Network Theory analyse the above case study. Who and what are the various actants? How are the interactions shaping and reshaping all the actants that are involved?
2. Think about the critique advanced by Lupton concerning how digital health technologies can individualise health and wellbeing. Is that occurring here? What other critiques of health technologies discussed above are possibly relevant here?

TAKING YOUR STUDIES FURTHER

This chapter will have helped you understand many of the key terms, concepts, theories and debates relating to health technologies. Listed below are journal articles and books that will provide deeper and more detailed discussions of the points raised in this chapter. You will also find additional resources on the companion website, including downloads of relevant material, links to useful websites, videos and other features. Please visit the companion website at https://study.sagepub.com/barryandyuill4e

RECOMMENDED READING

Faulkner, A. (2009) *Medical Technology into Healthcare and Society: A Sociology of Devices, Innovation and Governance*. London: Palgrave.

Prout, A. (1996) 'Actor-network theory, technology and medical sociology: an illustrative analysis of the metered dose inhaler,' *Sociology of Health & Illness*, 18(2): 198–219.

Timmermans, S. and Berg, M. (2003) 'The practice of medical technology', *Sociology of Health & Illness*, 25(3): 97–114.

Webster, A. (2007) *Health, Technology and Society: A Sociological Critique*. London: Palgrave.

GLOSSARY

A

Actant: within Actor-Network Theory each part of a network is referred to as an actant. There can be human actants and non-human actants, such as machines or technological devices.

Actor-Network Theory (ANT): the main tenet of this theory is that technology is not passive but plays an active role in shaping networks, relationships and power between humans and technology.

Ageism: a combination of a set of beliefs originating in biological variation related to the ageing process and the actions of corporate bodies and their agents, and the resulting views of ordinary people.

Agency: *see* **Structure**.

Alternative medicine: any medical practice that falls outside the boundaries of conventional medicine. Some commentators use the term 'complementary medicine' to imply that non-conventional medicine can be used in conjunction with western biomedicine rather than as a radical alternative.

Analysis: making sense of data and deriving conclusions that inform a research question.

B

Biographical disruption: the destabilisation, questioning and reorganisation of identity after the onset of chronic illness.

C

Civilised body: a concept developed by Norbert Elias to denote a historical and cultural shift whereby the body is subject to increasing restraints that appear to limit the 'natural' body. The development of rules around eating manners is an example of how the body has become 'civilised'.

Class: a complex stratification of society based on access to and control of power, status and economic resources.

Clinical autonomy: the freedom of clinicians to make decisions on the basis of their professional judgement and specialist knowledge. This definition implies the downgrading of other assessments of the same situation.

Community: a contested concept in sociology that basically refers to a group of people who possess, or create, a common identity.

Community care: the range of policies, procedures and legislation that is concerned with the planning, funding and delivery of services for older people, people with learning and physical difficulties and illness, people with mental health problems, people with HIV/AIDS, drug or alcohol problems and other progressive illnesses, and disabled children.

D

Dependency theory: this claims that older people's lives are restricted by poverty and by being unable to access social and cultural resources.

Digital health technologies: usually associated with web-based and internet applications that seek to improve health and wellbeing. Given that these technologies are constantly and rapidly developing, what constitutes a digital health technology is not a stable definition.

Discourse: a specific way of thinking about and conceptualising a particular subject. The essence of a discourse is the language used to express thoughts. Science is an example of a discourse that rules out some kinds of explanation (for example, spiritual) and only allows for others (for example, rational and evidenced 'facts').

Discrimination: acting in a way that treats people from another race or ethnic group unequally.

Disengagement theory: the theory that older people relinquish their roles in society so as to minimise social disruption as they approach their final years.

Dissemination: making the results and conclusions of research known to a wider audience.

E

Embodiment: the experience of living through and with the physical body. Our experiences are essentially embodied. For example, we experience pleasure and pain through the body. Feelings of happiness and sadness are as physical as they are emotional.

Enlightenment, The: a body of thought developed in the eighteenth century, which challenged explanations of the world based on religious or superstitious explanations. Enlightenment thought, by contrast, was based on a commitment to rational, secular and scientific explanations.

Ethics: guiding principles and considerations concerning the conduct of the researcher in ensuring that no harm is done to the physical and emotional wellbeing of those who participate in their research.

Ethnicity: the cultural heritage and identity of a group of people.

Ethnoization: where a particular disease or illness is mistakenly associated with one specific ethnic group.

F

Feminist Theory (Feminism): a broad concept that explains social structures as fundamentally based on inequalities between women and men. In general, feminist sociologists have challenged the traditional preoccupation of the discipline with the effects of industrialisation and the world of paid work and institutional politics. Such an approach, it is argued, has ignored the significant elements of society, such as the family and gender relationships.

Fifth wave of public health: a speculative set of policies and approaches that are needed to deal with the health problems created by living in the unequal and consumerist societies of late modernity.

Functionalism: a theory of human society as a collection of interrelated substructures, the purpose of which is to sustain the overarching structure of society. As such, functionalism provides a 'consensual' representation of society based on, first, an agreement to sustain society as it is and, second, shared norms and beliefs.

G

Gender: the social, cultural and psychological differences between men and women.

Gini coefficient: a standard way of measuring income inequality within a nation state. It can be measured on a scale of 0 to 1, or 0 to 100. Basically, the lower the score the more equal the country in terms of income.

H

Hegemonic masculinity: the dominant form of masculinity in society. Currently, this refers to men who are healthy, wealthy, white and powerful and act in a 'macho' manner. Very few men live up to this expectation but it exerts a strong influence over both men and women.

I

Iatrogenesis: harm caused by doctors. In its most literal sense it refers to the harmful consequences of medical intervention. Illich also uses the concept to draw attention to our cultural dependence on medicine and medical practitioners, such that we do not seek alternative explanations or alternative remedies for ill health.

Ideology: a set of beliefs that informs action or the making of policy by politicians.

Informal care: a combination of service and affection provided on the basis of kinship or friendship. It is mainly unpaid.

Institutional racism: the intentional or unintentional actions of a public or private body that result in people from ethnic minority backgrounds being discriminated against.

L

Life course: a way of conceptualising the passage of life that better recognises the increasing fluidity and fragmentation of contemporary society, and the interaction of individual agency and social structure.

Life cycle: a concept borrowed from natural science, implying a series of set rigid stages that humans move through in their lives.

Literature review: a systematic analysis of all published material that is of interest or relevant to the research.

M

Macro: the larger, structural aspects of society. In terms of criminal activities, this might refer to an analysis of the economic circumstances of criminals, and an analysis of law making and law enforcement, as well as of the role of the state in regulating such behaviour.

Marxist Theory(Marxism): a theory that explains social phenomena as primarily determined by the economic structure of society. Social change, it argues, is the product of changes in economic relationships. In the context of the modern period, the advent of capitalism and industrialisation is seen as producing social divisions based on the ownership or non-ownership of property.

Medical model of disability: a model that places a strong emphasis on seeing disability as an individual tragedy where, by a quirk of fate, either genetic or accidental, someone becomes disabled and their life is in many ways ruined.

Medical model of health: a specific way of thinking about and explaining disease based on biological factors.

Medicalisation: a concept used to describe a tendency to explain behaviour and experiences in medical terms.

Method: the way in which actual data are gathered.

Micro: the small-scale aspects of human behaviour; for example, why individuals embark on criminal activities.

Micropolitics: how individuals or organisations can realise their aims or exert their power in a specific defined context.

N

Neoliberalism: a disputed term, but seen as both an economic and ethical ideology that stresses the free market and individual responsibility.

P

Paradigm: a systematic way of thinking.

Passing: attempts to conceal a potential stigma and prevent its disclosure.

Patriarchy: male domination in society, expressed both privately and publicly in culture, economics and politics and through physical violence. Matriarchy refers to a society that is female dominated.

Postmodernist theories: these veer away from all-embracing theories that attempt to explain all social phenomena. Instead, the emphasis is on the impossibility of uncovering the 'truth' about society. Postmodernism draws our attention to how our knowledge of the social world is constructed, and offers a critical and questioning approach to understanding the world around us. Also *see* **Discourse**.

Power: a subject of much debate within sociology. In the context of this discussion, the concept refers to (a) the ability to ensure that a particular point of view prevails in a disputed situation, (b) the capacity to ensure that someone acts in a certain way, and (c) the ability to stifle opposition to a particular perspective.

Prejudice: a negative attitude towards someone from another race or ethnic group.

Private provision or private sector: the situation when individuals are responsible for organising and purchasing their own health and social care. This is achieved by taking out insurance and other policies with private for-profit companies. The extent and level of coverage are decided by what the individual can and wishes to spend. This approach is common in the United States.

Psycho-social perspectives: explanations of class and health inequality that emphasise the negative emotional experiences of living in an unequal society, particularly feelings of stress, shame and powerlessness.

Public provision or public sector: the situation when health and social care is organised and provided by the state through a network of different services at a national and local level. Funding usually comes from taxation or some form of national or social insurance. This approach is common in European countries.

Q

Qualitative research: mainly interview-based research that seeks to find out the meanings that people attach to their experiences and actions.

Quantitative research: mainly statistics-based research that is useful for answering research questions that focus on measuring the extent and range of particular phenomena.

R

Race: a highly contested concept that categorises people by reference to biological differences between people based on skin colour and other physical features. The genetic differences between so-called races are extremely small and many social scientists prefer not to use the term.

Racism: the belief that one race is superior to another.

Research question: the aspect of the social world that is to be investigated.

S

Secularisation: the acceptance of non-religious explanations of the world.

Sex: the biological differences between men and women.

Sick role: a functionalist theory that outlines the privileges and expectations associated with being legitimately sick in contemporary society.

Social constructionism: a theory that emphasises the extent to which 'society' is actively and creatively produced by human beings.

Social model of disability: the argument that prejudicial attitudes, disabling environments and cultural barriers socially create disability.

Social model of health: the view that health is multidimensional with social factors, such as class, gender and ethnicity, influencing and patterning health and illness.

Social policy: how governments organise the meeting of the health and social needs of their population.

Socialisation: the process whereby we become aware of the values and beliefs of society.

Society: a range of external factors that influence our beliefs and behaviours.

Sociological imagination: a concept developed by C. Wright Mills, referring to a specific way of thinking about the world, characterised by a willingness to think beyond our own experiences and to challenge common-sense or obvious explanations of human society and human behaviour.

Sociology: the study of the interaction between groups and individuals in human society.

Stigma: an attribute that 'discredits', or prevents, someone's full acceptance in a particular situation.

Structure: a similar term to 'society' in so far as it draws our attention to those factors that help determine our experiences through the establishment of expected ways of behaving.

The contrasting concept of agency means that individuals do not simply act out predetermined roles but 'interpret' those roles in a way unique to them.

Surveillance: a form of scrutiny and observation that does not necessarily depend directly on the physical proximity of the watcher and the watched. Subtle forms of surveillance are said to characterise modern society, as typified by the tendency of individuals to act in ways that they think they 'ought' to.

Symbolic interactionism: a theory of social phenomena from the perspective of its participants. An essential element of this theoretical perspective is the unique nature of the social world as made up of the actions of participants motivated by human consciousness. The meaning of human action cannot, therefore, be observed or assumed, but is 'interpreted' by studying the meanings that people attach to their behaviour.

T

Telemedicine/telecare: technologies that allow people to live with greater independence or at a distance from a healthcare provider.

Theory: within sociology, this refers to attempts to provide systematic and consistent explanations of social phenomena.

Third Age theory: the theory that old age is a 'golden age' where enriching and rewarding experiences are available due to freedom from family and work commitments made possible by a consumerist society.

Traditional medicine: approaches to health and healing that are deeply woven into the culture and heritage of a specific society. Typically, these approaches do not conform to western or orthodox biomedical understandings of health.

REFERENCES

Aakster, C.W. (1993) 'Concepts in alternative medicine', in A. Beattie, M. Gott, L. Jones and M. Sidell (eds), *Health and Well-being: A Reader*. London: Macmillan/Open University.

ACE (Age Concern England) (2002a) *Issues Facing Older Lesbians, Gay Men and Bisexuals*. Policy Position Paper 15. London: ACE.

ACE (Age Concern England) (2002b) *Ageism*. Policy Position Paper. London: ACE.

Acheson, D. (1998) *Independent Inquiry into Inequalities in Health*. London: Stationery Office.

Acheson, D., Barker, D., Chambers, J., Marmot, H. and Whitehead, M. (1998) *Independent Inquiry into Inequalities in Health: Report to the Secretary of State for Health*. London: Stationery Office.

Adams, R., Dominelli, L. and Payne, M. (eds) (1998) *Social Work: Themes, Issues and Critical Debates*. Basingstoke: Palgrave.

Age UK (2010) *Lesbian, Gay or Bisexual: Planning for Later Life*. London: Age UK.

Agyemang, C., Kunst, A.E., Bhopal, R., Zaninotto, P., Nazroo, J., Unwin, N., van Valkengoed, I., Redekop, W.K. and Stronks, K. (2012) 'A cross-national comparative study of metabolic syndrome among non-diabetic Dutch and English ethnic groups', *The European Journal of Public Health*, 23(3): 447–52.

Ahmad, W.I.U. (2000) *Ethnicity, Disability and Chronic Illness*. Buckingham: Open University Press.

Alkhuzai, A.H., Ahmad, I.J., Hweel, M.J., Ismail, T.W., et al. (2008) 'Violence-related mortality in Iraq from 2002 to 2006', *The New England Journal of Medicine*, 358(2): 484–93.

Allsop, J. (2003) 'Health care', in P. Alcock, A. Erskine and M. May (eds), *The Student's Companion to Social Policy*, 2nd edn. Oxford: Blackwell.

Alvarez-Rosete, A., Bevan, G., Mays, N. and Dixon, J. (2005) 'Effect of diverging policy across the NHS', *British Medical Journal*, 331: 946–50.

Angermeyer, M.C. and Matschinger, H. (1999) 'Lay beliefs about mental disorders: a comparison between the western and the eastern parts of Germany', *Social Psychiatry and Psychiatric Epidemiology*, 34(5): 275–81.

Angus, J., Kontos, P., Dyck, I., McKeever, P. and Poland, B. (2005) 'The personal significance of home: habitus and the experience of receiving long-term home care', *Sociology of Health & Illness*, 27(2): 161–87.

Annandale, H. and Hunt, K. (eds) (2000) *Gender Inequalities in Health*. Buckingham: Open University Press.

Arber, S.L. and Ginn, J. (1992) 'Class and caring: a neglected dimension', *Sociology*, 26(4): 619–34.

Archibald, B. (2011) 'Police report massive rise in Scottish gay hate crime', *Scotland on Sunday*, 6 February.

Ariès, P. (1974) *Western Attitudes toward Death: From the Middle Ages to the Present*. Baltimore, MD: Johns Hopkins University Press.

Ariès, P. (1982) *The Hour of Our Death*. London: Vintage.

Ataguba, J.E., Akazili, J. and McIntyre, D. (2011) 'Socioeconomic-related health inequality in South Africa: evidence from General Household Surveys', *International Journal for Equity in Health*, 10(28): 1–10.

Atkin, K., Ahmad, W.I.U. and Jones, L. (2002) 'Young South Asian deaf people and their families: negotiating relationships and identities', *Sociology of Health & Illness*, 24(1): 21–45.

Atwoli, L., Stein, D.J., Williams, D.R., Mclaughlin, K.A., Petukhova, M., Kessler, R.C. and Koenen, K.C. (2013) 'Trauma and posttraumatic stress disorder in South Africa: analysis from the South African stress and health study', *BMC Psychiatry*, 13(1): 182.

Audit Commission (1986) *Making a Reality of Community Care*. London: Stationery Office.

Baggott, R. (2015) *Public Health: Policy and Politics*, 3rd edn. Basingstoke: Palgrave Macmillan.

Bagguley, P. and Hussain, Y. (2008) *Riotous Citizens: Ethnic Conflict in Multicultural Britain*. Aldershot: Ashgate Publishing.

Baker, S. and MacPherson, J. (2000) *Counting the Cost: Mental Health in the Media*. London: MIND.

Banks, I. (2001) 'No man's land: men, illness, and the NHS', *British Medical Journal*, 323: 1058–60.

Banning, T. (2010) *The Romantic Revolution*. London: Weidenfeld & Nicolson.

Barnes, C., Mercer, G. and Shakespeare, T. (1999) *Exploring Disability: A Sociological Introduction*. Cambridge: Polity Press.

Barnett, R. (2008) *Sick City: Two Thousand Years of Life and Death in London*. London: Strange Attractor.

Bartley, M. (2003) *Health Inequality: An Introduction to Concepts, Theories and Methods*. Cambridge: Polity Press.

Bauman, Z. (1990) *Thinking Sociologically*. Oxford: Basil Blackwell.

BBC (2015) Will a robot take your job? http://www.bbc.co.uk/news/technology-34066941 [Accessed 06/05/2016]

BBC News (2000) 'Washing up bowls "a health hazard"'. http://news.bbc.co.uk/1/hi/health/1056364.stm

BBC News (2001) 'Naomi Klein: "Know logo"'. http://news.bbc.co.uk/hi/english/health/newsid_1312000/1312479.stm

BBC News (2002) 'Britain "a racist society" – poll'. http://news.bbc.co.uk/1/hi/uk/1993597.stm

Bebbington, P. (1996) 'The origins of sex differences in depressive disorder: bridging the gap', *International Review of Psychiatry*, 8: 295–332.

Bécares, L., Nazroo, J., Jackson, J. and Heuvelman, H. (2012) 'Ethnic density effects on health and experienced racism among Caribbean people in the US and England: a cross-national comparison', *Social Science & Medicine*, 75(12): 2107–15.

Beck, U. (2002) 'The cosmopolitan society and its enemies', *Theory, Culture & Society*, 19: 17–44.

Becker, H. (1974) 'Labelling theory reconsidered', in P. Rock and M. McIntosh (eds), *Deviance and Social Control*. London: Tavistock.

Bell, C. and Newby, H. (1976) 'Communion, communalism, class and community action: the sources of the new urban politics', in D. Herbert and R. Johnston (eds), *Social Areas in Cities*, vol. 2. Chichester: Wiley.

Bellina, J. and Wilson, J. (1986) *The Fertility Handbook: A Positive and Practical Guide*. Harmondsworth: Penguin.

Bendelow, G., Birke, L. and Williams, S.J. (eds) (2003) *Debating Biology: Sociological Reflections on Health, Medicine and Society*. London: Routledge.

Benson, S. (1997) 'The body, health and eating disorders', in K. Woodward (ed.), *Identity and Difference*. London: SAGE.

Bernal, M. (1991) *Black Athena. Afro-Asiatic Roots of Classical Civilization: The Fabrication of Ancient Greece, 1785–1985*, vol. 1. London: Vintage.

Bernal, M. (2001) *Black Athena Writes Back: Martin Bernal Responds to His Critics*. Durham, NC: Duke University Press.

Berney, L., Blane, D., Smith, G.D., Gunnell, D.J., Holland, P. and Montgomery, S.M. (2000) 'Socioeconomic measures in early old age as indicators of previous lifetime exposure to environmental health hazards', *Sociology of Health & Illness*, 22(4): 415–30.

Beveridge, W. (1942) *Social Insurance and Allied Services*. London: Her Majesty's Stationery Office.

Bhaskar, R. (2007) *A Realist Theory of Science*, 2nd edn. London: Verso.

Bilton, T., Bonett, K., Jones, P., Lawson, T., Skinner, D., Stansworth, M. and Webster, A. (1996) *Introductory Sociology*, 3rd edn. London: Macmillan.

Birch, K. (2016) *We Have Never Been Neoliberal: A Manifesto for a Doomed Youth*. Arlesford: Zero Books.

Birke, L. (1992) 'Transforming human biology', in H. Crowley and S. Himmelweit (eds), *Knowing Women: Feminism and Knowledge*. Cambridge: Polity Press/Open University.

Black, D., Morris, J., Smith, C. and Townsend, P. (1980) *Inequalities in Health: Report of a Research Working Group*. London: Department of Health and Social Security.

Blackburn, R. (1998) *The Making of New World Slavery: From the Baroque to the Modern, 1492–1800*. London: Verso.

Blamey, A., Hanlon, P., Judge, K. and Muirie, J. (eds) (2002) *Health Inequalities in the New Scotland*. Glasgow: Public Health Institute of Scotland.

Blane, D., Higgs, P., Hyde, M. and Wiggins, R.D. (2004) 'Life course influences on quality of life in early old age', *Social Science & Medicine*, 58(11): 2171–9.

Blau, P.M. (1963) *The Dynamics of Bureaucracy*, 2nd edn. Chicago, IL: University of Chicago Press.

Blaxter, M. (1990) *Health and Life Styles*. London: Routledge.

BMA (British Medical Association) (1993) *Complementary Medicine: New Approaches to Good Practice*. Oxford: Oxford University Press.

BMA (British Medical Association) (2000) *Eating Disorders, Body Image and the Media*. London: BMJ Books.

Boeije, H., Duijnstee, M.S.H., Grypdonck, M.H.F. and Pool, A. (2002) 'Encountering the downward phase: biographical work in people with multiple sclerosis living at home', *Social Science & Medicine*, 55: 881–93.

Bok, S. (2004) *Rethinking the WHO Definition of Health*. Working Paper Series, vol. 14, no. 7. Cambridge, MA: Harvard Center for Population and Development Studies.

Bond, J., Coleman, P. and Peace, S. (eds) (1993) *Ageing in Society: An Introduction to Social Gerontology*, 2nd edn. London: SAGE.

Bond, J., Coleman, P. and Peace, S. (eds) (2007) *Ageing in Society: An Introduction to Social Gerontology*, 2nd edn. London: SAGE.

Bond, R. and Rosie, M. (2002) 'National identities in post-devolution Scotland'. www. institute-of-governance.org/onlinepub/bondrosie.html.

Booth, C. (1902) *Life and Labour of the People in London. Final Volume. Notes on Social Influences and Conclusions*. London: Macmillan.

Bordo, S. (1990) 'Reading the slender body', in M. Jacobs, E.F. Keller and S. Shuttleworth (eds), *Body/Politics: Women and the Discourse of Science.* New York: Routledge.

Bourdieu, P. (1984) *Distinction: A Social Critique of the Judgement of Taste.* London: Routledge and Kegan Paul.

Bradby, H. (1995) 'Ethnicity: not a black and white issue. A research note', *Sociology of Health & Illness*, 17(3): 405–17.

Bradby, H. (2012) 'Race, ethnicity and health: The costs and benefits of conceptualising racism and ethnicity', *Social Science & Medicine*, 75(6): 955–8.

Braveman, P. (2012) 'Health inequalities by class and race in the US: What can we learn from the patterns?', *Social Science & Medicine*, 74(5): 665–7.

Braybrooke, D. & Lindholm, C. (1963) *A Strategy of Decision.* New York: Free Press.

Breast Cancer Care (2011) *Lesbian and Bisexual Women and Breast Cancer: A Policy Briefing.* London.

Brondolo, E., Hausmann, L.R.M., Jhalani, J., Pencille, M., Atencio-Bacayon, J., Kumar, A., Kwok, J., Ullah, J., Roth, A., Chen, D., Crupi, R. and Schwartz, J. (2011) 'Dimensions of perceived racism and self-reported health: examination of racial/ethnic differences and potential mediators', *Annals of Behavioral Medicine*, 42(1): 14–28. doi: 10.1007/s12160-011-9265-1.

Brown, G.W. and Harris, T. (1978) *Social Origins of Depression: A Study of Psychiatric Disorder in Women.* Cambridge: Cambridge University Press.

Bruce, S. (1999) *Sociology: A Very Short Introduction.* Oxford: Oxford University Press.

Bruce, S. and Glendinning, T. (2010) 'When was secularization? Dating the decline of the British churches and locating its cause', *The British Journal of Sociology*, 61: 107–26.

Bryson, L., Warner-Smith, P., Brown, P. and Fray, L. (2007) 'Managing the work–life roller-coaster: private stress or public health issue?', *Social Science & Medicine*, 65(6): 1142–53.

Buquet-Marcon, C., Charlier, P. and Samzun, A. (2009) 'A possible Early Neolithic amputation at Buthiers-Boulancourt (Seine-et-Marne), France', *Antiquity*, 83(322).

Burawoy, M. (2004) '2004 presidential address: for public sociology', *American Sociological Review*, 70(Feb.): 4–28.

Burnham, G., Lafta, R., Doocy, D. and Roberts, L. (2006) 'Mortality after the 2003 invasion of Iraq: a cross-sectional cluster sample survey', *The Lancet*, 368: 1421–8.

Bury, M. (1991) 'The sociology of chronic illness: a review of research and prospects', *Sociology of Health & Illness*, 13(4): 451–68.

Bury, M. (1997) *Health and Illness in a Changing Society.* London: Routledge.

Bury, M. (2000) 'Health, ageing and the lifecourse', in S.J. Williams, J. Gabe and M. Calnan (eds), *Health, Medicine and Society: Key Theories, Future Agendas.* London: Routledge.

Busfield, J. (2000) 'Introduction: rethinking the sociology of mental health', *Sociology of Mental Health & Illness*, 22: 543–88.

Busia, K. (2005) 'Medical provision in Africa – past and present', *Phytotherapy Research*, 19(11): 919–23.

Butler, J. (2004) *Undoing gender.* Boca Raton, FL: Routledge, Taylor & Francis Group.

Bytheway, B. (1995) *Ageism.* Buckingham: Open University Press.

Bytheway, B. and Johnson, J. (1990) 'On defining ageism', *Critical Social Policy*, 27: 27–39.

Bywaters, P. (1999) 'Social work and health inequalities', *British Journal of Social Work*, 29: 811–16.

Carpenter, M. (2000) 'Reinforcing the pillars: rethinking gender', in H. Annandale and K. Hunt (eds), *Gender Inequalities in Health.* Buckingham: Open University Press.

Carricaburu, D. and Pierret, J. (1995) 'From biographical disruption to bio-graphical reinforcement: the case of HIV-positive men', *Sociology of Health & Illness*, 17(1): 65–88.

Carrington, B. (2010) *Race, Sport and Politics: The Sporting Black Diaspora*. London: SAGE.

Carter, B. and Dyson, S.M. (2011) 'Territory, ancestry and descent: the politics of sickle cell disease', *Sociology*, 45(6): 963–76.

Carter, B. and Dyson, S.M. (2015) 'Actor network theory, agency and racism: the case of sickle cell trait and US athletics', *Social Theory & Health*, 13(1): 62–77.

Carter, B. and Fenton, S. (2010) 'Not thinking ethnicity: A critique of the ethnicity paradigm in an over-ethnicised sociology', *Journal for the Theory of Social Behaviour*, 40(1): 1–18.

Cashmore, E. (2002) *Beckham*. Cambridge: Polity Press.

Cashmore, E. (2005) *Making Sense of Sport*, 4th edn. London: Routledge.

Cashmore, E. (2008) 'Tiger Woods and the new racial order', *Current Sociology*, 56: 621–34.

Castells, M. (1997) *The Power of Identity*. Oxford: Blackwell.

Castles, S., de Haas, H. and Miller, M.J. (2013) *The Age of Migration: International Population Movements in the Modern World*, 5th edn. Basingstoke: Palgrave Macmillan.

Chahal, K. (2004) *Experiencing Ethnicity: Discrimination and Service Provision*. York: York Publication Services.

Chahal, K. and Julienne, L. (1999) *'We Can't All Be White!' Racist Victimisation in the UK*. York: York Publication Services.

Chakraborty, A., McManus, S., Brugha, T. and Bebbington, P. (2011) 'Mental health of the non-heterosexual population of England', *The British Journal of Psychiatry*, 198: 143–8.

Charmaz, K. (1983) 'Loss of self: a fundamental form of suffering in the chronically ill', *Sociology of Health & Illness*, 5(2): 168–95.

Chimot, C. and Louveau, C. (2010) 'Becoming a man while playing a female sport: the construction of masculine identity in boys doing rhythmic gymnastics', *International Review for the Sociology of Sport*, 45(4): 436–56.

Clarke, J. (ed.) (1994) *A Crisis in Care? Challenges to Social Work*. London: SAGE.

Cochrane, K. (2011) 'Miriam O'Reilly: "Standing up to the BBC was the right thing to do"', *The Guardian*, 11 February.

Coker, N. (ed.) (2001) *Racism in Medicine: An Agenda for Change*. London: King's Fund.

Colgrove, J. (2002) 'The McKeown thesis: a historical controversy and its enduring influence', *American Journal of Public Health*, 92(5): 725–9.

Collins, C. and Levitt, I. (2016) 'The "modernisation" of Scotland and its impact on Glasgow, 1955–1979: "unwanted side effects" and vulnerabilities', *Scottish Affairs*, 25(3): 294–316.

Collins, M.F. and Kay, T. (2003) *Sport and Social Exclusion*. London: Routledge.

Colman, P. (1995) *Rosie the Riveter: Women Workers on the Home Front in World War II*. New York: Crown.

Commission on Social Determinants of Health (CSDH) (2008) *Closing the Gap in a Generation: Health Equity through Action on the Social Determinants of Health*. Final Report of the Commission on Social Determinants of Health. Geneva: World Health Organisation.

Connell, R. (2002) *Gender*. Cambridge: Polity Press.

Connell, R.W. (2005) *Masculinities*. Cambridge: Polity Press.

Connell, R. (2012) 'Gender, health and theory: Conceptualizing the issue, in local and world perspective', *Social Science & Medicine*, 74(11): 1675–83.

Courtenay, W.H. (2000) 'Constructions of masculinity and their influence on men's well-being: A theory of gender and health', *Social Science & Medicine*, 50(10): 1385–401.

Coward, R. (1993) 'The myth of alternative health', in A. Beattie, M. Gott, L. Jones and M. Sidell (eds), *Health and Well-being: A Reader*. London: Macmillan/Open University.

Craib, I. (1997) *Classical Social Theory*. Cambridge: Polity Press.

Crang, M. and Cook, I. (2007) *Doing Ethnographies*. London: SAGE.

Crinson, I. (2008) *Health Policy: A Critical Perspective*. London: SAGE.

Crinson, I. and Yuill, C. (2008) 'What can alienation theory contribute to an understanding of social inequalities in health?', *International Journal of Health Services*, 38(3): 455–70.

Crow, G., Allan, G. and Summers, M. (2002) 'Neither busybodies nor nobodies: managing proximity and distance in neighbourly relations', *Sociology*, 36(2): 127–45.

Cumming, E. and Henry, W. (1961) *Growing Old: The Process of Disengagement*. New York: Basic Books.

Cunningham, A. (1994) 'Blood', in C. Seale and S. Pattison (eds), *Medical Knowledge: Doubt and Certainty*. Buckingham: Open University Press.

Dearden, C. and Becker, S. (2000) *Young Carers' Transitions into Adulthood*. York: Joseph Rowntree Foundation.

Department for Business, Innovation and Skills (2014) *Trade Union Membership 2013: Statistical Bulletin*. London: Office of National Statistics.

Department of Health (1989) *Working for Patients*. London: Stationery Office.

Department of Health (1999a) *Saving Lives: Our Healthier Nation*. Cm 4386. London: Stationery Office.

Department of Health (1999b) *Reducing Health Inequalities: An Action Report*. London: Stationery Office.

Department of Health (2000) *The NHS Plan: A Plan for Investment, a Plan for Reform*. London: Stationery Office.

Department of Health (2001) *Valuing People: A New Strategy for Learning Disability for the 21st Century*. London: Stationery Office.

Department of Health (2003) *Tackling Health Inequalities: A Programme for Action*. London: Stationery Office.

Department of Health (2004) *Choosing Health: Making Healthier Choices Easier*. London: Stationery Office.

Department of Health (2005a) *Tackling Health Inequalities: Status Report on the Programme for Action*. London.

Department of Health (2005b) *Independence, Well-being and Choice*. Green Paper on Adult Social Care. London: Stationery Office.

Department of Health (2006) *Our Health, Our Care, Our Say: A New Direction for Community Services*. London: Stationery Office.

Department of Health (2011) *National Service Framework for Mental Health*. http://www.dh.gov.uk/en/Publicationsandstatistics/Publications/PublicationsPolicyAndGuidance/DH_4009598.

Derrida, J. (1993) *Aporias*. Stanford, CA: Stanford University Press.

DHSS (Department of Health and Social Security) (1989) *Caring for People: Community Care in the Next Decade and Beyond*. London: Stationery Office.

Doll, R. (1992) 'Health and the environment in the 1990s', *American Journal of Public Health*, 82: 933–41.

Donnelly, P. (2005) 'Sport and social theory', in B. Houlihan (ed.), *Sport and Society*, 2nd edn. London: SAGE.

Dorling, D. (2014) *Inequality and the 1%*. London: Verso.

Dossa, P. (2009) *Racialized bodies, Disabling Worlds: Storied Lives of Immigrant Muslim Women*. Toronto: University of Toronto Press.

Douglas, J.D. (1967) *The Social Meanings of Suicide*. Princeton, NJ: Princeton University Press.

Doyal, L. (1979) *The Political Economy of Health*. London: Pluto.

Doyal, L. (1994) *What Makes Women Sick? The Political Economy of Health*. London: Macmillan.

Doyal, L. (2001) 'Sex, gender and health: the need for a new approach', *British Medical Journal*, 323: 1061–3.

Drabble, L., Midanik, L.T. and Trocki, K. (2005) 'Reports of alcohol consumption and alcohol-related problems among homosexual, bisexual and heterosexual respondents: results from the 2000 National Alcohol Survey', *Journal of Studies on Alcohol*, 66: 111–20.

Dumazedier, J. (1967) *Towards a Society of Leisure*. New York: Free Press.

Durkheim, E. (1970 [1897]) *Suicide: A Study in Sociology*. London: Routledge and Kegan Paul.

Dyson, S.M. (2005) *Ethnicity and Screening for Sickle Cell/Thalassaemia: Lessons for Practice from the Voices of Experience*. Edinburgh: Elsevier Churchill Livingstone.

Easton, D. (1953) *The Political System*. New York: Knopf.

Elias, N. (1982) *The Civilising Process. Vol. 1: A History of Manners*. Oxford: Blackwell.

Emslie, C., Ridge, D., Ziebland, S. and Hunt, K. (2006) 'Men's accounts of depression: reconstructing or resisting hegemonic masculinity?', *Social Science & Medicine*, 62: 2246–57.

Engels, F. (2009) *The Condition of the Working Class in England*. Oxford: Oxford University Press.

Eriksson, K.H., Jäntti, M., Lindahl, L. and Torssander, J. (2014) 'Trends in life expectancy by income and the role of specific causes of death', *Swedish Institute for Social Research* , Working Paper (8/2014).

Eurostat (2013)

Faircloth, C.A., Boylstein, C., Rittman, M., Young, M.E. and Gubrium, J. (2004) 'Sudden illness and biographical flow in narratives of stroke recovery', *Sociology of Health & Illness*, 26(2): 242–61.

Fairhurst, E. (1998) '"Growing old gracefully" as opposed to "mutton dressed as lamb": the social construction of recognising older women', in S. Nettleton and J. Watson (eds), *The Body in Everyday Life*. London: Routledge.

Faris, R. and Dunham, H. (1939) *Mental Disorders in Urban Areas: An Ecological Study of Schizophrenia and Other Psychoses*. Chicago, IL: University of Chicago Press.

Faulkner, A. (2009) *Medical Technology into Healthcare and Society: A Sociology of Devices, Innovation and Governance*. London: Palgrave.

Faulkner, A. and Wyatt, S. (2008) *Medical Technology into Healthcare and Society: A Sociology of Devices, Innovation and Governance*. Edited by Andrew Webster. New York: Palgrave Macmillan.

Featherstone, M. (2007) *Consumer Culture and Postmodernism*, 2nd edn. London: SAGE.

Featherstone, M. and Hepworth, M. (1993) 'Images of ageing', in J. Bond, P. Coleman and S. Peace (eds), *Ageing in Society: An Introduction to Social Gerontology*, 2nd edn. London: SAGE.

Fenton, A. and Charsley, K. (2000) 'Epidemiology and sociology as incommensurate games: accounts from the study of health and ethnicity', *Health*, 4(4): 403–25.

Fenton, S. and Sadiq-Sangster, A. (1996) 'Culture, relativism and the experience of mental distress: South Asian women in Britain', *Sociology of Health & Illness*, 18(1): 66–85.

Ferrari, A.J., Charlson, F.J., Norman, R.E., Patten, S.B., Freedman, G., Murray, C.J.L., Vos, T. and Whiteford, H.A. (2013) 'Burden of depressive disorders by country, sex, age, and year: findings from the Global Burden of Disease Study 2010. *PLoS Med*, 10(11): e1001547.

Festinger, A., Riecken, H.W. and Schachter, S. (1956) *When Prophecy Fails*. New York: Harper & Row.

Field, D. (1992) 'Contemporary issues in relation to the elderly', in M. O'Donnell (ed.), *New Introductory Reader in Sociology*. Walton-on-Thames: Nelson.

Fink, J. (2004) *Care: Personal Lives and Social Policy.* Milton Keynes: Open University Press.

Fish, J. (2010) *Coming Out about Breast Cancer: Lesbian and Bisexual Women's Experiences of Breast Cancer.* Leicester: National Cancer Action Team and De Montfort University.

Fogel, C. (2011) 'Sporting masculinity on the gridiron: construction, characteristics and consequences', *Canadian Social Science*, 7(2): 1–14.

Foster, P. (1995) *Women and the Health Care Industry: An Unhealthy Relationship?* Buckingham: Open University Press.

Foucault, M. (1967) *Madness and Civilisation: A History of Insanity in the Age of Reason.* London: Tavistock.

Foucault, M. (1970) *The Order of Things: An Archaeology of the Human Sciences.* London: Tavistock.

Foucault, M. (1973) *The Birth of the Clinic: An Archaeology of Medical Perception.* London: Tavistock.

Foucault, M. (1979a) *Discipline and Punish: The Birth of the Prison.* Harmondsworth: Penguin.

Foucault, M. (1979b) *The Will to Knowledge: The History of Sexuality, Vol. I.* London: Allen Lane.

Foucault, M. (2008) *The Birth of Biopolitics: Lectures at the Collège de France, 1978–1979.* London: Palgrave Macmillan.

Fox, N.J. (2015) 'Personal health technologies, micropolitics and resistance: a new materialist analysis', *Health: An Interdisciplinary Journal for the Social Study of Health, Illness and Medicine.*

Frank, A.W. (1995) *The Wounded Storyteller: Body, Illness and Ethics.* Chicago, IL: University of Chicago Press.

Franklin, S. (1997) *Embodied Progress: A Cultural Account of Assisted Conception.* London: Routledge.

Fredrickson, B.L. and Harrison, K. (2005) 'Throwing like a girl: self-objectification predicts adolescent girls' motor performance', *Journal of Sport and Social Issues*, 29: 79–101.

Fulop, N., Elston, J., Hensher, M., McKee, M. and Walters, R. (1998) 'Evaluation of the implementation of *The Health of the Nation*', in Department of Health (ed.), *The Health of the Nation: A Policy Assessed.* London: Stationery Office.

Giddens, A. (1986) *Sociology: A Brief but Critical Introduction.* London: Macmillan.

Giddens, A. (1991) *Modernity and Self-Identity: Self and Society in the Late Modern Age.* Cambridge: Polity Press.

Giddens, A. (1994) *Sociology.* Cambridge: Polity Press.

Giddens, A. (1997) *Introductory Readings.* Cambridge: Polity Press.

Giddens, A. (ed.) (2001) *Sociology: Introductory Readings.* Cambridge: Polity Press.

Giddens, A. and Sutton, P. W. (2013) *Sociology*, 7th edn. Cambridge: Polity Press.

Ginn, J. and Arber, S. (1995) '"Only connect": gender relations and ageing', in S. Arber and J. Ginn (eds), *Connecting Gender and Ageing: A Sociological Approach.* Buckingham: Open University Press.

Giulianotti, R. (2005) *Sport: A Critical Sociology.* Cambridge: Polity Press.

Goffman, E. (1961) *Asylums: Essays on the Social Situation of Mental Patients and Other Inmates.* Harmondsworth: Penguin.

Goffman, E. (1968) *Stigma: Notes on the Management of a Spoiled Identity.* Harmondsworth: Penguin.

Goodley, D. (2001) '"Learning difficulties", the social model of disability and impairment: challenging epistemologies', *Disability & Society*, 16(2): 207–31.

Gorer, G. (1965) *Death, Grief and Mourning.* London: Cresset.

Gott, M. (2005) *Sexuality, Sexual Health and Ageing.* Maidenhead: Open University Press.

Gould, S.J. (1980) *The Panda's Thumb*. New York: W. W. Norton.

Gove, W.R. (1984) 'Gender differences in mental and physical illness: the effects of fixed roles and nurturant roles', *Social Science & Medicine*, 19(2): 77–91.

Graham, H. (1983) 'Caring: a labour of love', in J. Finch and D. Groves (eds), *A Labour of Love: Women, Work and Caring*. London: Routledge & Kegan Paul.

Graham, H. (1991) 'The concept of caring in feminist research: the case of domestic service', *Sociology*, 25(1): 61–78.

Graham, H. (1993) *Hardship and Health in Women's Lives*. New York: Wheatsheaf.

Green, J. and Thorogood, N. (2014) *Qualitative Methods for Health Research*, 3rd edn. London: SAGE.

Griffiths, F., Bendelow, G., Green, E. and Palmer, J. (2010) 'Screening for breast cancer: medicalization, visualization and the embodied experience', *Health: An Interdisciplinary Journal for the Social Study of Health, Illness and Medicine*, 14(6): 653–68.

Griffiths, R. (1988) *Community Care: An Agenda for Action*. London: Stationery Office.

Gupta, P., Sharma, V.K. and Sharma, S. (2014) *Healing Traditions of the Northwestern Himalayas*. London: Springer.

Gupta, S., de Belder, A. and O'Hughes, L. (1995) 'Avoiding premature coronary deaths in Asians in Britain: spend now on prevention or pay later for treatment', *British Medical Journal*, 311: 1035–6.

Hall, P., Brockington, I.F., Levings, J. and Murphy, C. (1993) 'A comparison of responses to the mentally ill in two communities', *British Journal of Psychiatry*, 162: 99–108.

Hall, S. (2003) 'Women still on 72% of men's pay', *The Guardian*, 17 October.

Ham, C. (2009) *Health Policy in Britain*, 6th edn. Basingstoke: Palgrave Macmillan.

Hankivsky, O. (2012) 'Women's health, men's health and gender and health: the implications of intersectionality,' *Social Science & Medicine*, 74(11): 1712–1720.

Hanlon, P., Carlisle, S., Hannah, M., D. Reilly, D. and Lyon, A. (2011) 'Making the case for a "fifth wave" in public health', *Public Health*, 125(1): 30–36.

Hanlon, P., Walsh, D., Buchanan, D., Redpath, A., Bain, M., Brewster, D., Chalmers, J., Muir, R., Smalls, M., Willis, J. and Wood, R. (2001) *Chasing the Scottish Effect: Why Scotland Needs a Step-Change in Health if it is to Catch Up with the Rest of Europe*. Glasgow: Public Health Institute of Scotland.

Hardey, M. (2002) '"The story of my illness": personal accounts of illness on the internet', *Health*, 6(1): 31–46.

Hardley, M. (1998) *The Social Context of Health*. Buckingham: Open University Press.

Harris, B. (2004) 'Public health, nutrition and the decline of mortality: the McKeown thesis revisited', *Social History of Medicine*, 17(3): 379–407.

Harris, R., Tobias, M., Jeffreys, M., Waldegrave, K., Karlsen, S. and Nazroo, J. (2006) 'Racism and health: the relationship between experience of racial discrimination and health in New Zealand', *Social Science & Medicine*, 63: 1428–41.

Harvey, J. (1997) 'The technological regulation of death: with reference to the technological regulation of birth', *Sociology*, 31(4): 719–35.

Hattersly, L. (1997) 'Expectation of life by social class', in F. Drever and M. Whitehead (eds), *Health Inequalities: Decennial Supplement*. London: Stationery Office.

Hawkes, G. (1996) *A Sociology of Sex and Sexuality*. Buckingham: Open University Press.

Heaphy, B., Yip, A. and Thompson D. (2004) 'Ageing in a non-heterosexual context', *Ageing and Society*, 24: 881–902.

Hewitt, P. and Warren, J. (1997) 'A self-made man', in A. Giddens (ed.), *Sociology: Introductory Readings*. Cambridge: Polity Press.

Hibbard, J.H. and Pope, C.R. (1986) 'Another look at sex differences in the use of medical care: illness orientation and the types of morbidities for which services are used', *Women and Health*, 11(2): 21–36.

Higginbottom, G.M.A. (2006) '"Pressure of life": ethnicity as a mediating factor in mid-life and older people's experiences of high blood pressure', *Sociology of Health & Illness*, 28(5): 583–610.

Higgs, P. and Gilleard, C. (2015) *Rethinking Old Age: Theorising the Fourth Age*. London: Palgrave Macmillan.

Hines, S. and Sanger, T. (eds) (2010) *Transgender Identities: Towards a Social Analysis of Gender Diversity*. London: Routledge.

Hochschild, A. (1983) *The Managed Heart: Commercialization of Human Feeling*. Berkeley, CA: University of California Press.

Hockey, J. and James, A. (2003) *Social Identities across the Life Course*. Basingstoke: Palgrave Macmillan.

Hodkinson, P. (2002) *Goth: Identity, Style and Subculture*. Oxford: Berg.

Holland, S. (2004) *Alternative Femininities: Body, Age and Identity*. Oxford: Berg.

Hollingshead, A. and Redlich, F. (1953) 'Social stratification and psychiatric disorders', *American Sociological Review*, 18(2): 163–9.

hooks, bell (1987) *Ain't I a Woman? Black Women and Feminism*, 7th edn. London: Pluto.

Hughes, T.L. and Jacobson, K.M. (2003) 'Sexual orientation and women's smoking', *Current Women's Health Reports*, 3: 254–61.

Hunt, R., Cowan, K. and Chamberlain, B. (2007) *Being the Gay One: Experiences of Lesbian, Gay and Bisexual People Working in the Health and Social Care Sector*. London: Stonewall.

Hunt, R. and Fish, J. (2008) *Prescription for Change: Lesbian and Bisexual Women's Health Check*. London: Stonewall.

Hunt, T. (2005) *Building Jerusalem: The Rise and Fall of the Victorian City*. London: Phoenix.

Hunter, D.J. (1994) 'From tribalism to corporatism: the managerial challenge to medical dominance', in J. Gabe, D. Kelleher and G. Williams (eds), *Challenging Medicine*. London: Routledge.

Hunter, M. (2001) 'Medical research under threat after Alder Hey scandal', *British Medical Journal*, 322(24 February): 448.

Hussain, Y. and Bagguley, P. (2015) 'Reflexive ethnicities: crisis, diversity and re-composition', *Sociological Research Online*, 20(3): 18.

Illich, I. (1976) *Limits to Medicine*. Harmondsworth: Penguin.

Illich, I. (1993) 'The epidemics of modern medicine', in N. Black, D. Boswell, A. Gray, S. Murphy and J. Popay (eds), *Health and Disease: A Reader*. Milton Keynes: Open University Press.

Institute for Fiscal Studies (2011) *Poverty and Inequality in the UK: 2011*. London: Institute for Fiscal Studies.

Institute for Fiscal Studies (2015) *Living Standards, Poverty and Inequality in the UK: 2015*. London: Institute for Fiscal Studies.

Iphofen, R. (1996) 'Coping with a "perforated life": a close study in managing the stigma of petit mal epilepsy', *Sociology*, 24(3): 447–63.

Irvine, B. and Ginsberg, I. (2004) *England versus Scotland: Does More Money Mean Better Health?* London: Civitas.

Jackson, L. (2014) *Dirty Old London: The Victorian Fight Against Filth*. New Haven, CT: Yale University Press.

James, M. (1994) 'Hysteria', in C. Seale and S. Pattison (eds), *Medical Knowledge: Doubt and Certainty*. Milton Keynes: Open University Press.

James, O. (1998) *Britain on the Couch. Why We're Unhappier Compared with 1950, Despite Being Richer: A Treatment for the Low-Serotonin Society*. London: Arrow.

Jenkins, R. (2004) *Social Identity*, 2nd edn. London: Routledge.

Jewson, N.D. (1976) 'The disappearance of the sick-man from medical cosmology, 1770–1870', *Sociology*, 10(2): 225–44.

Johnson, J.L., Oliffe, J.L., Kelly, M.T., Galdas, P. and Ogrodniczuk, J.S. (2011) 'Men's discourses of help-seeking in the context of depression', *Sociology of Health & Illness*, 34(3): 345–361.

Jorm, J.F. (2000) 'Mental health literacy: public knowledge and beliefs about mental disorder', *British Journal of Psychiatry*, 177: 396–401.

Kandrack, M., Grant, K. and Segall, A. (1991) 'Gender differences in health-related behaviour: some unanswered questions', *Social Science & Medicine*, 32(5): 579–90.

Kangas, I. (2001) 'Making sense of depression: perceptions of melancholia in lay narratives', *Health*, 5(1): 76–92.

Karasz, A. (2005) 'Cultural differences in conceptual models of depression', *Social Science & Medicine*, 60(7): 1625–35.

Karlsen, S. and Nazroo, J.Y. (2002a) 'Agency and structure: the impact of ethnic identity and racism on the health of ethnic minority people', *Sociology of Health & Illness*, 24(1): 1–20.

Karlsen, S. and Nazroo, J.Y. (2002b) 'The relationship between racial discrimination, social class and health among ethnic minority groups', *American Journal of Public Health*, 92(4): 624–31.

Karlsen, S. and Nazroo, J.Y. (2004) 'Fear of racism and health', *Journal of Epidemiology and Community Health*, 58: 1017–18.

Karlsen, S., Nazroo, J.Y. and Stephenson, R. (2002) 'Ethnicity, environment and health: putting ethnic inequalities in health in their place', *Social Science & Medicine*, 55(9): 155–69.

Kellehear, A. (2007) *A Social History of Dying*. Cambridge: Cambridge University Press.

Kellehear, A. (2008) 'Dying as a social relationship: a sociological review of debates on the determination of death', *Social Science & Medicine*, 66(7): 1533–44.

Kelly, L. (1988) *Surviving Sexual Violence*. Cambridge: Polity Press.

King, M. and McKeowan, E. (2003) *Mental Health and Social Wellbeing of Gay Men, Lesbians and Bisexuals in England and Wales*. London: MIND.

Kirby, M., Kidd, W., Koubel, F., Barter, J., Hope, T., Kirton, A., Madry, N., Manning, P. and Triggs, K. (2000) *Sociology in Perspective*. Oxford: Heinemann.

Kline, R. (2015) 'NHS interview panels must do more to encourage would-be BME leaders', *Nursing Standard*, 30(6): 30–30.

Koteyko, N., Hunt, D. and Gunter, B. (2015) 'Expectations in the field of the internet and health: an analysis of claims about social networking sites in clinical literature', *Sociology of Health & Illness*, 37(3): 468–84.

Krieger, N., Chen, J.T., Waterman, P.D., Rehkopf, D.H. and Subramanian, S.V. (2005) 'Painting a truer picture of US socioeconomic and racial/ethnic health inequalities: the Public Health Disparities Geocoding Project', *American Journal of Public Health*, 95: 312–23.

Kübler-Ross, E. (1969) *On Death and Dying*. London: Routledge.

Laing, W. and Buisson, E. (2003) *Laing's Healthcare Market Review 2003–2004*. London: LaingBuisson.

Langdon, S.A., Eagle, A. and Warner, J. (2007) 'Making sense of dementia in the social world: a qualitative study', *Social Science & Medicine*, 64(4): 989–1000.

Laslett, P. (1987) 'The emergence of the third age', *Ageing and Society*, 7(2): 133–60.

Laslett, P. (1989) *Fresh Map of Life: Emergence of the Third Age*. London: Weidenfeld & Nicolson.

Laslett, P. (1996) *A Fresh Map of Life: The Emergence of the Third Age*, 2nd edn. London: Macmillan.

Latour, B. (1992) 'Where are the missing masses? The sociology of a few mundane artifacts', in W.E. Bijker and John Law (eds), *Shaping Technology/Building Society: Studies in Sociotechnical Change*. Cambridge, MA: MIT Press, pp. 225–58.

Latour, B. (2005) *Reassembling the Social: An Introduction to Actor-Network-Theory*. Oxford: Oxford University Press.

Lawler, J. (1991) *Behind the Screens: Nursing, Somatology and the Body*. London: Churchill Livingstone.

Lawson, T. (1997) *Economics and Reality*. London: Routledge.

Lee, C. (1998) *Women's Health: Psychological and Social Perspectives*. London: SAGE.

Lee, R. (2008) 'Modernity, mortality and re-enchantment: the death taboo revisited', *Sociology*, 42(4): 745–75.

Lefebvre, H. (2008) *Critique of Everyday Life*. London: Verso.

Leon, D.A., Walt, G. and Gilson, L. (2001) 'Recent advances: international perspectives on health inequalities and policy', *British Medical Journal*, 322(7286): 591–4.

Levinson, R. (1998) 'Issues at the interface of medical sociology and public health', in G. Scambler and P. Higgs (eds) *Modernity, Medicine and Health*. London: Routledge.

LSE (London School of Economics) (2006) *The Depression Report: A New Deal for Depression and Anxiety Disorders*. London: LSE.

Lupton, D. (1996) *The Imperative of Health: Public Health and the Regulated Body*. London: SAGE.

Lupton, D. (2012a) *Medicine as Culture: Illness, Disease and the Body in Western Societies*. London: SAGE.

Lupton, D. (2012b) 'M-health and health promotion: the digital cyborg and surveillance society', *Social Theory & Health*, 10(3): 229–44.

Lupton, D. (2014) 'Critical perspectives on digital health technologies', *Sociology Compass*, 8(12): 1344–59.

Lutfey, K. (2005) 'On practices of "good doctoring": reconsidering the relationship between provider roles and patient adherence', *Sociology of Health & Illness*, 27(4): 421–47.

Lynch, J., Davey-Smith, G., Kaplan, G. and House, J. (2000) 'Income inequality and mortality: importance to health of individual income, psychosocial environment, or material conditions', *British Medical Journal*, 320: 1200–4.

MacDonald, L. (1988) 'The experience of stigma: living with rectal cancer', in R. Anderson and M. Bury (eds), *Living with Chronic Illness: The Experience of Patients and their Families*. London: Unwin Hyman.

Macintyre, S. (1997) 'The Black Report and beyond: what are the issues?', *Social Science and Medicine*, 44: 723–46.

Macintyre, S., Ford, G. and Hunt, K. (1999) 'Do women "over-report" morbidity? Men's and women's responses to structured prompting on a standard question on long-standing illness', *Social Science & Medicine*, 48: 89–98.

Macintyre, S., Hunt, K. and Sweeting, H. (1996) 'Gender differences in health: are things as simple as they seem?', *Social Science & Medicine*, 42: 617–24.

MacPherson, E.E., Sadalaki, J., Njoloma, M., Nyongopa, V., Nkhwazi, L., Mwapasa, V., Lalloo, D.G., Desmond, N., Seeley, J. and Theobald, S. (2012) 'Transactional sex and HIV: understanding the gendered structural drivers of HIV in fishing communities in southern Malawi', *Journal of the International AIDS Society*, 15(3), Suppl. 1.

Macpherson, W. (1999) *The Stephen Lawrence Inquiry: Report of an Inquiry by Sir William Macpherson of Cluny.* London: Stationery Office.

Malin, N., Manthorpe, J., Race, D. and Wilmot, S. (1999) *Community Care for Nurses and the Caring Professions.* Buckingham: Open University Press.

Mallett, S. (2004) 'Understanding home: a critical review of the literature', *Sociological Review*, 52(1): 62–89.

Mane, P. and Aggleton, P. (2001) 'Gender and HIV/AIDS: what do men have to do with it?', *Current Sociology*, 49(6): 23–37.

March, J. and Olsen, J. (eds) (1976) *Ambiguity and Choice in Organisations.* Oslo: Universitetsforlaget.

Marmot, M. (2004) *Status Syndrome: How Your Social Standing Directly Affects Your Health and Life Expectancy.* London: Bloomsbury.

Marmot, M. (2005) *The Status Syndrome: How Social Standing Affects Our Health and Longevity.* London: Bloomsbury.

Marmot, M. (2006) 'Health in an unequal world', *The Lancet*, 368(9552): 2081–94.

Marmot, M. (2012) *Status Syndrome: How Your Social Standing Directly Affects Your Health.* London: Bloomsbury.

Marmot, M. (2015) *The Health Gap: The Challenge of an Unequal World.* London: Bloomsbury.

Marshall, B.L. (2010) 'Science, medicine and virility surveillance: "sexy seniors" in the pharmaceutical imagination', *Sociology of Health & Illness*, 32(2): 211–24.

Marshall, G. (1998) *Oxford Dictionary of Sociology.* Oxford: Oxford University Press.

Marsland, D. (1996) *Welfare or Welfare State: Contradictions and Dilemmas in Social Policy.* Basingstoke: Macmillan.

Mayall, B. (1996) *Children, Health and the Social Order.* Buckingham: Open University Press.

McDonald, A. (1999) *Understanding Community Care: A Guide for Social Workers.* Basingstoke: Macmillan.

McEwen, B.S. (2000) 'Allostasis and allostatic load: implications for neuropsychopharmacology', *Neuropsychopharmacology*, 22(2): 108–24.

McKeown, T. (1976) *The Modern Rise of Population.* New York: Academic Press.

McKie, L. (1995) 'The art of surveillance or reasonable prevention? The case of cervical screening', *Sociology of Health & Illness*, 17(4): 441–57.

McLaren, L. and Johnson, M. (2004) 'Understanding the rising tide of anti-immigrant sentiment', in A. Park, J. Curtice, K. Thomson, C. Bromley and M. Phillips (eds), *British Social Attitudes: The 21st Report.* London: Sage, pp. 169–200.

McPherson, S. and Armstrong, D. (2006) 'Social determinants of diagnostic labels in depression', *Social Science & Medicine*, 62: 50–8.

McQuaide, M.M. (2005) 'The rise of alternative health care: a sociological account', *Social Theory and Health*, 3: 286–301.

Mead, M. (1930) *Growing Up in New Guinea.* New York: Harper and Collins.

Means, R., Richards, S. and Smith, R. (2003) *Community Care Policy and Practice*, 3rd edn. Basingstoke: Palgrave Macmillan.

Meyer, M. and Struthers, H. (eds) (2012) *(Un)covering Men: Rewriting Masculinity and Health in South Africa.* Chicago, IL: Jacana Media (Pty).

Mills, C. Wright (1970) *The Sociological Imagination.* Harmondsworth: Penguin.

MIND (1999) *Suicide.* London: MIND.

MIND (2000a) *Mental Health Statistics 1: How Common is Mental Distress?* London: MIND.

MIND (2000b) *The Mental Health of Irish-Born People in Britain.* London: MIND.

Minton, A. (2009) *Ground Control: Fear and Happiness in the Twenty-First-Century City*. London: Penguin.

Mitchell, R., Shaw, M. and Dorling, D. (2000) *Inequalities in Life and Death: What if Britain Were More Equal?* Bristol: Policy Press.

Moon, G. & Gillespie, R. (2005) *Society and Health: An Introduction to Social Science for Health Professionals*. London: Routledge.

Moor, L. (2007) 'Sport and commodification: a reflection on key concepts', *Journal of Sport and Social Issues*, 31(2): 128–42.

Moran, A. (2005) 'White Australia, settler nationalism and aboriginal Assimilation', *Australian Journal of Politics and History*, 51(2): 168–193.

Morgan, M., Calnan, M. and Manning, N. (1985) *Sociological Approaches to Health and Medicine*. London: Croom Helm.

Morris, J. (ed.) (1989) *Able Lives: Women's Experience of Paralysis*. London: Women's Press.

Mort, M., Roberts, C. and Callén, B. (2012) 'Ageing with telecare: care or coercion in austerity?', *Sociology of Health & Illness*, 35(6): 799–812.

Muntaner, C. (2004) 'Commentary: social capital, social class, and the slow progress of psychosocial epidemiology', *International Journal of Epidemiology*, 33: 674–80.

Musingarimi, P. (2008) *Health Issues Affecting Older Gay, Lesbian and Bisexual People in the UK: A Policy Brief*. London: ILC-UK.

Navarro, V. (1976) *Medicine under Capitalism*. New York: Prodist.

Navarro, V. (ed.) (2002) *The Political Economy of Social Inequalities: Consequences for Health and Quality of Life*. Amityville, NY: Baywood.

Navarro, V., Muntaner, C., Borrell, C., Benach, J., Quiroga, Á., Rodríguez-Sanz, M., Vergés, N. and Pasarín, M.I. (2006) 'Politics and health outcomes', *The Lancet*, 368(9540): 1033–37.

Nazroo, J. (2012) 'Ethnicity and health: the role of social and economic inequalities', British Sociological Association Annual Conference Leeds, 11–13 April.

Nazroo, J., Edwards, A. and Brown, G.W. (1998) 'Gender differences in the prevalence of depression: artefact, alternative disorders, biology or roles?', *Sociology of Health & Illness*, 20(3): 312–30.

Nazroo, J., Jackson, J., Karlsen, S. and Torres, M. (2007) 'The black diaspora and health inequalities in the US and England: does where you go and how you get there make a difference?', *Sociology of Health & Illness*, 29(6): 811–30.

Nazroo, J.Y. (1997) *The Health of Britain's Ethnic Minorities: Findings from a National Survey*. London: Policy Studies Institute.

Nazroo, J.Y. (1998) 'Genetic, cultural or socio-economic vulnerability? Explaining ethnic inequalities in health', *Sociology of Health & Illness*, 20: 710–30.

Nazroo, J.Y. (2001) *Ethnicity, Class and Health*. London: Policy Studies Institute.

Nazroo, J.Y. (ed.) (2006) *Health and Social Research in Multiethnic Societies*. Abingdon: Routledge.

Nettleton, S. (1995) *The Sociology of Health and Illness*. Cambridge: Polity Press.

Nettleton, S. (2013) *The Sociology of Health and Illness*, 3rd edn. Cambridge: Polity Press.

Nettleton, S. and Watson, J. (1998) *The Body in Everyday Life*. London: Routledge.

Netto, G., Gaag, S., Thanki, M., Bondi, L. and Munro, M. (2001) *A Suitable Space: Improving Counselling Services for Asian People*. York: Joseph Rowntree Foundation.

Noon, M. (1993) 'Racial discrimination in speculative applications: evidence from the UK's top 100 firms', *Human Resource Management Journal*, 3(4): 35–47.

O'Brien, R., Hart, G. and Hunt, K. (2007) '"Standing out from the herd": men renegotiating masculinity in relation to their experience of illness', *International Journal of Men's Health*, 6(3): 178–200.

O'Brien, R., Hunt, K. and Hart, G. (2005) 'It's caveman stuff, but that is to a certain extent how guys still operate', *Social Science & Medicine*, 61(3): 503–16.

O'Keeffe, M., Hills, A., Doyle, M., McCreadie, C., Scholes, S., Constantine, R., Tinker, A., Manthorpe, J., Biggs, S. and Erens, B. (2007) *UK Study of Abuse and Neglect of Older People: Prevalence Survey Report*. London: NatCen.

Oakley, A. (1984) *The Captured Womb: A History of the Medical Care of Pregnant Women*. Oxford: Blackwell.

Oakley, A. (1987) 'From walking wombs to test-tube babies', in M. Stanworth (ed.), *Reproductive Technologies: Gender, Motherhood and Medicine*. Cambridge: Polity Press.

Oliver, M. (1990) *The Politics of Disablement*. London: Macmillan.

Oliver, M. (1993) 'Redefining disability: a challenge to the research', in J. Swain, V. Finkelstein, S. French and M. Oliver (eds), *Disabling Barriers: Enabling Environments*. London: SAGE.

ONS (Office for National Statistics) (2003) *Health Statistics Quarterly No. 20: Winter 2003*. London: Stationery Office.

ONS (Office for National Statistics) (2004) *Focus on Social Inequalities*. London: Stationery Office.

ONS (Office for National Statistics) (2005a) *Focus on Older People*. London: Stationery Office.

ONS (Office for National Statistics) (2005b) *Focus on Ethnicity and Identity*. London: Stationery Office.

ONS (Office for National Statistics) (2006a) *Focus on Gender*. London: Stationery Office.

ONS (Office for National Statistics) (2006b) *Focus on Health*. London: Stationery Office.

ONS (Office for National Statistics) (2014) *UK Wages Over the Past Four Decades*. London: Stationery Office.

ONS (Office for National Statistics) (2015) *Trend in Life Expectancy at Birth and at age 65 by Socio-Economic Position Based on the National Statistics Socio-Economic Classification, England and Wales: 1982–1986 to 2007–2011*. London: Stationery Office.

Oxfam (2014) *Working for the Few: Political Capture and Economic Inequality*. Oxford: Oxfam International.

Palmer, G., Carr, J. and Kenway, P. (2005) *Monitoring Poverty and Social Exclusion in Scotland 2005*. York: New Policy Institute and Joseph Rowntree Foundation.

Paradies, Y. (2006) 'A systematic review of empirical research on self-reported racism and health', *International Journal of Epidemiology*, 35(4): 888–901.

Parker, G. (1993) *With This Body: Caring and Disability in Marriage*. Buckingham: Open University Press.

Parks, A., Curtice, J., Clery, E. and Bryson, C. (2010) *British Social Attitudes: The 27th Report*. London: SAGE.

Pedersen, I.K., Hansen, V.H. and Grünenberg, K. (2015) 'The emergence of trust in clinics of alternative medicine', *Sociology of Health & Illness*, 38(1), pp. 43–57. doi: 10.1111/1467-9566.12338.

Penny, L. (2013) *Cybersexism: Sex, Gender and Power on the Internet*. London: Bloomsbury.

Peterson, A. (1997) 'Risk, governance and the new public health', in A. Peterson and R. Bunton (eds), *Foucault: Health and Medicine*. London: Routledge.

Phillips, T. and Phillips, M. (1999) *Windrush: The Irresistible Rise of Multi-racial Britain*. London: HarperCollins.

Philo, G. (ed.) (1996) *Media and Mental Distress*. London: Longman.

Picardie, R. (1993) *Before I Say Goodbye*. London: Penguin.

Pietilä, I. and Rytkönen, M. (2008a) 'Coping with stress and by stress: Russian men and women talking about transition, stress and health', *Social Science & Medicine*, 66(2): 327–38.

Pietilä, I. and Rytkönen, M. (2008b) '"Health is not a man's domain": Lay accounts of gender difference in life-expectancy in Russia', *Sociology of Health & Illness*, 30(7): 1070–85.

Piketty, T. (2014) *Capital in the Twenty-First Century*. Cambridge, MA: Harvard University Press.

Pilgrim, D. and Rogers, A. (1994) 'Something old, something new … sociology and the organisation of psychiatry', *Sociology*, 28(2): 521–38.

Pilgrim, D. and Rogers, A. (2014) *A Sociology of Mental Health and Illness* (5th edn). Buckingham: Open University Press.

Plummer, K. (1981) *The Making of the Modern Homosexual*. New York: Barnes and Noble.

Pols, J. & Willems, D. (2011) 'Innovation and evaluation: taming and unleashing telecare technology', *Sociology of Health & Illness*, 33(3): 484–98.

Pormann, P.E. and Savage-Smith, E. (2007) *Medieval Islamic Medicine*. Edinburgh: Edinburgh University Press.

Porter, M. (1990) 'Professional–client relationships and women's reproductive health care', in S. Cunningham-Burley and N. McKeganey (eds), *Readings in Medical Sociology*. London: Tavistock.

Porter, R. (1999) *The Greatest Benefit to Mankind: A Medical History of Humanity from Antiquity to the Present*. Hammersmith: Fontana.

Porter, R. and Porter, D. (1985) 'Sickness and health in pre-modern England', in R. Porter and D. Porter (eds), *In Sickness and in Health: The British Experience 1650–1850*. London: Fourth Estate.

Pound, P., Britten, N., Morgan, M., Yardley, L., Pope, C., Daker-White, G. and Campbell, R. (2005) 'Resisting medicines: a synthesis of qualitative studies of medicine taking', *Social Science & Medicine*, 61: 133–55.

Pound, P., Gompertz, P. and Ebrahim, S. (1998) 'Illness in the context of older age: the case of stroke', *Sociology of Health & Illness*, 20(4): 489–506.

Priest, N., Paradies, Y., Trenerry, B., Truong, M., Karlsen, S. and Kelly, Y. (2013) 'A systematic review of studies examining the relationship between reported racism and health and wellbeing for children and young people', *Social Science & Medicine*, 95: 115–27.

Prior, F. (2004) *Britain BC: Life in Britain and Ireland before the Romans*. London: Harper Perennial.

Prior, L. (1993) *The Social Organization of Mental Illness*. London: SAGE.

Prout, A. (1996) 'Actor-network theory, technology and medical sociology: an illustrative analysis of the metered dose inhaler', *Sociology of Health & Illness*, 18(2): 198–219.

Pugh, S. (2005) 'Assessing the cultural needs of older lesbians and gay men: implications for practice', *Practice: A Journal of the British Association of Social Workers*, 17(3): 207–18.

Pullen, I. (2002) 'The Scottish scene', *Psychiatric Bulletin*, 26: 86–7.

Putnam, R. (2000) *Bowling Alone: The Collapse and Revival of American Community*. New York: Simon & Schuster.

Qureshi, H. and Walker, A. (1989) *The Caring Relationship: Elderly People and Their Families*. Basingstoke: Macmillan.

Race, D. (2002) 'The historical context', in D. Race (ed.), *Learning Disability: A Social Approach*. London: Routledge.

Radia, K. (1996) *Ignored, Silenced, Neglected: Housing and Mental Health Care Needs of Asian People*. York: York Publication Services for Joseph Rowntree Foundation.

Rahman, M., Palmer, G., Kenway, P. and Howarth, C. (2000) *Monitoring Poverty and Social Exclusion*. London: New Policy Institute.

Ramazanoglu, C. (1989) *Feminism and the Contradictions of Oppression*. London: Routledge.

Reissman, L. (1992) 'Women and medicalisation: a new perspective', in L. McDowell and R. Pringle (eds), *Defining Women: Social Institutions and Gender Divisions*. Cambridge: Polity Press/Open University.

Rich, A. (1980) 'Compulsory heterosexuality and lesbian existence', *Signs*, 5(4): 630–60.

Rishworth, A., Dixon, J., Luginaah, I., Mkandawire, P. and Tampah Prince, C. (2016) '"I was on the way to the hospital but delivered in the bush": maternal health in Ghana's upper west region in the context of a traditional birth attendants' ban', *Social Science & Medicine*, 148: 8–17.

Ristock, J. (2002) *No More Secrets: Violence in Lesbian Relationships*. London: Routledge.

Robinson, I. (1988) *Multiple Sclerosis*. London: Routledge.

Rooney, S. (2002) 'Social inclusion and people with profound and multiple disabilities: reality or myth?', in D. Race (ed.), *Learning Disability: A Social Approach*. London: Routledge.

Rose, S. (2005) *Lifelines: Life beyond the Gene*. London: Vintage.

Rose, S. (2006) *The 21st-Century Brain*. London: Vintage.

Rosenhan, D.L. (1973) 'On being sane in insane places', *Science*, 179: 250–8.

Roughhead, W. (2000) 'The body snatchers (1921)', in B.D. Osborne and R. Armstrong (eds), *Wicked Men and Fools: A Scottish Crime Anthology*. Edinburgh: Birlinn.

Sabat, S.R. (2001) *The Experience of Alzheimer's Disease*. Oxford: Blackwell.

Sailes, G.A. (1998) 'The African-American athlete', in G.A. Sailes (ed.), *African-Americans in Sport*. New Brunswick, NJ: Transaction.

Saks, M. (ed.) (1992) *Alternative Medicine in Britain*. Oxford: Clarendon Press.

Saks, M. (1994) 'The alternatives to medicine', in J. Gabe, D. Kelleher and G. Williams (eds), *Challenging Medicine*. London: Routledge.

Saks, M. (1998) 'Medicine and complementary medicine', in G. Scambler and P. Higgs (eds), *Modernity, Medicine and Health: Medical Sociology towards 2000*. London: Routledge.

Samson, C. (1995) 'Madness and psychiatry', in B. Turner with C. Samson, *Medical Power and Social Knowledge*. London: SAGE.

Sanders, C., Donovan, J. and Dieppe, P. (2002) 'The significance and consequences of having painful and disabled joints in older age: co-existing accounts of normal and disrupted biographies', *Sociology of Health & Illness*, 24(2): 227–53.

Sapolsky, R.M. (1992) *Stress: Aging Brain and the Mechanisms of Neuron Death*. Cambridge, MA: MIT Press.

Saracci, R. (1997) 'The World Health Organisation needs to reconsider its definition of health', *British Medical Journal*, 314: 1409.

Sato, A. (2012) 'Does socio-economic status explain use of modern and traditional health care services?', *Social Science & Medicine*, 75(8): 1450–9.

Savage, M., Bagnall, G. and Longhurst, B. (2005) *Globalisation and Belonging*. London: SAGE.

Sayer, A. (2015) *Why We Can't Afford the Rich*. Bristol: Policy Press.

Scambler, G. (2001) 'Critical realism, sociology and health inequalities: social class as a generative mechanism and its media of enactment', *Journal of Critical Realism*, 4: 35–42.

Scheff, T. (1966) *Being Mentally Ill: A Sociology Theory*. Chicago, IL: Aldine.

Schnittker, J. (2005) 'Chronic illness and depressive symptoms', *Social Science & Medicine*, 60: 13–23.

Scottish Executive (2000) *Our National Health: A Plan for Action, a Plan for Change*. Edinburgh: Stationery Office.

Scottish Executive (2001) *Health in Scotland 2000*. Report of the Chief Medical Officer for Scotland. Edinburgh: Stationery Office.

Scottish Executive (2003) *Improving Health in Scotland: The Challenge.* Edinburgh: Stationery Office.

Scottish Executive (2004a) *Building a Better Scotland. Spending Proposals 2005–2008: Enterprise, Opportunity, Fairness. Technical Notes.* Edinburgh: Stationery Office.

Scottish Executive (2004b) *Closing the Opportunity Gap.* Edinburgh: Stationery Office.

Scottish Executive (2004c) *Fair to All, Personal to Each: The Next Step for the NHS Scotland.* Edinburgh: Stationery Office.

Scottish Executive (2005) *Delivering for Health 2005.* Edinburgh: Stationery Office.

Scottish Government (2010) www.scotland.gov.uk/Topics/Health/care/JointFuture.

Scottish Office Department of Health (1999) *Towards a Healthier Scotland: A White Paper on Health.* Edinburgh: Stationery Office.

Scull, A. (1979) *Museums of Madness: The Social Organization of Insanity in Nineteenth Century England.* London: Allen Lane.

Seale, C. (1998a) *Constructing Death: The Sociology of Dying and Bereavement.* Cambridge: Cambridge University Press.

Seale, C. (1998b) 'Normal/pathological', in C. Jenks (ed.), *Core Sociological Dichotomies.* London: SAGE.

Seale, C. (2000) 'Changing patterns of death and dying', *Social Science & Medicine,* 51: 917–30.

Seale, C. (2005) 'New directions for critical internet health studies: representing cancer experiences on the web', *Sociology of Health & Illness,* 27(4): 515–40.

Seale, C. and Pattison, S. (1994) *Medical Knowledge: Doubt and Certainty.* Milton Keynes: Open University Press.

Seymour, J.E. (2001) *Critical Moments: Death and Dying in Intensive Care.* Buckingham: Open University Press.

Shakespeare, T. (2006) *Disability Rights and Wrongs.* London: Routledge.

Shakespeare, T. (2013) *Disability Rights and Wrongs Revisited.* London: Routledge.

Sharkey, P. (2007) *The Essentials of Community Care.* Basingstoke: Palgrave Macmillan.

Sharma, U. (1992) *Complementary Medicine Today: Practitioners and Patients.* London: Routledge.

Sharp, L. and Brewster, D. (1999) 'The epidemiology of lung cancer in Scotland: a review of trends in incidence, survival and mortality and prospects for prevention', *Health Bulletin,* 57(5): 318–31.

Shaw, A., McMunn, A. and Field, J. (eds) (2000) *The Scottish Health Survey 1998: A Survey Carried Out on Behalf of the Scottish Executive Health Department.* Edinburgh: Scottish Executive.

Shaw, M., Dorling, D., Gordon, D. and Davey-Smith, G. (1999) *The Widening Gap: Health Inequalities and Policy in Britain.* Bristol: Policy Press.

Shryock, R.H. (1979) *The Development of Modern Medicine: An Interpretation of the Social and Scientific Factors Involved.* Madison, WI: Wisconsin University Press.

Singer, E. (1974) 'Premature social ageing: the social psychological consequences of a chronic illness', *Social Science & Medicine,* 8: 143–51.

Smaje C. (1995) *Health, 'Race' and Ethnicity: Making Sense of the Evidence.* London: King's Fund Institute.

Smaje, C. (1996) 'The ethnic patterning of health: new directions for theory and research', *Sociology of Health & Illness,* 18(2): 139–71.

Small, N. (1997) 'Death and difference', in D. Field, J. Hockey and N. Small (eds), *Death, Gender and Ethnicity.* London: Routledge, pp. 202–21.

Smart, C. (1996) 'Deconstructing motherhood', in E. Bortolaia Silva (ed.), *Good Enough Mothering? Feminist Perspectives on Lone Motherhood.* London: Routledge.

Smith, G., Shaw, M., Mitchell, R., Dorling, D. and Gordon, D. (2000) 'Inequalities in health continue to grow despite government's pledges', *British Medical Journal*, 320: 582.

Sorensen, R. and Iedema, R. (2009) 'Emotional labour: clinicians' attitudes to death and dying', *Journal of Health Organization and Management*, 23(1): 5–22.

SPIU (Scottish Poverty Information Unit) (1997) *Defining Poverty*. Glasgow: Glasgow Caledonian University. http://spiu.gcal.ac.uk/briefing1.html.

SPIU (Scottish Poverty Information Unit) (2002) *Poverty in Scotland*. Glasgow: Glasgow Caledonian University.

Stacey, M. (1988) *The Sociology of Health and Healing*. London: Routledge.

Star, S. (1955) 'The public's idea about mental illness'. Paper presented at the National Association for Mental Health Meeting, Chicago, November.

Statistics SA (Statistics South Africa) (2014) *Poverty Trends in South Africa: An Examination of Absolute Poverty between 2006 and 2011*. Pretoria, SA: Statistics South Africa.

Steinbach, R., Green, J., Datta, J. and Edwards, P. (2011) 'Cycling and the city: a case study of how gendered, ethnic and class identities can shape healthy transport choices', *Social Science & Medicine*, 72(7): 1123–30.

Strauss, A.L. (1987) *Qualitative Analysis for Social Scientists*. Cambridge: Cambridge University Press.

Stryker, S. and Whittle, S. (2006) *The Transgender Studies Reader*. London: Routledge.

Sutton, S. (2014) *Stephen's Story: A 19-Year-Old's Life Lessons on Making the Most of Your Time*. Magic Future.

Sweeting, H. and Gilhooly, M. (1997) 'Dementia and the phenomenon of social death', *Sociology of Health & Illness*, 19(1): 93–117.

Szreter, S. (1988) 'The importance of social intervention in Britain's mortality decline *c*. 1850–1914: a reinterpretation of the role of public health', *Social History of Medicine*, 1: 1–38.

Szreter, S. (2002) 'Rethinking McKeown: the relationship between public health and social change', *American Journal of Public Health*, 92(5): 722–5.

Taylor, S. (1989) *Suicide*. London: Longman.

Taylor, S. (1990) 'Beyond Durkheim: sociology and suicide', *Social Studies Review*, 6(2): 70–4.

Thomas, B., Pritchard, J., Ballas, D., Vickers, D. and Dorling, D. (2009) *A Tale of Two Cities: The Sheffield Project*. Sheffield: University of Sheffield Press.

Timmermans, S. and Berg, M. (2003) 'The practice of medical technology', *Sociology of Health & Illness*, 25(3): 97–114.

Tinker, A. (1996) *Older People in Modern Society*. Harlow: Longman.

Tozer, R. (1999) *Supporting Families with Two or More Severely Disabled Children*. York: Joseph Rowntree Foundation.

Trägårdh, L. (1997) 'Statist individualism: on the culturality of the Nordic welfare state', in O. Sørensen and B. Stråth (eds), *The Cultural Construction of Norden*. Oslo: Scandanavian University Press, pp. 253–85.

Turner, B. with Samson, C. (1995) *Medical Power and Social Knowledge*. London: SAGE.

Turner, B.S. (1994) *Medical Power and Social Knowledge*. London: SAGE.

Twenge, J.M. and Campbell, W.K. (2010) *The Narcissism Epidemic: Living in the Age of Entitlement*. New York: Atria.

Twigg, J. (2006) *The Body in Health and Social Care*. Basingstoke: Palgrave Macmillan.

Twigg, J. (2007) 'Clothing, age and the body: a critical review', *Ageing and Society*, 27: 285–305.

Twigg, J. (2013) *Fashion and Age: Dress, the Body and Later Life*. London: Bloomsbury.

Twigg, J. and Atkin, K. (1994) *Carers Perceived: Policy and Practice in Informal Care*. Buckingham: Open University Press.

United Nations (2005) *Demographic Year Book 2002*. New York: United Nations.

United Nations (2013) *International Migration Report 2013*. New York: United Nations.

Üstün, B. and Jakob, R. (2005) 'Calling a spade a spade: meaningful definitions of health conditions', *Bulletin of the World Health Organization*, 83: 802.

Vargo, M. (2002) *Scandal: Infamous Gay Controversies of the Twentieth Century*. London: Routledge.

Virdee, S., Kyriakides, C. and Modood, T. (2006) 'Codes of cultural belonging: racialised national identities in a multi-ethnic Scottish neighbourhood', *Sociological Research Online*, 11(4).

Wade, D.T. (2001) 'Ethical issues in the diagnosis of permanent vegetative state', *British Medical Journal*, 322(10 February): 352–4.

Walby, S. (1989) 'Theorising patriarchy', *Sociology*, 23(2): 213–34.

Walby, S. (1990) *Theorizing Patriarchy*. Cambridge, MA: Blackwell.

Walby, S. and Allen, J. (2004) *Domestic Violence, Sexual Assault and Stalking: Findings from the British Crime Survey*. Home Office Research No. 276. London: Home Office. www.homeoffice.gov.uk/rds/violencewomen.html, accessed 13 May 2011.

Walter, T. (2004) *The Revival of Death*, 2nd edn. London: Routledge.

Warnock, M. (1985) *A Question of Life*. Oxford: Blackwell.

Watney, S. (2000) *Imagine Hope: AIDS and Gay Identity*. London: Routledge.

Watson, J. (2000) *Male Bodies: Health, Culture, and Identity*. London: Taylor & Francis.

Weber, J. and Wahl, J. (2006) 'Neurosurgical aspects of trepanations from Neolithic times', *International Journal of Osteoarchaeology*, 16(6): 536–45.

Weber, M. (1997) *Theory of Social and Economic Organization*. London: Free Press.

Weber, M. (2001) *The Protestant Work Ethic and the Spirit of Capitalism*. London: Routledge.

Webster, A. (2007) *Health, Technology and Society: A Sociological Critique*. Basingstoke: Palgrave Macmillan.

Weeks, J. (2003) *Sexuality*. London: Routledge.

West, P. (1998) *Perspectives on Health Inequalities: The Need for a Lifecourse Approach*. Glasgow: Medical Research Council Social and Public Health Sciences Unit, University of Glasgow.

West, R. (1993) 'Alternative medicine: prospects and speculation', in N. Black, D. Boswell, A. Gray, S. Murphy and J. Popay (eds), *Health and Disease: A Reader*. Milton Keynes: Open University Press.

Whitehead, S.M. (1987) 'The health divide', in P. Townsend, M. Whitehead and N. Davidson (eds), *Inequalities in Health: The Black Report and the Health Divide*. London: Penguin.

Whitehead, S.M. (2002) *Men and Masculinities: Key Themes and New Directions*. Cambridge: Polity Press.

Widgery, D. (1991) *Some Lives! A GP's East End*. London: Simon & Schuster.

Wigg, J.M. (2010) 'Liberating the wanderers: using technology to unlock doors for those living with dementia', *Sociology of Health & Illness*, 32(2): 288–303.

Wiles, R., Ashburn, A., Payne, S. and Murphy, C. (2004) 'Discharge from physiotherapy following stroke: the management of disappointment', *Social Science & Medicine*, 59: 1263–73.

Wilkinson, R. (1996) *Unhealthy Societies: The Afflictions of Inequality*. London: Routledge.

Wilkinson, R. (2005) *The Impact of Inequality: How to Make Sick Societies Healthier*. London: Routledge.

Wilkinson, R.G. (2002) 'Income inequality, social cohesion, and health: clarifying the theory: A reply to Muntaner and Lynch', in V. Navarro (ed.), *The Political Economy of Social Inequalities: Consequences for Health and Quality of Life*. Amityville, NY: Baywood Publishing Co., pp. 347–65.

Wilkinson, R.G. and Pickett, K. (2010) *The Spirit Level: Why Equality Is Better for Everyone*. London: Penguin.

Williams, D.R., Gonzalez, H.M., Williams, S., Mohammed, S.A., Moomal, H. and Stein, D.J. (2008) 'Perceived discrimination, race and health in South Africa', *Social Science & Medicine*, 67(3): 441–52.

Williams, S. (2001) 'Sociological imperialism and the profession of medicine revisited: Where are we now?', *Sociology of Health & Illness*, 23(2), pp. 135–158.

Williams, S.J. (1999) 'Is anybody there? Critical realism, chronic illness and the disability debate', *Sociology of Health & Illness*, 21(6): 797–819.

Williams, S.J. (2000) 'Chronic illness as biographical disruption or biographical disruption as chronic illness? Reflections on a core concept', *Sociology of Health & Illness*, 22(1): 40–67.

Williams, S.J. (2003) *Medicine and the Body*. London: SAGE.

Williams, S.J. (2004) 'Bio-attack or panic attack? Critical reflections on the ill-logic of bioterrorism and biowarfare in late/postmodernity', *Social Theory and Health*, 2: 67–93.

Williams, V.L. and Whiting, M.J. (2016) 'A picture of health? Animal use and the Faraday traditional medicine market, South Africa', *Journal of Ethnopharmacology*, 179: 265–73.

Wilton, T. (2000) *Sexualities in Health and Social Care: A Textbook*. Basingstoke: Open University Press.

Witz, A. (1992) *Professions and Patriarchy*. London: Routledge.

Wogan, P. (2004) 'Deep hanging out: reflections on fieldwork and multisided Andean ethnography', *Identities: Global Studies in Culture and Power*, 11: 129–39.

Wolf, S. and Bruhn, J.G. (1998) *The Power of Clan: The Influence of Human Relationships on Heart Disease*. United States: Transaction Publishers.

Wood, M., Hales, J. and Purdon, S. (2009) *A Test for Racial Discrimination in Recruitment Practice in British Cities*. London: Dept. for Work and Pensions.

Woodward, K. (2007) *Boxing, Masculinity and Identity: The 'I' of the Tiger*. London: Routledge.

World Bank (2015) Gender Data Portal. http://datatopics.worldbank.org/gender/

World Health Organisation (WHO) (1992) *Basic Documents*, 39th edn. Geneva: World Health Organisation.

World Health Organisation (WHO) (2008) *Global Burden of Disease: 2004 Update*. Geneva: World Health Organisation.

World Health Organisation (WHO) (2010) *Global Status Report on Noncommunicable Diseases*. Geneva: World Health Organisation.

World Health Organisation (WHO) (2011) *World Health Statistics*. Geneva: World Health Organisation.

World Health Organisation (WHO) (2013) *Traditional Medicine Strategy, 2014–2023*. Geneva: World Health Organisation.

World Health Organisation (2015) *Depression: Fact Sheet No. 369*. http://www.who.int/mediacentre/factsheets/fs369/en/ (accessed 2 March 2016).

Wouters, E. and De Wet, K. (2015) 'Women's experience of HIV as a chronic illness in South Africa: hard-earned lives, biographical disruption and moral career', *Sociology of Health & Illness*, DOI: 10.1111/1467-9566.12377

Young, I.M. (1980) 'Throwing like a girl: a phenomenology of feminine body comportment motility and spatiality', *Human Studies*, 3(1): 137–56.

Young, M. and Willmott, P. (1961) *Family and Kinship in East London.* Harmondsworth: Penguin.

Yuill, C. (2005) 'Marx: capitalism, alienation and health', *Social Theory and Health*, 3: 126–43.

Yuill, C. (2007) 'The body as weapon: Bobby Sands and the Republican hunger strikes', *Sociological Research Online*, 12(2). www.socresonline.org.uk/12/2/yuill.html.

Yuill, C. (2010) '"The Spirit Level": health inequalities and economic democracy', *International Journal of Management Concepts and Philosophy*, 4(2): 177–93.

Zsembik, B.A. and Fennell, D. (2005) 'Ethnic variation in health and the determinants of health among Latinos', *Social Science & Medicine*, 61(11): 53–63.

INDEX

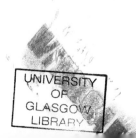